COVID-19: Diagnosis and Management-Part I

Edited by

Neeraj Mittal

*Department of Endocrinology
Postgraduate Institute of Medical Education and Research
Chandigarh-160012
India*

Sanjay Kumar Bhadada

*Department of Endocrinology
Postgraduate Institute of Medical Education and Research
Chandigarh-160012
India*

O. P. Katare

*University Institute of Pharmaceutical Sciences
UGC Centre of Advanced Studies
Punjab University
Chandigarh-160014
India*

&

Varun Garg

*Department of Medical Affairs
Cadila Healthcare Limited
Ahmedabad 382421
Gujarat
India*

COVID-19: Diagnosis and Management-Part I

Editors: Neeraj Mittal, Sanjay Kumar Bhadada, O. P. Katare and Varun Garg

ISBN (Online): 978-1-68108-808-2

ISBN (Print): 978-1-68108-809-9

ISBN (Paperback): 978-1-68108-810-5

© 2021, Bentham Books imprint.

Published by Bentham Science Publishers – Sharjah, UAE. All Rights Reserved.

BENTHAM SCIENCE PUBLISHERS LTD.
End User License Agreement (for non-institutional, personal use)

This is an agreement between you and Bentham Science Publishers Ltd. Please read this License Agreement carefully before using the ebook/echapter/ejournal (**"Work"**). Your use of the Work constitutes your agreement to the terms and conditions set forth in this License Agreement. If you do not agree to these terms and conditions then you should not use the Work.

Bentham Science Publishers agrees to grant you a non-exclusive, non-transferable limited license to use the Work subject to and in accordance with the following terms and conditions. This License Agreement is for non-library, personal use only. For a library / institutional / multi user license in respect of the Work, please contact: permission@benthamscience.net.

Usage Rules:

1. All rights reserved: The Work is 1. the subject of copyright and Bentham Science Publishers either owns the Work (and the copyright in it) or is licensed to distribute the Work. You shall not copy, reproduce, modify, remove, delete, augment, add to, publish, transmit, sell, resell, create derivative works from, or in any way exploit the Work or make the Work available for others to do any of the same, in any form or by any means, in whole or in part, in each case without the prior written permission of Bentham Science Publishers, unless stated otherwise in this License Agreement.
2. You may download a copy of the Work on one occasion to one personal computer (including tablet, laptop, desktop, or other such devices). You may make one back-up copy of the Work to avoid losing it.
3. The unauthorised use or distribution of copyrighted or other proprietary content is illegal and could subject you to liability for substantial money damages. You will be liable for any damage resulting from your misuse of the Work or any violation of this License Agreement, including any infringement by you of copyrights or proprietary rights.

Disclaimer:

Bentham Science Publishers does not guarantee that the information in the Work is error-free, or warrant that it will meet your requirements or that access to the Work will be uninterrupted or error-free. The Work is provided "as is" without warranty of any kind, either express or implied or statutory, including, without limitation, implied warranties of merchantability and fitness for a particular purpose. The entire risk as to the results and performance of the Work is assumed by you. No responsibility is assumed by Bentham Science Publishers, its staff, editors and/or authors for any injury and/or damage to persons or property as a matter of products liability, negligence or otherwise, or from any use or operation of any methods, products instruction, advertisements or ideas contained in the Work.

Limitation of Liability:

In no event will Bentham Science Publishers, its staff, editors and/or authors, be liable for any damages, including, without limitation, special, incidental and/or consequential damages and/or damages for lost data and/or profits arising out of (whether directly or indirectly) the use or inability to use the Work. The entire liability of Bentham Science Publishers shall be limited to the amount actually paid by you for the Work.

General:

1. Any dispute or claim arising out of or in connection with this License Agreement or the Work (including non-contractual disputes or claims) will be governed by and construed in accordance with the laws of the U.A.E. as applied in the Emirate of Dubai. Each party agrees that the courts of the Emirate of Dubai shall have exclusive jurisdiction to settle any dispute or claim arising out of or in connection with this License Agreement or the Work (including non-contractual disputes or claims).
2. Your rights under this License Agreement will automatically terminate without notice and without the

need for a court order if at any point you breach any terms of this License Agreement. In no event will any delay or failure by Bentham Science Publishers in enforcing your compliance with this License Agreement constitute a waiver of any of its rights.
3. You acknowledge that you have read this License Agreement, and agree to be bound by its terms and conditions. To the extent that any other terms and conditions presented on any website of Bentham Science Publishers conflict with, or are inconsistent with, the terms and conditions set out in this License Agreement, you acknowledge that the terms and conditions set out in this License Agreement shall prevail.

Bentham Science Publishers Ltd.
Executive Suite Y - 2
PO Box 7917, Saif Zone
Sharjah, U.A.E.
Email: subscriptions@benthamscience.net

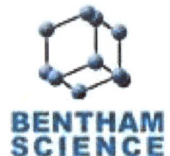

CONTENTS

FOREWORD	i
PREFACE	ii
LIST OF CONTRIBUTORS	iv
CHAPTER 1 HISTORY OF PANDEMICS	**1**
Sunishtha, Govind Singh and *Sanju Nanda*	
INTRODUCTION	1
THE ATHENIAN PLAGUE	3
PLAGUE OF JUSTINIAN	4
THE BLACK DEATH	4
SPANISH FLU	4
AIDS	5
SMALLPOX	5
SARS	6
SWINE FLU OR H1N1 PANDEMIC	6
EBOLA	6
COVID-19	7
ORIGIN OF CORONAVIRUS	7
TYPES OF CORONAVIRUSES	8
DISEASE ASSOCIATED WITH CORONAVIRUSES	11
MURINE HEPATITIS VIRUS (MHV)	11
Central Nervous System	11
Hepatitis	12
Pneumonitis	12
BOVINE CORONAVIRUS	12
HUMAN CORONAVIRUS	12
ABBREVIATIONS	13
CONSENT FOR PUBLICATION	13
CONFLICT OF INTEREST	13
ACKNOWLEDGEMENTS	14
REFERENCES	14
CHAPTER 2 INTRODUCTION TO COVID-19	**18**
Hitesh Malhotra, Anjoo Kamboj and *Peeyush Kaushik*	
INTRODUCTION	18
GENOMIC STRUCTURE OF CORONAVIRUS	21
STRUCTURAL PROTEINS	21
Spike Protein	22
Small Membrane Protein	23
Membrane Protein	24
Hemagglutinin-Esterase	24
Nucleocapsid and Internal Proteins	24
Replicase Protein	25
VIRAL CYCLE	25
OUTBREAKS OF CORONAVIRUS	27
Porcine Coronavirus	27
Avian Coronavirus	28
Feline Coronavirus	28
Bovine Coronavirus	28

Murine Coronavirus	29
Human Coronavirus	29
SARS-CoV	29
MERS-CoV	31
COVID-19	**32**
Introduction	32
Chronology of COVID-19	33
Symptoms	34
Transmission	36
Treatment	36
LIST OF ABBREVIATIONS	**37**
CONSENT FOR PUBLICATION	**39**
CONFLICT OF INTEREST	**39**
ACKNOWLEDGEMENTS	**39**
REFERENCES	**39**
CHAPTER 3 COVID-19: EPIDEMIOLOGY	**42**

Kamya Goyal, Shammy Jindal, Tarun Kumar, Jugnu Goyal, Reena Sharma, Ravinder Singh and *Samir Mehndiratta*

INTRODUCTION	**43**
GEOGRAPHICAL DISTRIBUTION	**44**
GLOBAL EPIDEMIOLOGY OF COVID-19	**45**
Effect of Age, Sex and other Factors on Covid-19-Related Deaths	54
COVID-19 CASE COMPARISONS IN DIFFERENT REGION OF WORLD (WORLD HEALTH ORGANIZATION, 2020)	**55**
COVID-19 IN INDIA	**58**
REPORT BY ICMR ON COVID-19 ABOUT CONTAINMENT ZONE IN INDIA	**60**
NATIONAL RESPONSES ON COVID-19 WORLDWIDE	**61**
Asia	61
China	62
South Korea	63
Middle Eastern	64
Iran	64
Europe	65
Spain	65
France	66
North America	66
United States	67
South America	68
Africa	68
Oceania	69
EFFECT OF LOCKDOWN ON COVID-19 CASES IN TOP TEN MOST AFFECTED COUNTRIES OF WORLD	**69**
THE ROLE OF WHO AND INGOS FOR PROVIDING DATA IN COVID-19	**73**
OUTCOMES FROM SOME PUBLISHED REPORTS ON COVID-19 EPIDEMIOLOGY	**74**
Herd Immunity-COVID-19	76
CONCLUSION	**77**
LIST OF ABBREVIATIONS	**77**
CONSENT FOR PUBLICATION	**77**
CONFLICT OF INTEREST	**77**
ACKNOWLEDGEMENTS	**77**

| REFERENCES | 78 |

CHAPTER 4 PATHOPHYSIOLOGY ... 83
Anirban Ghosh and *Shamsher Singh*

INTRODUCTION	83
TRANSMISSION OF COV	84
Virus Life Cycle	85
Role of Structural Proteins in The Pathogenesis	86
A. Spike Protein	86
B. Hemagglutinin-Esterase (HE) Protein	88
C. Membrane (M) Protein	89
D. Small Envelop (E) Protein	91
E. Nucleocapsid (N) Protein and Internal (I) Protein	92
F. Replicase Proteins	93
G. CoV Associated Protein	99
Pathophysiology from a Cell Biology Perspective	100
Phase I. Asymptomatic Stage (First 1-2 Days of Infection)	100
Phase II. Upper Airway and Conducting Airway Response (Next Few Days)	101
Phase III. Hypoxia, Ground-glass Infiltrates, Progression to ARDs	102
CONCLUSION	104
LIST OF ABBREVIATIONS	104
CONSENT FOR PUBLICATION	105
CONFLICT OF INTEREST	105
ACKNOWLEDGEMENTS	105
REFERENCES	105

CHAPTER 5 CLINICAL PRESENTATION AND COMORBIDITIES ... 117
Jasleen Kaur, Baljinder Singh, Bikash Medhi and *Gurpreet Kaur*

INTRODUCTION	118
CLINICAL PRESENTATIONS OF COVID-19 INFECTION	118
INTER-INDIVIDUAL VARIATIONS IN CLINICAL PRESENTATIONS DUE TO DIFFERENTIAL SUSCEPTIBILITY TOWARDS COVID-19	120
Neonates or Newborns (Upto 1 Month); Infants (1 Month-2 Years), Children (2-10 Years)	120
Adolescent (11-19 Years), Young (20-35 Years) and Middle Aged (36-59 Years) Patients	128
Elderly (>60 Years) and Older (>80 Years) Patients	143
ACE2	148
Gender	149
Blood Group	150
Previous Immunization	151
COMORBIDITY	152
CONCLUSION	152
LIST OF ABBREVIATIONS	153
CONSENT FOR PUBLICATION	154
CONFLICT OF INTEREST	154
ACKNOWLEDGEMENTS	154
REFERENCES	154

CHAPTER 6 DIAGNOSIS ... 164
Richa Deshpande, Aishwarya Joshi, Nikunj Tandel and *Rajeev K. Tyagi*

COVID-19: A PANDEMIC DISEASE	165
COVID-19: EARLY DETECTION BASED ON SYMPTOMS	166
Clinical Analysis	166

Hematological Analysis	167
Chest CT	168
COVID-19: MOLECULAR DETECTION OF VIRUS	**169**
RT-PCR Based Assays	170
Loop Mediated Isothermal Amplification (LAMP)	172
CRISPR-Isothermal Amplification Based Assays	174
Microarrays	175
Metagenomic Sequencing Based Methods	175
Gold Nanoparticles-Based Colorimetric Assay	176
COVID-19: SEROLOGICAL AND IMMUNOLOGICAL BASED DETECTION	**179**
BIOMARKER IDENTIFICATION: APPROACH OF SEROLOGICAL PLATFORM	**181**
Antibody Biomarkers	181
Antigen Biomarkers	182
Procalcitonin and Interleukin-6 as Prognostic COVID-19 Biomarkers	183
SEROLOGICAL AND IMMUNOLOGICAL ASSAYS	**184**
Enzyme-linked Immunosorbent Assay (ELISA)	184
Lateral Flow Immunoassay	185
Neutralization Assays	187
Luminescence-based Immunoassays	188
Biosensor Tests	188
Rapid Antigen Tests	189
CONCLUDING REMARKS	**190**
LIST OF ABBREVIATIONS	**191**
CONSENT FOR PUBLICATION	**192**
CONFLICT OF INTEREST	**192**
ACKNOWLEDGEMENTS	**192**
REFERENCES	**193**
SUBJECT INDEX	**200**

FOREWORD

It is my proud privilege to introduce the book "COVID-19: Diagnosis and Management", which is authored by a group from PGIMER, Chandigarh. The timing of this monograph is very apt as it has been about 9 months since the start of the COVID-19 pandemic, and it is now that we are starting to unravel the various mechanisms of disease pathogenesis and treatment modalities for this viral infection which has infected 29 million people, out of which about 1 million have died till date globally.

It has been the need of the hour to come up with a treatment for this pandemic disease. Moreover, it is of utmost importance that all the information related to COVID -19 should be compiled in one place, a goal which this book will fulfill.

Though the tests for diagnosis of the infection have been developed in the start of the pandemic, there are still some issues in diagnosis, including the sensitivity of the best test available, *i.e.*, Real-Time Polymerase Chain Reaction.

The book is very well organized and has been divided into two parts; each part is comprised of 6 chapters and covers all the aspects of COVID-19 from the history to the treatment of the disease. Based on the best scientific studies available, the editors and authors have used their vast professional experience to discuss the all clinical aspects of COVID-19, including clinical presentation to diagnosis in the first part and treatment of COVID-19 in the second part, and I am very sure that this compendium will become the benchmark to refer to for any information required on COVID-19.

Whenever we write books, we must have in our minds, as clearly as possible, the affirmation of Carlyle Guerra de Macedo, who was the Director of Pan American Health Organization, relative to the responsibility of what is being published: "It must be remembered that behind each table, every report or material examined, there are lives, there are people, there is suffering, waiting for our efforts and human solidarity." Both the parts of the book are very well organized, and the readers will get a mine of information available to date on COVID-19 in one place, and it would be helpful to both the clinicians and the lab professionals for day-to-day guidance in various matters. The monograph is comprehensive but is written in a lucid manner that is easy to grasp, and even complex topics are made simple for understanding.

I am also sure that as the knowledge of the virus evolves further, the authors will certainly keep updating the work from time to time, further adding to the importance of the book. I would like to congratulate the editors/authors for this tremendous effort, and I am very sure that this book will surely be of use to readers around the world and help them in the diagnosis and management of patients with COVID-19 and will also go a long way in the efforts to help fight the pandemic, which is being faced by the humanity now.

Prof. R. Sehgal
Department of Medical Parasitology
Chairperson Group D Departments
Postgraduate Institute of Medical Education & Research
Chandigarh-160012
India

PREFACE

The coronavirus disease 2019 (COVID-19) outbreak has spread throughout the globe and has been declared as a pandemic by the World Health Organization (WHO) on 11th March 2020. To date, *i.e.*, 1st September 2020, there are more than 25, 327, 098 confirmed cases of COVID-19 worldwide, and around 848, 255 deaths have been reported. Clinicians and scientists across the globe need all the information on this pandemic disease on one platform. This book, "COVID-19: Diagnosis and Management", is a concise and visual reference for this viral disease. This book has been divided into two parts I and II.

Part I will provide a comprehensive knowledge which will cover all the aspects related to COVID-19, such as: 1) History of coronaviruses, 2) epidemiology of COVID-19 3) clinical presentation of this viral disease, 4) how to diagnose it, whereas part II of the book covers the prevention and treatment methodology of this communicable disease.

Key Features:

1. Chapter wise description and segregation of all the areas from pathophysiology to diagnosis and management of COVID-19 in two different parts of the book.
2. Six chapters in the first part that begin with the history of the coronaviruses and their introduction.
3. Multiple tables and figures which summarize and highlight important points.
4. Covering all the aspects of COVID-19, making this a perfect textbook for virologists and medical students.
5. A summary of the current standards for the evaluation and diagnosis of COVID-19.
6. A detailed list of references, abbreviations, and symbols.

This book is an essential reference for practicing and training virologists, pulmonologists, medical students, scientists working in various research labs, pharmaceutical and biotechnology industries on COVID-19.

Neeraj Mittal
Department of Endocrinology
Postgraduate Institute of Medical
Education and Research,
Chandigarh-160012
India

Sanjay Kumar Bhadada
Department of Endocrinology
Postgraduate Institute of Medical
Education and Research,
Chandigarh-160012
India

O. P. Katare
University Institute of Pharmaceutical Sciences
UGC Centre of Advanced Studies
Panjab University
Chandigarh-160014
India

Varun Garg
Department of Medical Affairs
Cadila Healthcare Limited
Ahmedabad 382421
Gujarat
India

List of Contributors

Aishwarya Joshi	Institute of Science, Nirma University, Ahmedabad, Gujarat, India
Anirban Ghosh	Department of Pharmacology, ISF College of Pharmacy, Moga, Punjab, India
Anjoo Kamboj	Chandigarh College of Pharmacy, Landran, Mohali, Punjab, India
Baljinder Singh	MM School of Pharmacy, MM University, Sadopur, Ambala, Haryana, India
Bikash Medhi	Department of Pharmacology, PGIMER, Chandigarh, India
Govind Singh	Department of Pharmaceutical Sciences, Maharshi Dayanand University, Rohtak, India
Gurpreet Kaur	Department of Pharmaceutical Sciences and Drug Research, Punjabi University, Patiala, Punjab, India
Hitesh Malhotra	Chandigarh College of Pharmacy, Landran, Mohali, Punjab, India
Jasleen Kaur	Department of Pharmaceutical Sciences and Drug Research, Punjabi University, Patiala, Punjab, India
Jugnu Goyal	Swami Dayanand Institute of Pharmaceutical Sciences, UHS, Rohtak, Haryana, India
Kamya Goyal	Laureate Institute of Pharmacy, Kathog, Distt, Kangra, India
Nikunj Tandel	Institute of Science, Nirma University, Ahmedabad, Gujarat, India
Peeyush Kaushik	Chandigarh College of Pharmacy, Landran, Mohali, Punjab, India
Rajeev K. Tyagi	Department of Medicine, Vanderbilt University Medical Center, Nashville, TN, USA Biomedical Parasitiology and Nano-immunology Lab, CSIR Institute of Microbial Technology (IMTECH), Chandigarh, India
Ravinder Singh	Department of Chemistry, National Taiwan University, Taipei, Taiwan
Reena Sharma	Agricultural Biotechnology Research Center, Academia Sinica, Taipei, Taiwan
Richa Deshpande	Institute of Science, Nirma University, Ahmedabad, Gujarat, India
Samir Mehndiratta	School of Pharmacy, University of Southern California, Los Angeles, USA School of Pharmacy, Taipei Medical University, Taipei, Taiwan
Sanju Nanda	Department of Pharmaceutical Sciences, Maharshi Dayanand University, Rohtak, India
Shammy Jindal	Laureate Institute of Pharmacy, Kathog, Distt- Kangra, H.P., India
Shamsher Singh	Department of Pharmacology, ISF College of Pharmacy, Moga, Punjab, India
Sunishtha	Department of Pharmaceutical Sciences, Maharshi Dayanand University, Rohtak, India
Tarun Kumar	Department of ECE, Deenbandhu Chhotu Ram University of Science and Technology, Haryana, India

CHAPTER 1

History of Pandemics

Sunishtha[1], **Govind Singh**[1] and **Sanju Nanda**[1,*]

[1] *Department of Pharmaceutical Sciences, Maharshi Dayanand University, Rohtak, India*

Abstract: Pandemic is the term coined for the widespread of a disease or infection on a very large scale and across borders. COVID-19, an outcome of the spread of coronavirus, reportedly started from China and spread to almost all the countries of the world. Though it is not for the first time that there was an outbreak of a disease at such a high magnitude but the duration for which it has continued to grapple the world with its virulence and contagious nature, it has become important to take a peek into the history of other pandemics of the world too. Before COVID -19, about 20 major outbreaks of infectious diseases took place and claimed millions of lives in a sweep. The awareness of government bodies, WHO, and non-government organizations grew better with every pandemic. Understanding the role of basic hygiene, self-immunity, social distancing, living in coherence with other living and non-living components of the planet are some positive outcomes of these pandemics. These pandemics also necessitated the need for discovering new drugs and vaccines.

This chapter describes the major pandemics in the history of mankind, the origin and types of coronaviruses, the association of different types of coronaviruses with the ranges and severity of infections, and the origin of COVID-19.

Keywords: AIDS, Black Death, Contagious, Corona, COVID-19, Ebola, Epidemic, Flu, H1N1, Host, Outbreaks, Pandemic, Plague, SARS, Swine flu, Vaccine, Virulence, WHO, Yellow fever.

INTRODUCTION

The terms pandemic, epidemic, outbreak are primarily categorized based on the number of cases of a condition often used to describe infections. These terms have described the comparison of the expected number of cases in a particular time and how far-off cases have spread in the geographical area. Some conditions, such as cancer, hypertension, violence, beneficial behaviors, or even positive behaviors, can also be defined in the same way (Morens *et al.*, 2009).

---

[*] **Corresponding author Sanju Nanda:** Department of Pharmaceutical Sciences, Maharshi Dayanand University, Rohtak, India; E-mail: sn_mdu@rediffmail.com

Neeraj Mittal, Sanjay Kumar Bhadada, O. P. Katare and Varun Garg (Eds.)
All rights reserved-© 2021 Bentham Science Publishers

The term 'pandemic', has its origin derived from the Greek words *pan* (meaning "all") and *demos* (meaning "the people"). Pandemic refers to a spread of contagious illness that spreads across the countries or world, usually affecting a larger area than an 'epidemic'. It is important to note that a disease that is affecting a large number of people or widespread cannot be said to be a pandemic till it is contagious (Fig. **1**). For example, cancer kills many people, but it is not a contagious disease, so not included as a pandemic (WHO, 2011).

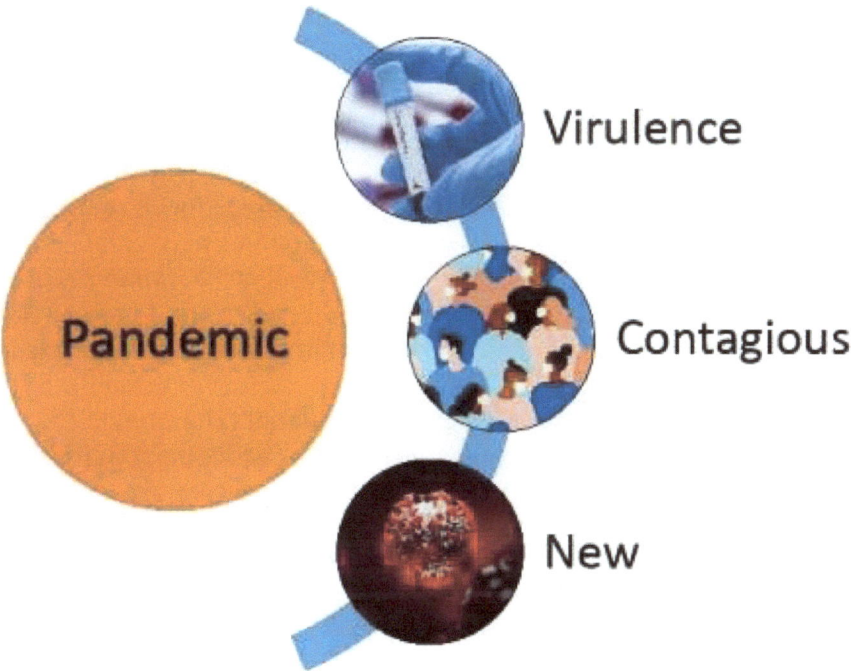

Fig. (1). The essentials of a pandemic.

The word "epidemic" is derived from the two Greek words *epi* meaning "upon or above", and *demos* "the people". An *epidemic* is an outbreak of disease that rapidly spread to a large population in a short period of time. For example, severe acute respiratory syndrome (SARS) took the lives of approx. 800 people worldwide during the epidemic of 2003 (Morens *et al*, 2009). An *outbreak* is an increase beyond expectation in the number of cases of a disease or condition occurring among a specified population in a limited geographic location and period of time (Gregg, 2002). The multi-state outbreak of *Salmonella Muenchen* in 1981 is an example of the outbreak.

Evidence suggested that the human population has suffered from many pandemics throughout history, be it the earlier form of smallpox or Spanish flu or the recent incidence of Ebola or Covid. In world history, we can see a number of significant pandemics like cholera, dengue, plague, smallpox, AIDS, tuberculosis, influenza, West Nile disease, and severe acute respiratory syndrome (Rewar *et al*., 2015; Qiu *et al*., 2016). In 1999, WHO issued a printed paper on pandemic readiness overview, which was further revised in 2005 and 2009 while planning for an influenza pandemic. In this guidance, WHO defined different phases of pandemic and required appropriate actions for each phase. The revision includes the explanation of a pandemic and declaration of its leading phases (WHO, 2011). There have been many pandemics declared at different times as enlisted in Table 1.

THE ATHENIAN PLAGUE

The plague has been responsible for three pandemics in history, including the 6th, 14th, and 19th centuries. The Athenian plague occurred during 430–26 B.C. It originated from Ethiopia, after that, it was distributed in Egypt and Greece. It is a well-known infectious disease primarily affecting rodents. *Yersinia pestis* bacteria is a causative agent of Athenian plaque that is related to the Enterobacteriaceae family. It is transferred in humans from rodents through skin-piercing by infected fleas. Transmission of bacteria in an uninfected person is possible by droplet contact, direct or indirect contact with infected material (Huremovic *et al*., 2017). Initial observed symptoms of the plague were headache, conjunctivitis, rashes on the whole body, and fever. After that patients showed severe symptoms like cough up blood, severe stomach cramps along with vomiting, and attacks of "ineffectual retching". Generally, on the seventh or eighth-day infected persons die (Thucydides, 2017). Approximately 75000 to 100000 people died due to the plague of Athens (Litteman *et al*., 2009).

Table 1. Chronology of pandemics.

Serial No.	Name of Pandemic Event	Year	Origin
1	Plague of Athens	430 B.C.	Ethiopia
2	Antonine Plague	165-190 A.D.	Italian peninsula
3	Justinian Plague	541-750 A.D.	Egypt
4	Japanese Smallpox	735-737 A.D.	Japan
5	Black Death	1347-1351	China
6	Aztecs Disease	1519-1520	Aztecs, America
7	London Plague	1665-1666	London
8	The Great Plague	1738	Central and Eastern Europe
9	Cholera 6 Outbreak	1817-1923	India

(Table 1) cont.....

Serial No.	Name of Pandemic Event	Year	Origin
10	The Third Plague	1885	Yunnan, China
11	Yellow Fever	1648-1800	Africa
12	Russian Flu	1889-1890	The first cases were observed at three separate and distant locations, Bukhara in Central Asia (Turkestan), Athabasca in northwestern Canada, and Greenland.
13	Spanish Flu	1918-1920	Europe
14	Asian Flu	1957-1958	The Chinese province of Guizhou
15	Hong Kong Flu	1968-1970	Hong Kong
16	HIV/AIDS	1980 – present	The Democratic Republic of the Congo
17	SARS	2003	China
18	Swine flu	2009-2010	Mexico
19	MERS	2012	Saudi Arabia
20	EBOLA	2014-2016	Zaire, Africa
21	COVID-19	2019 – present	Wuhan, China

PLAGUE OF JUSTINIAN

The Justinian plague is the first recorded pandemic that began in 541 AD, killed over 100 million people. The Justinian plague, the name given after the 6th century by Justinian I, Roman emperor of the Byzantine Empire at that time (Rosen, 2007). It was a "real plague" pandemic that originated in the mid-sixth century AD. The first recorded outbreak of this disease began in Egypt. Further, it spread in the capital of Turkey Constantinople caused the death of 10000 people per day, and killed around 40% of the city population. It reduced drop by drop European population by 50% between 550 AD and 700 AD (Horgan, 2014).

THE BLACK DEATH

The second pandemic was a global explosion of bubonic plague, widely known as the Great Plague, which originated from China in 1334, after that in 1347 it spread in Europe. After 50 years of its origin global population reduced from 450 million and caused approx 17 to 28 million deaths in Europe during the 14th century (Huremovic, 2016; DeWitte, 2014).

SPANISH FLU

The "Spanish" influenza pandemic of 1918-1919 first appeared in the USA. Dominating impression was mainly found in Europe, Asia, and North America, also appeared in New Zealand, India, and South Africa. It killed around 50 million people worldwide and remained a threat to public health. Around one-third of the world's population was infected and had clear symptoms of illness. This virus-derived in toto from an unknown source appeared as an avian-like influenza virus. It appeared quite ordinary, with mild symptoms. But it was not autopsies on victims that showed unusual hemorrhagic edema in the lungs, and it affected young adults more than others (Taubenberger, 2006). In 1918, this pandemic was caused by the venomous and pestilent influenza virus, a strain of the subtype H1N1 that mostly killed young adults. Examination of the virus proved it particularly deadly, as it activates overproduction, uncontrolled production of immune cells that destroy the immune system, and death of youngster. In 1918, the French bacteriologist Charles Nicole and his colleague Lebailly C concluded that the strain was found in mammals. The causative agent of Spanish flu is a virus of the "Orthomyxoviridae" family, which was recognized by Richard Edwin Scope (Tsoucalas *et al.*, 2016).

AIDS

AIDS (acquired immunodeficiency syndrome) is an autoimmune disease caused by the human immunodeficiency virus (HIV). The causative virus was firstly identified in the early 1980s in the United States, after that scientists observed some cases in Africa and Europe, and at the same time all over the world. AIDS spreads through blood, vaginal secretions, semen, breast milk and mainly transmitted through unprotected mating with an HIV-positive partner. AIDS is a fatal disease, whereas a less number of infected people remain alive with AIDS around 20 years. It is the leading infectious cause of adult death around the world. AIDS was first recognized in the 1980s, public health officers try to prevent spreading disease by providing knowledge about the virus-like how the virus transferred from person to person and how could be protected ourselves from it (Farmer and Walton 2000; Lampatey and Merywen 2002).

SMALLPOX

Smallpox is one the most devastating diseases known to humankind, indigenous to Europe, Arabia, and Asia for centuries, responsible for the death of three infected individuals out of ten infectious patients, and the rest remain with pocky scars on the whole body. Evidence suggested that during the 20th century the global death toll from smallpox have been estimated at around 300 million. The native people of the United States and modern-day Mexico had nil natural immunity power against smallpox and the virus deducted them below by the tens of millions. Smallpox is the first virus epidemic cured by vaccination. During the 18th century, the vaccine of smallpox was discovered by a British doctor named Edward Jenner. Around 50 million people were infected by the smallpox virus in one year- which was equal to the population of South Africa. After that WHO was established in 1948. In India, until the 1950s, annually more than a million people died due to smallpox. In 1980, WHO declared that smallpox had been eliminated from the Earth (Fenner and Henderson 1988; Gupta and Mahajan 2003; Roos, 2020).

SARS

The first case of Severe Acute Respiratory Syndrome (SARS) appeared in China in November 2002. After that, it was recognized as a global threat in March 2003. In the next few months, SARS disease spread over many continents such as North America, Europe, South America, and Asia. In the 21st century, it emerges as the first severe and readily transmissible disease. It is a viral respiratory illness caused by a coronavirus commonly known as SARS-associated coronavirus, having an incubation period of 2 to 10 days. The primary mode of transmission is respiratory droplets and direct contact. SARS-CoV has been detected mainly in stool, also detected in blood, urine, and conjunctival secretions but to a lesser extent (Christian and Poutanen 2004; Hui, 2005; WHO, 2013).

SWINE FLU OR H1N1 PANDEMIC

Swine flu is a respiratory disease of the pig, commonly known as Hog or Pig Flu. Infection caused by type A influenza virus subtype of H1N1that belongs to the Orthomyxoviridae family. The novel H1N1strain is the main reason for the explosion of swine flu, the origin of this new strain is unknown. It was first identified in April 2019 at the border region of the United States and Mexico. It emerged out as the first pandemic of the 21st century in a short term of two months, involving more than 170 countries and approximately 1.7 lakh infected individuals all over the world. Globally, the illness rate of swine flu was highest in children and young adults but the hospitalization rate was higher in children below one year of age (Mir *et al.*, 2009; Sebastian *et al.*, 2009).

EBOLA

It is defined as a neglected tropical disease (NTD), killed thousands of people. It is the largest and longest recorded pandemic in human history. The Ebola virus was the first point out in 1976 in Zaira, Yambuku, and Nzara, South Sudan as an outbreak of hemorrhagic fever. Ebola outburst started through zoonotic transmission, caused more than 30 outbreaks since 1976, with less than 1600 deaths before 2014, and since 2014 thousands of people killed in West Africa. The incubation period of the Ebola virus is 5 to 7 days. In most of the cases, it started from rural background controlled by following regular community health measures like having a view on several infected people and the patient was isolated to break the chain of virus (Troncoso, 2015; Richardson et al., 2016).

COVID-19

Coronavirus disease (COVID-19) is a highly contagious respiratory illness that was quickly spread globally within the short term after finding the first case of COVID-19 (in Wuhan, China) in December 2019. WHO announced it as a life threat worldwide on 30 January and a pandemic on 11 March 2020, caused by the novel coronavirus, subsequently named SARS-CoV-2. In this respiratory disease, a person has mild symptoms like cold and cough after some time it emerged out as a critical illness with blockage of respiratory track and high fever. It has an overall low fatality rate in youngsters and a much higher rate in older persons. The causative agent of COVID-19 (SARS-CoV-2) spread very easily by respiratory droplets generated during talking, sneezing, and coughing by an infected person. It has 5 to 6 days incubation period (Balkhair, 2020).

ORIGIN OF CORONAVIRUS

"Coronavirus" word originated in 1968, given to the crown projections on their surfaces observed in the electron microscope. "Corona" in Latin means "halo" or "crown". Coronaviruses mainly attack the respiratory system and give rise to some manifestations like cough and difficulty in breathing. Some people, including older adults, are at risk of severe illness from these viruses. Coronavirus is a single positive-sense RNA virus; identified in 1960. Since 1970 pathogenesis and molecular mechanisms of replication of several coronaviruses have been actively studied. International Committee established the Coronaviridae family on Taxonomy of viruses in 1975. Coronaviruses have been described for more than 50 years, infect many species of animals including humans, and primarily affect the respiratory, gastroenteritis, and nervous system (Weiss and Navas-Martin, 2005).

Coronavirus species had been categorized into three groups. Group I and II infect mammals whereas group III is exclusively found in birds. SARS-CoV has been proposed as the first member of the fourth group of coronaviruses, separated from a child affected by bronchiolitis and conjunctivitis, and causes life-threatening pneumonia. HCoV-229E and HCoV-OC43 were identified to cause the common cold. There are only three types of coronaviruses have been studied that affect human, after addition of SARS-CoV; supplementary feature of HCoV-NL63 as the fourth member will supply a significant understanding of the variation among human coronaviruses. HCoV-NL63 is an arm of the group 1 coronaviruses similarly to HCoV-229E, but the dissimilarities between them are important. These are as follows:

i. They have around 65% sequence similarities.
ii. In HCoV-NL63, a single gene ORF3 takes the place of the 4A and 4B genes in HCoV-229E.
iii. In HCoV-NL63, the 5' region of the S gene contains a large in-frame insertion of 537 nucleotides.
iv. With a narrow host range, HCoV-229E is fastidious in cell culture. But, efficient replication of HCoV-NL63 in monkey kidney cells has been observed.
v. In infants and immunocompromised patients, HCoV-229E can cause severe respiratory disease whereas HCoV-NL63 causes acute respiratory disease (Hoek et al., 2004).

In December 2019, an extended number of pneumonia cases were found in China, caused by a newly recognized β-coronavirus, which is enveloped in a non-segmented positive-sense RNA virus. Initially, on 12 January 2020, WHO officially named this virus 2019- novel coronavirus (2019-nCoV) and disease as coronavirus disease 2019 (COVID-19). Coronavirus Study Group of the International Committee suggested the name to the new coronavirus as SARS-CoV-2 on February 11, 2020.

TYPES OF CORONAVIRUSES

All coronaviruses have a single-stranded RNA, size of genome up to 30kb in length and have similar morphology features. They have been united in the subfamily Coronavirinae within the family Coronaviridae which belongs to the Nidovirales order. The family consists of two subfamilies, Coronavirinae and Torovirinae. The Coronavirinae subfamily further divided into four genera, Alphacoronavirus, Betacoronavirus, Gammacoronavirus and Deltacoronavirus as summarized in Table **2**. Genera further classified into various species, containing various viruses that cause infections of cattle, horses, pigs, goats, and cats. Although, to date, it is not proven that the Torovirinae subfamily infects humans. Betacoronaviruses and Alphacoronaviruses are mainly originated from mammals, while Gammacoronaviruses and Deltacoronaviruses primarily began from avian (Wertheim et al., 2013).

Table 2. Types of coronaviruses.

Genus	Abbreviation used for the Virus	Species Affected	Disease Name or Organ System Affected
Alphacoronavirus	PEDV	Porcine	Porcine epidemic diarrhea virus
	TGEV	Porcine	Transmissible gastroenteritis virus
	FIPV	Feline	Feline coronavirus
	CCoV	Canine	Canine coronavirus
	PRCV	Porcine	Porcine respiratory coronavirus
	HCoV-229E	Human	Common cold
	HCoV-NL63	Human	Common cold
	Rh-BatCoV-HKU2	Bat	-
	Mi-BatCoV 1A	Bat	-
	Mi-BatCoV 1B	Bat	-
	Mi-BatCoV-HKU8	Bat	-
	Sc-BatCoV-512	Bat	-
Betacoronavirus	HCoV-OC43	Human	Common cold
	BCoV	Bovine	Calf diarrhea, winter dysentery
	PHEV	Porcine	Chronic wasting, encephalomyelitis
	AntelopeCoV	Antelope	-
	GiCoV	Giraffe	-
	ECoV	Equine	Enteric infection
	MHV	Mouse	Hepatic infection
	HCoV-HKU1	Human	Respiratory infections
	RCoV	Rat	-
	SARS CoV	Human	Severe acute respiratory syndrome
	SARSr-CiCoV	Human	Severe acute respiratory syndrome
	SARSr-Rh-BatCoV HKU3	Bat	-
	SARSrCoV CFB	Human	Severe acute respiratory syndrome
	Ty-BatCoV-HKU4	Bat	-
	Pi-BatCoV-HKU5	Bat	-
	Ro-Bat-CoV HKU9	Bat	-
Gammacoronavirus	IBV	Chickens	Avian infectious bronchitis virus
	TCoV	Turkey	Bluecomb, turkey coronavirus
	BWCoV-SW1	Whale	Beluga whale CoV

(Table 2) cont.....

Genus	Abbreviation used for the Virus	Species Affected	Disease Name or Organ System Affected
Deltacoronavirus	BuCoV HKU11	Avian	Bulbul coronavirus
	ThCoV HKU12	Avian	Thrush coronavirus
	MunCoV HKU13	Avian	Munia coronavirus
	PorCoV HKU15	Porcine	Porcine coronavirus
	WECoV HKU16	-	White eye coronavirus
	SpCoV HKU17	Avian	Sparrow coronavirus
	MRCoV HKU18	Avian	Magpie robin coronavirus
	NHCoV HKU19	Avian	Night heron coronavirus
	WiCoV HKU20	-	Wigeon coronavirus
	CMCoV HKU21	Avian	Common moorhen

The genus Alphacoronavirus includes several animal coronaviruses (PEDV, TGEV, FIPV) and human coronaviruses (HCoV-229E, HCoV-NL63). The genus Betacoronavirus comprise numerous animal coronaviruses BCoV, PHEV, GICoV, and three types of human coronaviruses *i.e.* HCoV-HKU1, HCoV-OC43, SARS-HCoV, and the MERS (Middle Eastern respiratory syndrome) coronavirus, SARS-related coronavirus.

Based on antigenic similarity Coronaviruses are classified into four groups, viruses in all groups can affect a large number of different host species. Several recognized human coronaviruses 229E, NL63, OC43, and HKU1 are common human viruses that easily infect immunocompromised and elder patients. These are responsible for approximately 10% mortality by causing common cold and self-limiting upper respiratory disease. MERS-CoV, SARS-CoV, and SAR-Co--2 are also human coronaviruses but these occur less frequently than common human viruses. These viruses cause severe respiratory disease and cause up to 35% of death (Cascella *et al.*, 2020).

Alphacoronaviruses form a distinct monophyletic group in the Coronavirinae subfamily, having similar phylogenetic properties to other coronaviruses. General characteristics make it different among coronaviruses. Alphacoronavirus having an exclusive type of nsp1, specific size, and sequence from the nsp1 protein of betacoronavirus. Gammacoronavirus is similar to the other coronaviruses only in phylogenetic relation, there are no similarities in virion morphology, genome organization, and gene composition. These characteristics make it different from other coronaviruses. Viruses of the species avian coronavirus lack an nsp1 moiety. The genus Gammacoronavirus related to the third group of human coronavirus include viruses that were segregated from birds and whales. The genus

Deltacoronavirus is comprised of viruses isolated from pigs and birds. Until now various types of novel coronaviruses have been separated from bats. Many researchers suggested that human respiratory coronaviruses, MERS coronavirus, SARS coronavirus originated from an ancestor of bat viruses.

DISEASE ASSOCIATED WITH CORONAVIRUSES

Coronaviruses mainly strike on the respiratory system of mammals, birds, and humans. These are associated with pneumonia, common cold, bronchitis, severe acute respiratory syndrome (SARS), and coronavirus disease 2019 (COVID-19). From the last few years' studies, researchers concluded that these viruses can also infect rats, mice, dogs, cats, pigs, horses, and cattle. In most cases, animals transfer the viruses to humans.

Coronavirus is a significant pathogen that mainly affects the human respiratory tract and also attacks the gut of humans. The earlier outburst of coronaviruses having severe acute respiratory syndrome (SARS) and the Middle East respiratory syndrome (MERS) is earlier recognized as factors that are a major threat to public health. At the end of December 2019, numerous patients having pneumonia with unknown etiology entered hospitals.

MURINE HEPATITIS VIRUS (MHV)

Murine hepatitis virus is a commonly used laboratory strain that belongs to betacoronavirus genera; primarily infect the liver and brain. There are many strains of murine coronavirus exhibiting neurotropic and cause encephalitis with subsequent CNS demyelination. Although, the virus found in lasting infection of astrocytes, in most of the animals causes death by infecting oligodendrocytes and neurons. The animals that survive with acute infection develop a chronic progressive neurologic disease identified by outspread demyelinating lesions and CNS infiltration of lymphocytes and macrophages (Kyuwa and Stohlman 1990). It is one of the best animal models for encephalitis, hepatitis, and multiple sclerosis (Perlman, 1998).

Central Nervous System

The most frequently studied MHV strains are JHM and A59. The first time JHM was isolated from a paralytic mouse that was intensely neurovirulent producing encephalomyelitis with massive demyelination (Bailey *et al.*, 1949; Cheever *et al.*, 1949).

Hepatitis

MHV-induced hepatitis has been studied through several hepatovirulent strains including MHV-3, MHV-2, and the moderately hepatotropic A59. The most commonly used strain for the pathogenic study of MHV-induced hepatitis is the MHV-3 strain. It was separated from an offspring mouse that developed acute hepatitis following inoculation with the serum of an acute hepatitis patient (Dick et al., 1956).

Pneumonitis

MHV-1 strain is primarily pneumovirulent. MHV-1-induced pneumonitis is highly dependent on mouse strain; inbred albino strain, resistant to MHV-3 induced hepatitis is highly sensitive. Whereas other species of mice such as Balb/c and C57Bl/6 are resistible for MHV-1- induced pulmonary disease. MHV-1 infection of albino mice provides a mouse model for the pathogenic study of SARS-CoV in human beings (De Albuquerque et al., 2006).

BOVINE CORONAVIRUS

It is a non-segmented, positive-sense, single-stranded RNA virus that belongs to the Coronaviridae family and was first identified during an outbreak of diarrhea among neonatal calves in 1970 (Fauquet et al., 2005; Mebus et al., 1974). It was commonly identified in the respiratory system and gut of cattle where they used to shed fecal matter, nasal secretions and affect the lungs (Hasoksuz et al., 2002; Saif, 2010). It causes various diseases in cattle like winter dysentery, calf diarrhea in young cattle, and respiratory illness in the different age groups of cattle (Saif, 1990, 2007, 2010). It is also related to bovine respiratory disease in growing beef calves involved in the feedlots or grazing field (Fulton et al., 2011). To date, Bovine coronavirus monitoring programs might be included in the live attenuated virus or killed vaccines but there is no USFDA-approved bovine coronavirus vaccine in The United States to control bovine respiratory disease (North American Compendiums, 2010). Modified live vaccines can be used in newborn calf to prevent gastroenteric disease, also used for a pregnant cow. Antibodies of Bovine coronavirus transfer in neonates after calving to control BoCV (Fulton et al., 2011).

HUMAN CORONAVIRUS

In the mid-1960s, human coronaviruses were first recognised. To date, there are seven types of coronaviruses identified which can cause infections in the majority of people. There are seven mentioned types of human coronaviruses and these are

NL63 (alpha coronavirus), 229E (alpha coronavirus), HKU1 (beta coronavirus), OC43 (beta coronavirus), MERS-CoV (beta coronavirus that causes MERS), SARS-CoV (beta coronavirus that causes SARS), and SARS-CoV-2 (the new coronavirus which gives rise to COVID-19) (CDC, 2020).

Human coronaviruses are the respiratory pathogens that present an important group of coronaviruses linked with several respiratory diseases such as pneumonia, bronchitis, common cold, and respiratory disease (Pene *et al.*, 2003). Evolution of HCoVs has been expedited through the regular combination of species by crossing of species barrier and genetic recombination of these viruses. Many of these are widely spread in the human population and globally hit one-third of common cold infections in human beings (Lim *et al.*, 2016).

ABBREVIATIONS

AD	Anno Domini
AIDS	Acquired immunodeficiency syndrome
B.C	Before Christ
BoCV	Bovine coronavirus
CDC	Centers for Disease Control and prevention
CNS	Central nervous system
CoV	Coronavirus
COVID-19	Coronavirus disease 2019
HIV	Human immunodeficiency virus
MERS-CoV	Middle East respiratory syndrome coronavirus
MHV	Murine Hepatitis Virus
NTD	Neglected tropical disease
RNA	Ribonucleic acid
SARS-CoV	Severe acute respiratory syndrome coronavirus
USDA	United States Departments of Agriculture
WHO	World Health Organization

CONSENT FOR PUBLICATION

Not applicable.

CONFLICT OF INTEREST

The author declares no conflict of interest, financial or otherwise.

ACKNOWLEDGEMENTS

Declared none.

REFERENCES

Albuquerque, ND, Baig, E, Ma, X, Zhang, J, He, W & Rowe, A (2006) Murine hepatitis virus strain 1 produces a clinically relevant model of severe acute respiratory syndrome in A/J mice. *J Virol,* 80, 10382-94.
[http://dx.doi.org/10.1128/JVI.00747-06] [PMID: 17041219]

Balkhair, AA (2020) COVID-19 pandemic: a new chapter in the history of infectious diseases. *Oman Med J,* 35, e123.
[http://dx.doi.org/10.5001/omj.2020.41] [PMID: 32328297]

Bailey, OT, Pappenheimer, AM, Cheever, FS & Daniels, JB (1949) A murine virus (JHM) causing disseminated encephalomyelitis with extensive destruction of myelin. II. pathology. *J Exp Med,* 90, 195-212.
[http://dx.doi.org/10.1084/jem.90.3.195] [PMID: 19871701]

Bogoch, II, Watts, A, Thomas-Bachli, A, Huber, Kraemer MUG & Khan, K (2020) Pneumonia of unknown etiology in Wuhan, China: potential for international spread *via* commercial air travel. *J Travel Med,* 27, taaa008.

Cascella, M, Rajnik, M, Cuomo, A, Cascella, M, Scott, CD & Raffaela, DN (2020) *Features, Evaluation, and Treatment of Coronavirus (COVID-19).* StatPearls Publishing, Treasure Island, FL.

CDC (2020) https://www.cdc.gov/coronavirus/types.html

Centers for Disease Control and Prevention (CDC) (2008) Outbreak of Salmonella serotype Saintpaul infections associated with multiple raw produce items--United States, 2008. *MMWR Morb Mortal Wkly Rep,* 57, 929-34.
[PMID: 18756191]

Cheever, FS, Daniels, JB, Pappenheimer, AM & Baily, OT (1949) 'A murine virus (JHM) causing disseminated encephalomyelitis with extensive destruction of myelin. I. Isolation and biological properties of the virus'. *J Travel Med,* 90, 181-94.

Chen, CJ & Makino, S (2004) Murine coronavirus replication induces cell cycle arrest in G0/G1 phase. *J Virol,* 78, 5658-69.
[http://dx.doi.org/10.1128/JVI.78.11.5658-5669.2004] [PMID: 15140963]

Christian, MD & Poutanen, SM (2020) Severe Acute Respiratory Syndrome. *Emerg Infect CID,* 2004, 38.

Colwell, RR (1996) Global climate and infectious disease: the cholera paradigm. *Science,* 274, 2025-31.
[http://dx.doi.org/10.1126/science.274.5295.2025] [PMID: 8953025]

DeWitte, SN (2014) Mortality risk and survival in the aftermath of the medieval black death. *PLoS One,* 9, e96513.
[http://dx.doi.org/10.1371/journal.pone.0096513] [PMID: 24806459]

Dick, GWA, Niven, JSF & Gledhill, AW (1956) A virus related to that causing hepatitis in mice (MHV). *Br J Exp Pathol,* 37, 90-8.
[PMID: 13304245]

Farmer, PE, Walton, DA & Furin, JJ (2000) In the emergency of aids: the impact on immunology, microbiology and public health. *The Changing Face of AIDS: Implications for Policy and Practice* American Public Health Association 139-61.

Fauquet, CM, Mayo, MA, Maniloff, J, Desselberger, U & Ball, LA (2005) *Virus Taxonomy, Eighth Report of the International Committee on Taxonomy of Viruses.* Elsevier, Academic Press, London.

Fenner, F, Henderson, DA, Isao, A, Zdenek, J & Danilovich, LI (1988) *Smallpox and its Eradication.* World Halth Organization.

Fulton, RW, Step, DL, Wahrmund, J, Burge, LJ, Payton, ME, Cook, BJ, Burken, D, Richards, CJ & Confer, AW (2011) Bovine coronavirus (BCV) infections in transported commingled beef cattle and sole-source ranch calves. *Can J Vet Res,* 75, 191-9.
[PMID: 22210995]

Gregg, MB *Field Epidemiology, Emerging Infectious Disease.* Oxford University Press, New York 280.

Gupta, MC & Mahajan, BK (2003) *Textbook of Preventive and Social Medicine.* Jaypee Brothers Medical Publishers, New York.

Hasoksuz, M, Hoet, AE, Loerch, SC, Wittum, TE, Nielsen, PR & Saif, LJ (2002) Detection of respiratory and enteric shedding of bovine coronaviruses in cattle in an Ohio feedlot. *J Vet Diagn Invest,* 14, 308-13.
[http://dx.doi.org/10.1177/104063870201400406] [PMID: 12152810]

Hoek, LVD, Pyrc, K, Jebbink, MF, Vermeulen-Oost, W, Berkhout, RJM, Wolthers, KC, Wertheim-van Dillen, PM, Kaandorp, J, Spaargaren, J & Berkhout, B (2004) Identification of a new human coronavirus. *Nat Med,* 10, 368-73.
[http://dx.doi.org/10.1038/nm1024] [PMID: 15034574]

Horgan, J (2014) Ancient history encyclopedia. *Justinian's Plague (541–542 CE).*

Hui, DSC (2005) An overview on severe acute respiratory syndrome (SARS). *Monaldi Arch Chest Dis,* 63, 149-57.
[http://dx.doi.org/10.4081/monaldi.2005.632] [PMID: 16312205]

Huremovic, D (2019) Brief history of pandemics (pandemics throughout history). *Psychiatry of Pandemics: A Mental Health Response to Infection Outbreak,* 7-35.
[http://dx.doi.org/10.1007/978-3-030-15346-5_2]

Kyuwa, S & Stohlman, S (1990) Background paper. advances in the study of MHV infection of mice. *Adv Exp Med Biol,* 276, 555-6.
[http://dx.doi.org/10.1007/978-1-4684-5823-7_76] [PMID: 1966448]

Lamptey, P & Merywen, W (2002) Facing the HIV/AIDS Pandemic. *Popul Bull,* 57(3).

Lim, YX, Ng, YL, Tam, JP & Liu, DX (2016) Human coronaviruses: a review of virus-host interactions. *Diseases,* 4, 26.
[http://dx.doi.org/10.3390/diseases4030026] [PMID: 28933406]

Littman, RJ (2009) The plague of athens: epidemiology and paleopathology. *Mt Sinai J Med,* 76, 456-67.
[http://dx.doi.org/10.1002/msj.20137] [PMID: 19787658]

Lu, H, Stratton, CW & Tang, YW (2020) Outbreak of pneumonia of unknown etiology in Wuhan, China: The mystery and the miracle. *J Med Virol,* 92, 401-2.
[http://dx.doi.org/10.1002/jmv.25678] [PMID: 31950516]

Lu, R, Zhao, X, Li, J, Niu, P, Yang, B, Wu, H, Wang, W, Song, H, Huang, B, Zhu, N, Bi, Y, Ma, X, Zhan, F, Wang, L, Hu, T, Zhou, H, Hu, Z, Zhou, W, Zhao, L, Chen, J, Meng, Y, Wang, J, Lin, Y, Yuan, J, Xie, Z, Ma, J, Liu, WJ, Wang, D, Xu, W, Holmes, EC, Gao, GF, Wu, G, Chen, W, Shi, W & Tan, W (2020) Genomic characterisation and epidemiology of 2019 novel coronavirus: implications for virus origins and receptor binding. *Lancet,* 395, 565-74.
[http://dx.doi.org/10.1016/S0140-6736(20)30251-8] [PMID: 32007145]

Mebus, CA, Stair, EL, Rhodes, MB & Twiehaus, MJ (1973) Neonatal calf diarrhea: propagation, attenuation, and characteristics of a coronavirus-like agent. *Am J Vet Res,* 34, 145-50.
[PMID: 4568246]

Mir, SA, Tandon, VR & Abbas, Z (2009) History of swine flu. *JKScience,* 4, 161-2.

Morens, DM, Folkers, GK & Fauci, AS (2009) What is a pandemic? *J Infect Dis,* 200, 1018-21.
[http://dx.doi.org/10.1086/644537] [PMID: 19712039]

North American Compendiums (2010) *Compendium of Veterinary Products.* North American Compendiums,

Port Huron, MI.

Pene, F, Merlat, A, Vabret, A, Rozenberg, F, Buzyn, A, Dreyfus, F, Cariou, A, Freymuth, F & Lebon, P (2003) Coronavirus 229E-related pneumonia in immunocompromised patients. *Clin Infect Dis,* 37, 929-32.
[http://dx.doi.org/10.1086/377612] [PMID: 13130404]

Perlman, S (1998) Pathogenesis of coronavirus-induced infections. Review of pathological and immunological aspects. *Adv Exp Med Biol,* 440, 503-13.
[http://dx.doi.org/10.1007/978-1-4615-5331-1_65] [PMID: 9782322]

Qiu, WR, Mao, A & Chu, C (2016) The pandemic and its impact. *Heal Cult Soc,* 9-10.

Rewar, S, Mirdha, D & Rewar, P (2015) Treatment and prevention of pandemic H1N1 influenza. *Ann Glob Health,* 81, 645-53.

Richardson, ET, Barrie, MB, Kelly, JD, Dibba, Y, Koedoyoma, S & Farmer, PE (2016) Biosocial approaches to the 2013-2016 ebola pandemic. *Health Hum Rights,* 18, 115-28.
[PMID: 27781004]

Roos, D (2020) How 5 of history's worst pandemics finally ended. *History.* https://www.history.com/news/pandemics-end-plague-cholera-black-death-smallpox

Rosen, W (2007) *Justinian Flea: The First Great Plague and the End of the Roman Empire.*Viking Penguin.

Saif, LJ (1990) A review of evidence implicating bovine coronavirus in the etiology of winter dysentery in cows: an enigma resolved? *Cornell Vet,* 80, 303-11.
[PMID: 2170075]

Saif, LJ (2007) The nidoviruses. In: S, Perlman, T, Gallagher, EJ, Snijder, (Eds.), *Coronaviruses of Domestic Livestock and Poultry: Interspecies Transmission, Pathogenesis, and Immunity* ASM Press, Washington, DC 279-96.

Saif, LJ (2010) Bovine respiratory coronavirus. *Vet Clin North Am Food Anim Pract,* 26, 349-64.
[http://dx.doi.org/10.1016/j.cvfa.2010.04.005] [PMID: 20619189]

Sebastian, MR, Lodha, R & Kabra, SK (2009) Swine origin influenza (swine flu). *Indian J Pediatr,* 76, 833-41.
[http://dx.doi.org/10.1007/s12098-009-0170-6] [PMID: 19802552]

Spaan, WJM Family coronaviridae. *Virus Taxonomy: Eight Reports of the International Committee on Taxonomy of Viruses* Elsevier, San Diego, CA 947-64.

Taubenberger, JK & Morens, DM (2006) 1918 influenza: the mother of all pandemics. *Emerg Infect Dis,* 12, 15-22.
[http://dx.doi.org/10.3201/eid1209.05-0979] [PMID: 16494711]

Taylor, DN, Wachsmuth, IK, Shangkuan, YH, Schmidt, EV, Barrett, TJ, Schrader, JS, Scherach, CS, McGee, HB, Feldman, RA & Brenner, DJ (1982) Salmonellosis associated with marijuana: a multistate outbreak traced by plasmid fingerprinting. *N Engl J Med,* 306, 1249-53.
[http://dx.doi.org/10.1056/NEJM198205273062101] [PMID: 7070444]

Thucydides (2017) History of the peloponnesian war' trans. *Crawley R,* 89-100.

Troncoso, A (2015) Ebola outbreak in West Africa: a neglected tropical disease. *Asian Pac J Trop Biomed,* 5, 255-9.
[http://dx.doi.org/10.1016/S2221-1691(15)30340-3]

Tsoucalas, G, Kousoulis, A & Sgantzos, M (2016) The 1918 spanish flu pandemic, the origins of the H1N1-virus strain, a glance in history. *European Journal of Clinical and Biomedicial Sciences,* 2, 23-8.

Weiss, SR & Navas-Martin, S (2005) Coronavirus pathogenesis and the emerging pathogen severe acute respiratory syndrome coronavirus. *Microbiol Mol Biol Rev,* 69, 635-64.
[http://dx.doi.org/10.1128/MMBR.69.4.635-664.2005] [PMID: 16339739]

Wertheim, JO, Chu, DKW, Peiris, JSM, Kosakovsky Pond, SL & Poon, LLM (2013) A case for the ancient

origin of coronaviruses. *J Virol,* 87, 7039-45.
[http://dx.doi.org/10.1128/JVI.03273-12] [PMID: 23596293]

WHO (2011) Comparative analysis of national pandemic influenza preparedness plans. https://www.who.int/influenza/resources/documents/comparative_analysis_php_2011_en/en/

WHO (2003) Severe acute respiratory syndrome (SARS): Status of the outbreak and lessons for the immediate future. Geneva. https://www.who.int/csr/media/sars_wha.pdf

CHAPTER 2

Introduction to COVID-19

Hitesh Malhotra[1,*], Anjoo Kamboj[1] and Peeyush Kaushik[1]

[1] *Chandigarh College of Pharmacy, Landran, Mohali, Punjab, India*

Abstract: In the mid 20th century, virologists identified a new category of the virus, which has a fringe of projections on its surface that appears like a crown and named coronavirus. Coronavirus belongs to the family of pleomorphic spherical viruses recognized by bulbous surface projection and ssRNA. As the virus belongs to the family of RNA-virus, the chances of mutation are very high, which further increases its pathogenicity. The coronavirus mainly attacks the respiratory tract and ultimately leads to respiratory failure. Recent outbreaks of coronaviruses are severe acute respiratory syndrome and the Middle East respiratory syndrome, which cause a great threat to human health with a high mortality rate. Later on, in late 2019, a new form of coronavirus appears in Wuhan, China where numbers of people are recognized with pneumonia-like symptoms. The condition was entitled with COVID-19 by WHO on Feb 2020, which was declared to be pandemic by the same agency in Mar 2020. The COVID-19 is considered to be originated from bats, which then transmit to humans due to the consumption of contaminated animal raw. The virus is highly contagious and spread at a very high rate, which produces global health risks. Further various existing treatment is used for treating the infection but still the precise and accurate treatment yet to be investigated.

Keywords: ACE-II, Air droplets, Breathlessness, China, Chronology, Coronavirus, COVID-19, Genome, Helicase, Membrane protein, MERS, Pneumocytes, Pneumonia, Replicase, Respiratory distress syndrome, SARS, Structural proteins, Virus, World, Transmission.

INTRODUCTION

The coronavirus belongs to a family of viruses that mainly affects the respiratory tract infection with prime symptoms, such as hyperthermia, pneumonia, breathlessness, and acute or chronic pulmonary infections. The coronavirus mainly affects animals, but recent investigations in the late 20th century reported some human cases. In 1930, the first coronavirus case was reported in chickens recognized by pneumonia-like symptoms and termed as avian infectious bronchitis virus. Further, in late 1960, the first human coronavirus case was

---

[*] **Corresponding Author Hitesh Malhotra:** Chandigarh College of Pharmacy, Landran, Mohali, Punjab, India; Tel: 98 9637 1903; E-mail: hiteshmalhotra03.hm@gmail.com

Neeraj Mittal, Sanjay Kumar Bhadada, O. P. Katare and Varun Garg (Eds.)
All rights reserved-© 2021 Bentham Science Publishers

reported (Pyrc *et al.*, 2007). In 1968, electron microscopy of the virus was done and termed as **"Coronavirus"** due to its crown-like appearance, clearly depicted in Fig. **1(A & B)**. Later on, in 1975, the International Committee on the Taxonomy of Viruses introduced a family Coronaviridae. In 2005, the family Coronaviridae was further split into two subfamilies, the Coronaviruses, and the Toroviruses (Tyrrel *et al.*, 1968).

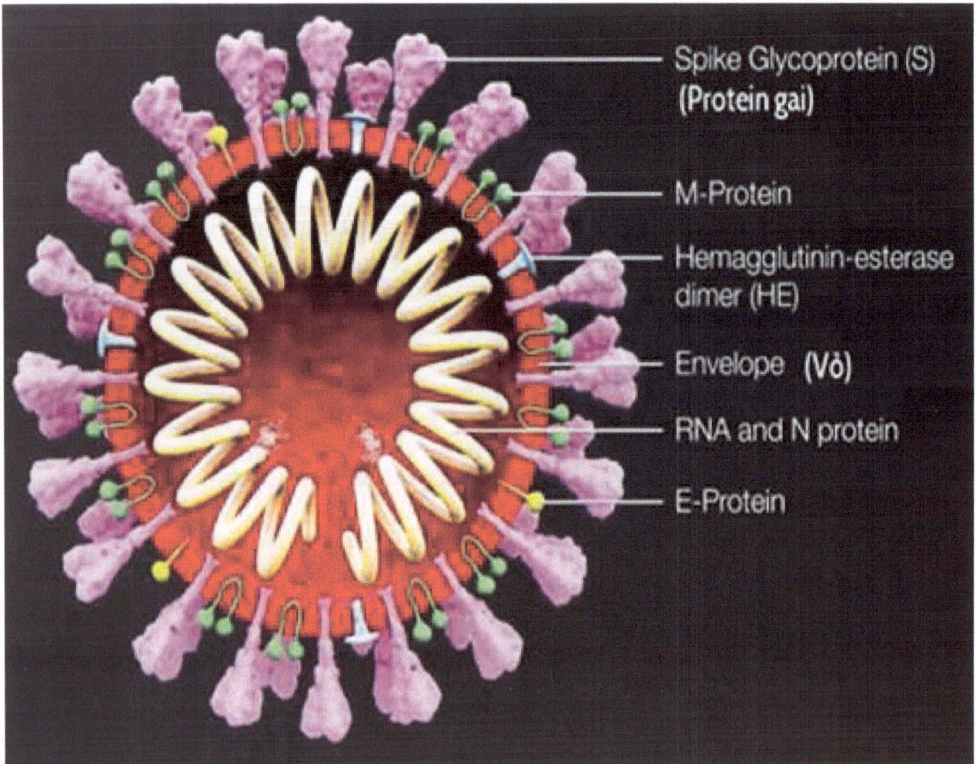

Fig. (1). Structure of Coronoavirus **(A)** Electron Microscopy and **(B)** Model of CoV.

Based on serological reactions, the coronavirus is divided into three groups or genera *i.e.* Group-I, Group-II, and Group-III (McIntosh *et al.*, 1974). Group-I includes viruses that cause infection in animals only, like the Porcine epidemic diarrhea virus and feline infectious peritonitis virus. It also includes the viruses that produce respiratory infections in humans, such as Human Coronavirus 229E (HCoV-229E) and KHU1. The Group-II viruses are Porcine hemagglutinating encephalomyelitis virus, bovine coronavirus, and equine coronavirus, which shows pathogenicity in animals, while HCoV-OC43 and HCoV-NL63 produce pneumonia-like conditions in humans. Group-II viruses that cause infections in rodents are murine hepatitis virus (MHV) and Rat sialodacryoadenitis CoV, which produce enteritis, hepatitis, and encephalitis in addition to respiratory infections.

Lastly, infectious bronchitis virus (IBV), Turkey coronavirus, and pheasant coronavirus are classified under Group-III viruses. Table 1 summarizes the types of CoV (Cavanagh *et al.*, 2020). All the CoV possess some common characteristics, which are as follows:

1. The shape of coronavirus is spherical with an average size of 80-220 nm.
2. The virus is covered with an envelope having club-shaped peplomers.
3. It all contains a tubular nucleocapsid structure with helical symmetry.
4. All are composed of single-stranded RNA with a genomic size of 27-32 kb.
5. The coronavirus contains numerous structural proteins, but some are present in all, such as nucleoprotein, peplomer glycoprotein, a transmembrane glycoprotein, and hemagglutinin esterase.
6. While some non-structural proteins are also present in CoV, such as RNA dependent RNA polymerase.
7. The newly-formed viruses *i.e.* virions are generally assembled in the endoplasmic reticulum and Golgi cisternae.
8. The mutation is very common in CoV and due to this reason, a diverse host range was exhibited (Enjuanes *et al.*, 2000).

Table 1. Different types of coronavirus.

Group	Virus	Host	System Affected
I	229E	Human	Respiratory Infection
	TGEV	Pig	Respiratory & Enteric Infection
	PRCoV	Pig	Respiratory Infection
	Canine coronavirus	-	Enteric infection
	FeCoV	-	Enteric infection
	FIPV	Cat	Respiratory, enteric & neurologic infection
	NL-63	Human	Respiratory Infection
II	OC43	Human	Respiratory & enteric infection
	MHV	Mouse	Intestinal & neurological infection
	Sialodacryoadenitis CoV	Rat	Neurological infection
	Hemaagglutinating encephalomyocarditis virus	Pig	Respiratory, enteric & neurological infection
	BCoV	Cow	Enteric infection
	HKU1	Human	Respiratory infection
	SARS-CoV	Human	Life-threatening respiratory infection
III	IBV	Chicken	Respiratory infection, Hepatitis
	Turkey CoV	Turkey	Respiratory & Enteric infection

GENOMIC STRUCTURE OF CORONAVIRUS

Coronavirus is known to possess the largest genomic structure of around 30kb having single-stranded RNA. The genomes of CoV are arranged with replicase loci encoded within the 5'-end while within the 3'-end of the genome encoded the structural proteins arranged in the sequence hemagglutinin esterase, spike protein, small membrane protein, membrane, and nucleocapsid protein. The genomic RNA is generally present along with nucleocapsid protein to form a helical structure found within the virus-cell membrane. Apart from nucleocapsid protein, some other proteins are also found in the virus. For instance, the spike protein, which is a type-I glycoprotein, forms peplomer on the surface of virion which reveals the crown-like appearance on microscopic examination. Further another protein present in the virus is termed as membrane protein which spans three times the viral membrane. The membrane protein possesses a short N-terminal domain and a cytoplasmic tail. Apart from spike and membrane protein, a hydrophobic protein is commonly known as small membrane protein, also exists having a short domain, transmembrane domain, and cytoplasmic tail. The hydrophobic protein present as a bi-layered structure around the viral membrane with N-terminal and C-terminal in the inner face. Heamglutinin esterase protein is supposed to help the virus to gain entry in the cell but usually not present in each CoV.

The two-third of the genome is covered by 5'-end which encodes for a replicase gene that comprises open reading frame -1a (ORF) and open reading frame-1b. The gene is translated into two large proteins *i.e.* pp1a and pp1ab. The proteins are further split into small fragments of around 16 proteins having an enzymatic activity like proteases, RNA modification enzymes, polymerase, and helicase as depicted in Fig. (**2**). Additionally, certain non-structural genes are also present in the genome of the virus which encodes accessory proteins whose function, sequence, and number varies in each virus belongs to coronavirus (Brian *et* al., 2005).

STRUCTURAL PROTEINS

Structural proteins in the coronavirus, such as membrane-spanning proteins play a crucial role in the pathogenicity and replication as well as assembly of the virus. This section covers the different structural proteins.

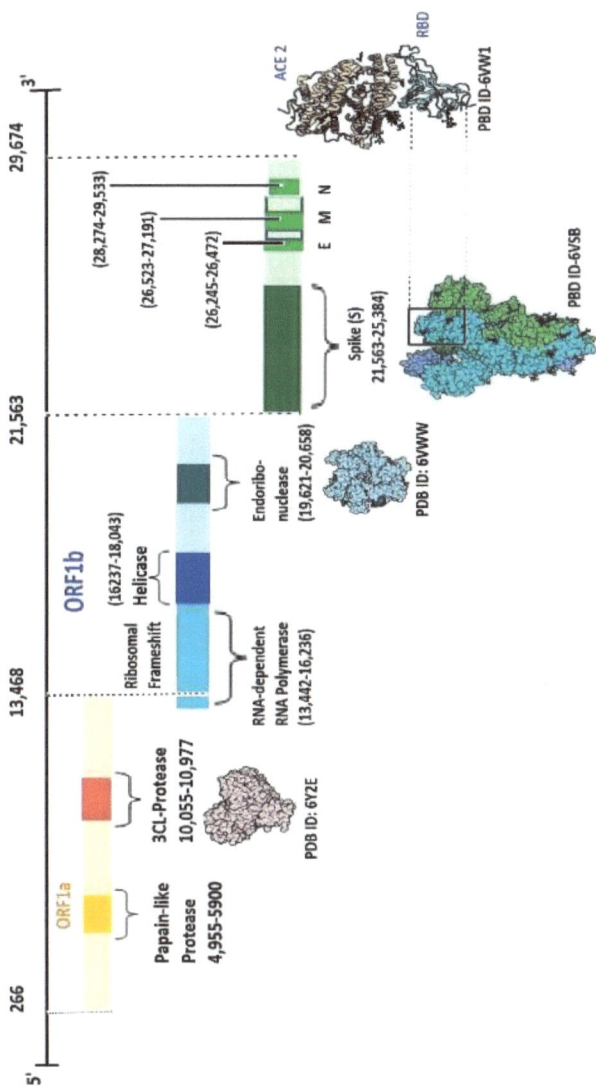

Fig. (2). Genomic Structure of COVID-19.

Spike Protein

The spike protein with a molecular weight of 180 kb belongs to Type-I glycoprotein enclosed in the outer membrane of the virus and form the peplomers. The arrangement of these peplomers is such that a crown-like morphology appears and also promotes the interaction of viral and host receptors to facilitate the viral entry into the cell by inducing membrane diffusion. The protein may further cleave to form subunits, the C-terminal S2, and N-terminal S1, with an approximate weight of 90 kb (Frana *et al.*, 1985). The reaction is catalyzed by a furan like a protease enzyme. The S1 subunit forms the globular head like structure while S2 subunit for a trans-membrane tail. At the time viral encounter to the host cell, the subunits of the protein interact with the host receptor and mediate the virus entry. The S1 subunit normally contains β-sandwich galectins similar to humans, which additionally promotes binding to the receptor. The spike protein influence mainly viral tropism and pathogenic phenotype (Sturman *et al.*, 1980).

In the case of SARS-CoV apart from cellular receptors, the Angiotensin-Converting Enzyme-II (ACE-II) is another major determinant of infection. SARS-CoV is the only type in the category which infects nearly all animals and humans. Also, the receptor binding domain of SARS-virus contains a 192-amino acid spanning residue which is mainly responsible for the interaction with the human ACE-II receptor. Unlike all CoV, the SARS CoV spike protein does not cleaved into S1 and S2 subunits. However, the entry of the virus is mainly mediated through Cathepsin-L in acidic pH as in the case of other CoV. The spike protein also regulates the renin-angiotensin system by the down-regulation of ACE-II expression on the plasma membrane which ultimately results in SARS-CoV infection as ACE-II possesses pneumo-protective property (Li *et al.*, 2006).

Small Membrane Protein

The small membrane proteins are generally integral transmembrane proteins and composed of 75-110 amino acid residues. The protein is composed of three domains, hydrophilic C-terminal domain, N-terminal domain, and a transmembrane domain. The palmitoylation and ubiquination of protein are necessary for proper assembly of the virus. Thus for efficient virus assembly, the small membrane protein, as well as the membrane protein, are the key proteins in every CoV. The interaction of both proteins is mediated through the cytoplasmic tails. In addition to assembly, this protein also aids in the release of the virion. Various studies demonstrated that the majority of the protein is localized near the nuclear membrane (Boscarino *et al.*, 2008). But in certain cases like SARS-CoV, the protein is present along with Golgi complexes. The arrangement of this protein in the membrane varies in each type of CoV. For instance, in TGEV, the C-terminal is oriented towards the lumen of intracellular membranes with its N-terminal in the cytoplasm. While in the case of IBV, the N-terminal is in the lumen of the membrane while C-terminal exposes to the cytoplasm. Both C-terminal and N-terminal are exposed in the cytoplasm of MHV and forms a hairpin-like structure. In SARS, dual arrangement occurs, one hairpin loop structure and second with a single membrane-spanning domain with C-terminal in the cytoplasm and N-terminal oriented towards the lumen. The over-expression of small membrane protein induces apoptosis through the activation of Bcl-2 and Bcl-xL and thus responsible for SARS virus-induced alveolar damage (Cohen *et al.*, 2011).

Membrane Protein

The membrane protein is the most abundant protein found in a viral envelope, which normally has 221-262 amino acid residues. The protein composed of short hydrophilic N-terminal chain exposed on the outer surface of the virus, long C-terminal tail located inside the virus, and both connected by three transmembrane domains. The long C-terminal domain is further subdivided into two domains, one near to the third trans-membrane domain termed as amphipathic domain, and the second is the short hydrophilic domain. The N-terminal domain is either N-glycosylated or O-glycosylated, depending upon the type of CoV. The amphipathic is linked with the viral membrane and plays a significant role in virus assembly and budding (Armstrong *et al.*, 1984). The membrane protein interacts with other proteins like spike proteins and small membrane proteins for enhancing the assembly and budding of virions. In the host, the membrane protein also stimulates the release of interferon-α and thus the protein is said to possess interferogenic property (Rottier *et al.*, 1984).

Hemagglutinin-Esterase

In addition to spike protein, some viruses carry hemagglutinin esterase protein on the envelope. The protein is a glycosylated polypeptide with a molecular weight of 65 kDa and exists in the form of a homodimer linked by a disulfide bond. The major constituents of the protein are sialic acid and acetyl esterase which potentially play a role in viral entry or budding. In some viruses like MHV, the protein initiates the binding process of the virus with the host cell surface receptor while spike protein is responsible for binding to specific glycoprotein receptors. Additionally, the protein aids in the release of the virus. Hemagglutinin esterase suggested possessing the entero-pathogenic property and responsible for the spread of disease to non-infected cells. To cause infection in the gastrointestinal tract, the esterase component of the virus plays a significant role by allowing the movement of virions through the mucous of the infected cells (Brian *et al.*, 1995).

Nucleocapsid and Internal Proteins

The nucleocapsid protein is an RNA binding protein that encodes in the 3'-end of the genome, having multiple roles in conjunction with other proteins. The nucleocapsid protein interacts with the membrane protein for the efficient assembly of the virions. The protein is also associated with replication and transcription of the virus in infected host cells as these proteins are localized to the nucleus of infected cells. The nucleocapsid protein has a significant role in the pathogenesis of CNS disease and hepatitis. Nucleocapsid protein in the neurons interferes with the axonal transport mechanism. Furthermore, the protein also antagonizes the interferon in the host cells. The protein in the host induces the release of fibrinogen like protein-2, which possesses the pro-coagulant and immuno-suppressive activity and thus causes liver damage. The genome of group-II CoV contains internal ORF in the nucleocapsid gene. The internal protein possesses very little role in pathogenesis (Verheije et al., 2010).

Replicase Protein

The replicase proteins are the key determinants of viral replication which may influence pathogenesis and tropism of the virus. It mainly interacts with non-coding 5' and 3' sequence in the viral genome *via* the cell specific or immune response factors. The enzymes that have been encoded in ORF 1a and 1b mainly concerned with subverting the host cell metabolism (Zhu et al., 2004).

VIRAL CYCLE

The cycle of CoV is shown in Fig. (3). Coronavirus binds to specific host cell receptor by spike proteins, which initiates the structural change in the spike protein. As a result of conformational change in spike proteins, a fusion of the host cell membrane with viral envelope occurs, which causes the release of nucleocapsid protein into the cell. After gaining the entry of the virus into the host cell, the 5' end of the genome RNA is translated into pp1a and pp1ab. Further, ORF 1a encodes papain-like proteases and 3C-like protease that converts pp1a and pp1ab into replicase proteins. The X domain of ORF-1a encodes for ADP-ribose-1-phosphatase activity while ORF-1b encodes RNA dependent RNA polymerase, helicase, exonuclease, endoribonuclease, and S-adenosylmethionin--dependent ribose methyltransferase. Additionally, ORF-2a encodes for cyclic phosphodiesterase. The enzymes play a crucial role in the metabolism of CoV and interact with host cell mechanisms to induce pathogenicity (Bond et al., 1979).

As the virus gains entry in the host cell, replication of genome and transcription of mRNA initiates, which results in the synthesis of negative-strand and positive strand RNAs through unique discontinuous transcription phenomenon. The negative strand RNA serves as a template for full length genomic RNA and sub-genomic RNA. The multiple sub-genomic RNA so formed acts as an mRNA having leader sequence at 5'-end. The mRNA synthesis is regulated by transcription-regulating sequences, present at the transcriptional initiating sites in the genomic RNA. The sub-genomic negative strand RNA having anti-leader sequences will be added onto the 3'-end of negative strand RNA that acts as a template for the synthesis of mRNA. Further, the viral proteins are translated from specific mRNA. For instance, replicase is translated from genomic RNA mainly at 5'-end. While in the case of spike protein, which is translated from ORF-5b on mRNA and subsequently translation of ORF-5b is mediated through the ribosome (Bredenbeek *et al.*, 1990).

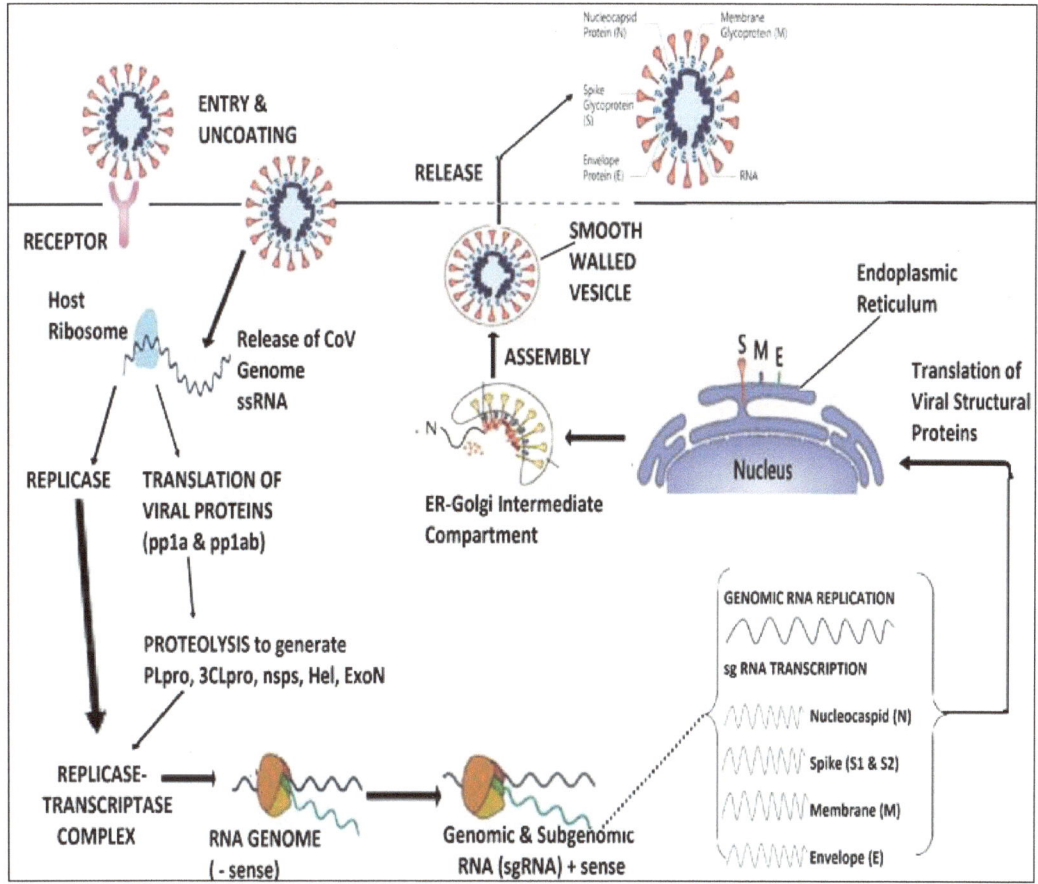

Fig. (3). Schematic Model of Viral Replication in Host Cell.

After the completion of the translation of membrane and spike proteins, the proteins are localized to the endoplasmic reticulum Golgi intermediate compartment and then to Golgi intracellular membranes from where actually budding takes place. The proteins and other viral factors determine the site of budding of virions. The spike proteins are uniformly present on plasma membranes as well as the intracellular membrane. At the time of assembly, the spike proteins interact with the transmembrane region of the membrane protein.

The spike protein sometimes mediates the fusion of cells and thus syncytium is formed and the virus is transmitted. Nucleocapsid protein forms a complex with RNA to form a helical structure. As a result of the interaction of nucleocapsid proteins with membrane proteins, the budding of virions occurs in the form of vesicles. Lastly, the virus arrives at the cell surface from where it exits the host cell (Lee et al., 1991).

OUTBREAKS OF CORONAVIRUS

Generally, coronavirus replicates in epithelial cells of the enteric or respiratory system of animals, including humans. Due to the presence of an envelope around the virus, the stability is very poor as compared to non-enveloped viruses. The SARSCoV is transmitted through direct contact and despite the envelope; it has high stability on environmental surfaces. The enveloped SARS CoV has the potential to cause infection even in the presence of proteolytic enzymes and bile in the gastric tract. The glycosylated glycoprotein present on the envelope makes them resistant to proteolytic degradation. Infections caused by flu CoV results in ciliostatsis *i.e.* loss of ciliary action and degeneration of cilia of the respiratory tract. SARS CoV generally targets type-I and type-II alveolar epithelial cells of the lower respiratory tract. The desquamation of alveolar epithelial cells causes the formation of the hyaline membrane in the alveoli, which ultimately results in acute respiratory distress syndrome.

The mechanism of infection and the immune reaction of the host cell would be demonstrated in the animals. For instance, MHV mainly affects the enteric system, lower respiratory organs, nervous system, and hepatic cells. The neurological manifestations mainly include multiple sclerosis, demyelination, neuronal degeneration and sometimes also involve oligodendrocytes, microglia, and astrocytes. The degree of neurological manifestation depends upon the strain and type of virus. Demyelination occurs due to virus-mediated immune reaction in the host through the activation of virus-specific T-cells. Further, due to demyelination, macrophages infiltrates and microglia cells start accumulated into the white matter. Moreover, the innate immune reaction is also a key determinant of viral replication in host cells. But certain CoV encounters the innate immune attack by producing certain proteins like ORF6 and ORF3b which inhibits interferon release mainly by preventing the nuclear translocation of proteins responsible for the production of interferons (Coleman *et al.,* 2014).

Porcine Coronavirus

In 1946, the first case was reported in porcine by the Transmissible gastroenteritis virus which majorly causes viral enteritis and diarrhea with a high mortality rate. The virus mainly attacks epithelial cells of the small intestine which leads to life-threatening enteritis especially in neonates. In certain cases, the virus invades mainly the upper respiratory tract, which rarely reaches the lungs. Another virus that infects is the Porcine respiratory virus (PRCoV) which is an attenuated strain of TGEV. PRCoV mainly infects epithelial cells of lungs mainly in type-I and type-II pneumocytes, alveolar macrophages, and ultimately in interstitial fluid. The genome of both the virus is similar but differs in the 5' region of the spike gene which results in different pathogenic outcomes. In the late 1970s, group-I porcine coronavirus PEDV emerged in Europe, which later spreads to Asia. PEDV somewhat resembles human CoV mainly HCV-229E. Last but not least; another porcine CoV is hemagglutinating enteric CoV having an entirely different genomic structure than other porcine viruses (Saif 2004a and Saif 2004b).

Avian Coronavirus

IBV contributes to the majority of deaths in chickens whose mode of transmission is through air droplets and poses an economic burden on the poultry industry. IBV mainly multiplies in the upper respiratory tract and invades the entire bronchi tissue to cause severe and life-threatening ailment. In some cases, IBV also causes severe systemic infections such as nephritis, decreased egg production, and gastric disturbances. The B-cells mediated antibodies/immunoglobulins produced due to viral encounter in the respiratory tract prevents systemic manifestation in the host. Even maternal antibodies also possess the activity against the IBV (Saif 2004a and Saif 2004b).

Feline Coronavirus

There are two main types of feline CoV, FeCoV and FIPV. FeCoV (Feline Enteric Coronavirus) mainly transmitted from different components of the environment to produce an asymptomatic condition which, when converts into an active form in plasma produce virulent consequences. FIPV, on the other hand, concentrates and replicates in macrophages to cause a life-threatening condition. In the initial phase, FIPV replicates in pharyngeal or intestinal cells and further systemic outcomes appear when the virus starts invading the macrophages. The systemic manifestations are inflammation of the abdominal and thoracic cavity, ocular, and neurological disorders. One of the biggest challenges to treat FIVP is immune-mediated pathology. The FIVP induced immune system stimulation sometimes becomes the major cause of death (Addie, 2004).

Bovine Coronavirus

Bovine coronavirus attacks both respiratory as well as enteric systems and produces symptoms like diarrhea, winter dysentery, shipping fever, and respiratory infections (Saif, 2004a).

Murine Coronavirus

A vast variety of strains of coronavirus infects murine exhibits different characteristics and degrees of virulence. MHV mainly infects hepatic cells and neurons, where the prime manifestations of infection involve encephalitis, immune-mediated demyelination, multiple sclerosis, and hepatitis. MHV encounters the host immune system *via* variable viral gene products. The degree of virulence and tropism depends on the interaction of viral gene products and host immune response. The presentation of viral molecules activates both antibody and cell-mediated immunity. The CD8+ and CD4+ T-cells are the key immune cells responsible for encountering the virus during acute infection. Apart from T-cells, interferon-gamma is also responsible for the clearance of viruses from neuroglial cells of the nervous system. The CD8+ T-cells retard viral replication and thus limit the spread of the virus. It also decreases the amount of demyelination of neurons. On the other hand, B-cell mediated antibodies are required to prevent the re-occurrence of infection by the MHV in the CNS after the initial clearance by the T-cells (Barthold *et al.*, 1993 and Glass *et al.*, 2002).

The second prominent infection in murine is caused by JHM, in which mass release of INF-α/β and chemotaxis agents like CCL3, CCL4, CXCL2, CXCL10, and CXCL5 occurs. The elevated levels of chemokines in the host result in the release of macrophages and neutrophils and thus represents acute infection. The neurovirulent JHM is unable to initiate significant T-cell activity and thus delays viral clearance, which accounts for a high mortality rate (Perlman, 1998).

Human Coronavirus

The first emerging CoV infection in humans is caused by OC43 and 229E, with a common sign of a common cold. Later on, SARS-CoV was identified, which likely to cause severe acute respiratory syndrome. Furthermore, two more strains were isolated from humans, one is HKUI and HCoV-NL63, with the prime symptom of pneumonia and bronchiolitis and conjunctivitis respectively. The main manifestations of HCoV-NL63 include respiratory syndrome, respiratory infections, bronchiolitis, and pneumonia. In Fig. (**4**), different human CoV are shown with their potential source of origin (Van der Hoek *et al.*, 2005).

SARS-CoV

In 2003, a documentary was released from China which reports that new respiratory illness in the form of atypical pneumonia emerged in some patients. Later on, a detailed investigation was done by isolating the sample from the lungs of the patients, which demonstrates that a new coronavirus starts invading the society with a prime indication of respiratory distress (WHO, 2003). SARS is characterized by hyperthermia, dyspnea, lymphopenia, and infections in the bronchioles. Later on, gastric symptoms such as epigastric distress, diarrhoea, and intestinal infection appear due to active replication of SARS-CoV. In a later stage, the virus and its products were also seen in the kidney, liver, and small intestine. Mainly the transmission occurs through air-droplets, blood, and fecal-oral route. SARS endemic ends with a toll death of around 778 out of 8000 infected persons. The SARS declared to be endemic in Singapore, Taiwan, and Beijing, with a mode of transmission is mainly *via* airborne droplets or through fomites (Nie *et al.*, 2003).

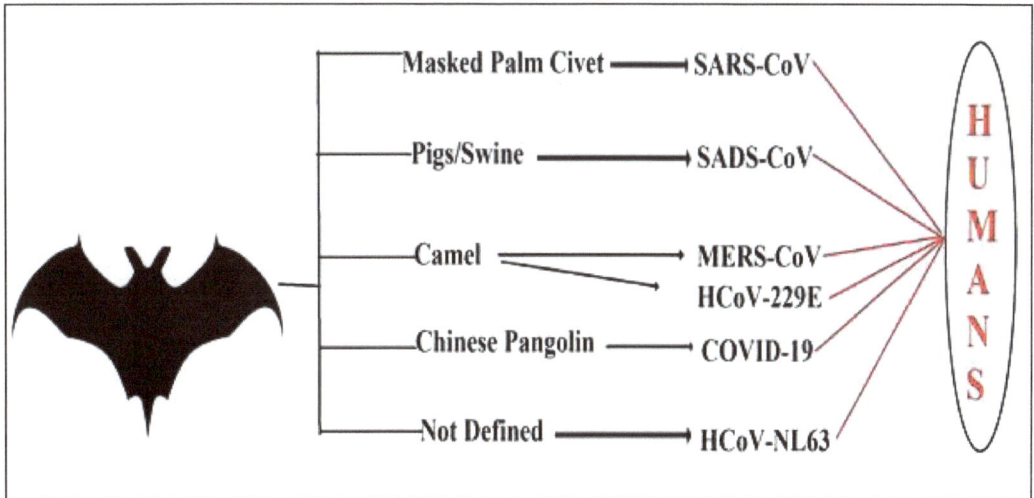

Fig. (4). Origin of Different Types of CoV.

The SARS patient normally exhibits a tri-phasic pattern of disease where patients initially have signs of flu such as hyperthermia, dry cough, sore throat, myalgia, and breathlessness, which persist for around 7-14 days. After around 14 days, the above signs become more severe, and additionally hypoxia and diarrhea also become prominent. The respiratory status of the patient deteriorates continuously and ultimately developed a condition termed as acute respiratory distress syndrome and maximum patients require an artificial respiratory system to overcome such conditions. By the end of approximately 21 days, the second phase ends up. The last phase involves systemic manifestations in which the virus sheds out from the respiratory tract and subsequently invades the gastrointestinal tract. The mortality rate is normally low but considered to be 50% for patients for more than 60 years. The histological examination revealed that the lungs contained a hyaline membrane, edema, fibrin exudates, thrombus in blood vessels, and sloughing of pneumocytes. Additionally, there is the infiltration of lymphocytes, macrophages, and polymorphonuclear leukocytes, and pneumocytes appear abnormally as multinucleated giant cells. At the end of the second phase, the histological image indicates pneumonitis, which can be compensated by type-II pneumocyte hyperplasia, squamous metaplasia, and bronchiolitis. Further, the viral load decline as the immune system activates but it also worsens the disease due to the abrupt release of cytokines. Various pro-inflammatory cytokines released are MCP-1, MIP-1, RANTES, MCP-2, TNF-α, and IL-6 (Zhong et al., 2003).

The receptor binding domain (RBD) for SARS on the host cells is an angiotensin converting enzyme-II receptor (ACE2R). As the CoV binds to ACE2R, the structure of the receptor is transformed which enables the virus to initiates the course of infection. As the disease progresses, the expression of ACE2R on the cell surface is downregulated. The downregulation occurs due to two main reasons, the internalization of ACE2R during the viral entry and over expression of tumor necrosis factor converting enzyme commonly termed as metalloproteases. The metalloproteases cause cleavage of the ACE2 extracellular domain from its transmembrane domain and thus results in shedding of the domain. Since ACE2R possesses pneumoprotective activity, the disappearance of the receptor after CoV-RBD interaction additionally increases the severity of acute lung injury. Moreover, the downregulation of ACE2R also produces a detrimental effect on the myocardium, for instance, myocarditis and infection in the myocardium. Also, infection with the virus initiates a series of humoral and cellular immune responses in the host. In the plasma, high titers of immunoglobulins are found, mainly IgG and IgM, and also cytotoxic T-cells are also detected. The levels of immune cells in host plasma correlates with the infection period and recovery from the disease. It is believed that the more the count of immune cells in the host, the more will be recovery rate and thus immune cells are considered to be crucial for the clearance of the SARS-CoV. Till now, there is no treatment of the SARS-CoV, but the vaccine is supposed to be a suitable measure to eradicate the disease (Tsui et al., 2003). Below mentioned Table **2** compares different characteristics of SARS-CoV and SARS-CoV-2.

MERS-CoV

Furthermore, another infection in humans caused by the member of CoV is the Middle East Respiratory Virus (MERS-CoV). The first case of MERS was reported in June 2012, in Jeddah, Saudi Arabia. The patients suffering from MERS-CoV present mainly acute pneumonia and renal failure. Later on WHO declared MERS-CoV as a pandemic as the disease affects around twenty-seven countries in Asia with a death rate of 36%. The preliminary manifestations include flu-like conditions or pneumonia, acute respiratory distress syndrome (ARDS), septicemia, shock-like condition, and lastly, organ failure, which lead to death. Generally, the condition appears with hyperthermia, chills, dry cough, sore throat, arthralgia, myalgia, and breathlessness. The infection further progresses to life-threatening pneumonia, diarrhea, and vomiting. The progression rate of disease is very fast that within 7-11 days the infection presents with systemic manifestations. As in other cases, MERS-CoV invades the innate immune cells and thus, in immuno-compromised patients, the condition becomes life-threatening. Unlike SARS, MERS-CoV acts through CD26 receptors *i.e.* a dipeptyl peptidase (PLOS Currents Outbreaks 2013).

Table 2. Comparison of SARS-CoV and SARS-CoV-2.

Characteristic	SARS-CoV	SARS-CoV-2
Target receptor	ACE-2	ACE-2
Nucleocapsid protein	IFN-γ inhibitor	Unknown
Chest X-ray	Ground glass opacities	Bilateral, multilobar ground glass opacities
Chest CT-scan	Lobar consolidation Nodular opacities	No nodular opacities
Prevention	Hand hygiene, coughetiquette	Possibly hand hygiene, cough etiquette
Transmission	Droplets Contact with infected individuals	Droplets Contact with infected individuals, even asymptomatic ones
Case fatality rate (overall)	9.6%	2.3%

COVID-19

Introduction

As per the WHO, viral diseases continuously appear and produce a serious concern for societal health. In the last two decades, numerous epidemics or pandemics have been recorded due to viruses, for instance, SARS-CoV in 2002, H1N1 influenza in 2009, and MERS-CoV in 2012.

In a timeline that reaches the present day, an epidemic of cases with lower respiratory tract infection was detected in China. Initially, due to the unavailability of data and unidentified causative organism, the first case was designated as "pneumonia of unknown etiology" (Bogoch *et al.*, 2020). After that, the Chinese Center for Disease Control and Prevention (CDC) conducted a thorough investigation program. After completing the investigation, it was concluded that a new virus belongs to the coronavirus family responsible for such illness. Thus at the end of 2019, a cluster of pneumonia cases was reported in Wuhan, China, whose etiology was considered to be a new member of the β-coronavirus subfamily. This member of the β-coronavirus subfamily was initially designated as a 2019-novel coronavirus (2019-nCoV) on 12 January 2020 by WHO. But on 11 February 2020, WHO re-designate the virus as COVID-19 (Coronavirus disease 2019), and Coronavirus Study Group of the International Committee termed it as SARS-CoV-2. The SARS-CoV-2 is highly contagious and spreads globally at a very high rate. International Health Regulation of WHO, in his meet on 30 January 2020, declared a report that the virus was spread to around 18 countries, with four countries reporting community transmission. Further, an alarming situation occurs; a case was reported on 26 February 2020 in the United States having no history of travelling from China (Zhao *et al.,* 2020).

The coronavirus has become one of the major pathogens which mainly attacks the respiratory tract and produces the pneumonia-like condition. Till now there is a big question on how these viruses can overcome the species barrier and successfully produce illness which ranges from common flu-like condition to severe respiratory distress syndrome as in the case of SARS and MERS. The former condition was possibly originated from bats virus and then enters into the mammalian hosts while the latter originates from dromedary camels.

Despite the origin of coronaviruses, these viruses have the potential to grow and transmit at a very high rate which causes a worldwide pandemic and seems to be a serious health issue. On 28 February 2020, the WHO declared the COVID-19 epidemic to a very high-level emergency. As the disease spread outside China to around 114 countries and the number of cases crosses one lakh, WHO declared the COVID-19 a pandemic.

The governments of all the countries try to build a plan of work to stem possible devastating effects. For this various international health, organizations flow out various information and guidelines used to lessen the impact of this virus. At the same time, further investigations are done to explore the mechanism of transmission, the clinical course of the disease, advanced diagnosis guidelines, prevention, and treatment strategies. Currently, no targeted drug is available to treat COVID-19. So at the moment, only supportive treatment is available and preventive measures are aimed to reduce community transmission. For instance, in China, aggressive isolation measures led to a great reduction in COVID-19 cases (Ren *et al.,* 2020).

Chronology of COVID-19

The chronology of COVID-19 infection is mentioned as follows. In December 2019, the first case of COVID-19 was reported. From 18 December 2019 till 29 December 2019 five cases were reported with ARDS and the number increases to 41 till 2 January 2020. Later on, it was diagnosed that less than half of the patients have a history of diabetes, hypertension, and ischemic heart disease. Thus it was presumed that patients got infected mainly due to hospital-acquired infection. Further, till 22 January 2020, the number of cases increases to 571 in various cities of China, with a total death of 17 patients. But suddenly within the next three days, the total cases were jumped to 1975 with the death of around 56 infected patients. Whereas some reports suggest that the number of cases increases to 5502 till 24 January 2020 in China.

Furthermore, till 30 January 2020, 7734 cases were confirmed in China and a total of 90 cases reported from different countries such as Germany, France, Canada, Australia, India, United States, Japan, Singapore, Sri Lanka, Nepal, Malaysia, Thailand, Taiwan, and United Arab Emirates. The toll death rate is found to be 2.2% (170/7824). On 19 January 2020, the first case was reported in Washington, United States, who presents with a four-day history of cough and fever and recently returned from Wuhan, China (Du, 2020). On 30 January 2020, the first case of human-human transmission was reported in the US. Moreover, a report was issued on 7 February 2020, which declares a total of 31,161 cases with the death of more than 630 people. World health organization globally released a report on 16, February 2020 which confirmed 51,587 cases in around 25 countries.

Till the end of February 2020, the infected cases reach 88,000 worldwide (Holshue et al., 2020). Further, the cases of COVID-19 increase exponentially which creates serious health issues, as mentioned in Fig. **5(A & B)**.

In India, the first case was reported on 30 January 2020. While WHO released the first report on 14 Mar 2020, which said that a total of 84 COVID-19 patients are present in different territories of India, out of which two die. The first death was reported in Karnataka of a 76-year-old man and the second death occurs in Delhi of a 68-year-old female. By the end of May 2020, the total cases reported in India were around 191,000, with total death of 5,300 patients.

Symptoms

The signs of viral invasion come after an incubation period of around 4-6 days. Generally, the symptoms appear after 6 days of entry of the virus in the body and range to a maximum of 41 days. The period depends upon the patient's age and the immune system of the host. The commonly recognized symptoms (Fig. **6**) are excessive sputum production, hyperthermia, fatigue, cough, headache, breathlessness, lymphopenia, and hemoptysis. Computed tomography of the chest reveals unusual features such as pneumonia, RNAaemia, ARDS, cardiac injury, and multiple peripheral ground-glass opacities in the subpleural region, which is the main cause of death.

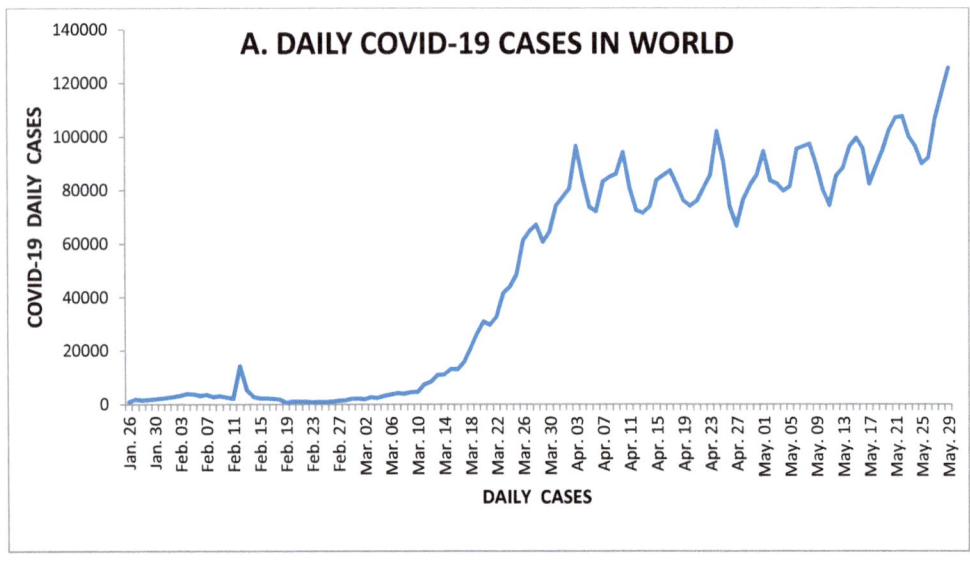

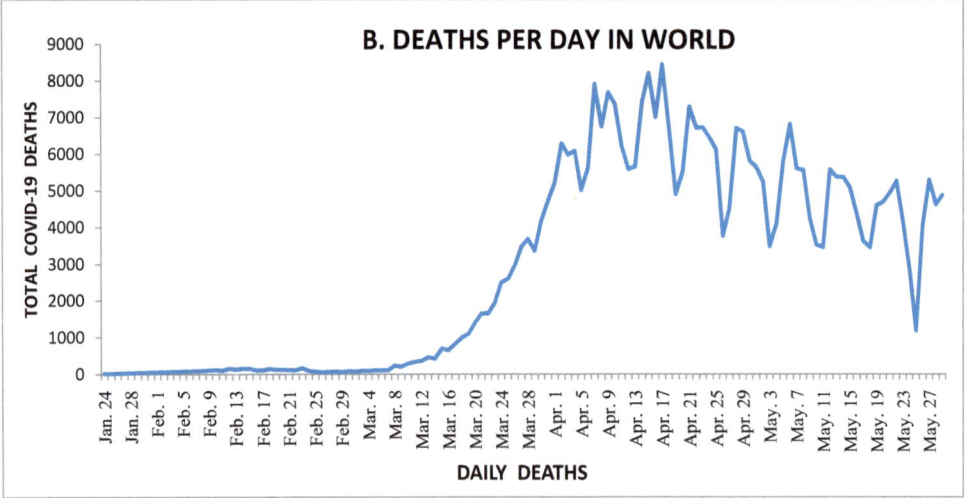

Fig. (5). Chronology of COVID-19 **(A)** Daily COVID-19 cases & **(B)** Deaths due to COVID-19.

The clinical features of COVID-19 and other human coronavirus are somewhat similar such as fever, cough, breathlessness, and ground-glass opacity in the subpleural region. However, certain unique clinical features of COVID-19 infection include rhinorrhoea, sneezing, and sore throat. The chest radiography reveals the infiltration in the upper lobe of the lungs that leads to profound dyspnoea and hypoxemia. Also, the chances of developing gastrointestinal manifestations such as diarrhea are more in COVID-19 as compared to MERS-

CoV and SARS-CoV. From this, a new diagnostic tool is recognized where fecal and urine samples to exclude a potential alternative route of transmission (Rothana *et al.*, 2020).

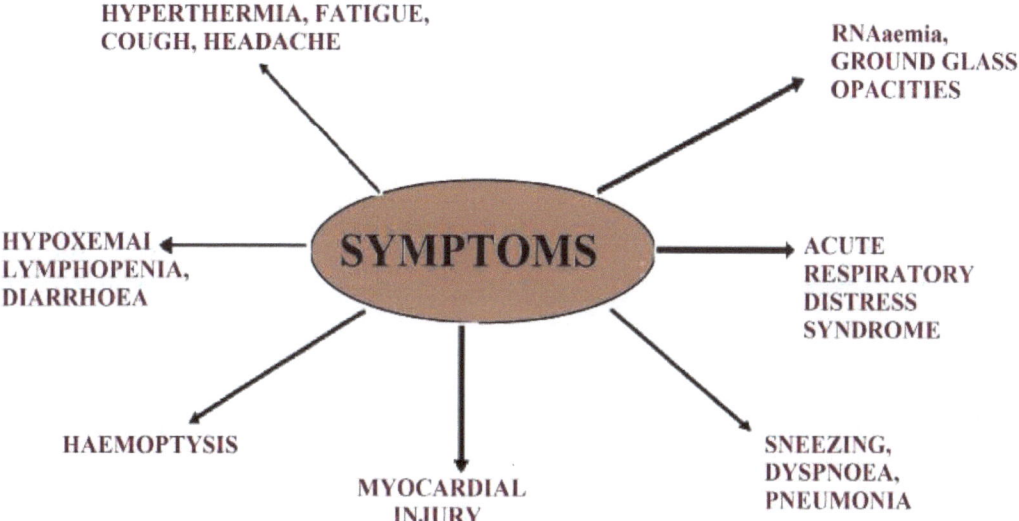

Fig. (6). Clinical features of COVID-19.

Transmission

As we know, around all the infected people were exposed to the animal market in Wuhan, it might be concluded that COVID-19 originates through the zoonotic source. Further investigation will be done to search out the reservoir host or intermediate carrier from which the infection may transfer to humans. The genomic analysis of COVID-19 showed approximately 90% similarity with SARS-like coronaviruses, which were derived from bats. This report indicates that only mammals are the connecting link between humans and COVID-19.

But human to human transmission is the fastest mode of transmission of infection. The transmission occurs either by direct contact or air droplets spread due to coughing or sneezing from a COVID-19 patient, as depicted in Fig. (7). Fortunately, it was confirmed that if pregnant women infected with COVID-19, no placental transmission occurs from infected mother to child (Rothana *et al.*, 2020).

Treatment

Currently, no antiviral drug is available for COVID-19, and no vaccine is introduced till now. The treatment recommended includes supportive therapy, symptomatic therapy, and oxygen therapy. In case of respiratory failure, mechanical ventilation is required, whereas for managing septic shock, hemodynamic support is mandatory. The evidence-based precise guidelines were released by WHO on 28 January 2020 for sorting the patients based on their respiratory conditions; method of prevention and control; supportive therapy; diagnosis; management of respiratory distress and septic shock; prevention of complications; and treatment (Lu, 2020).

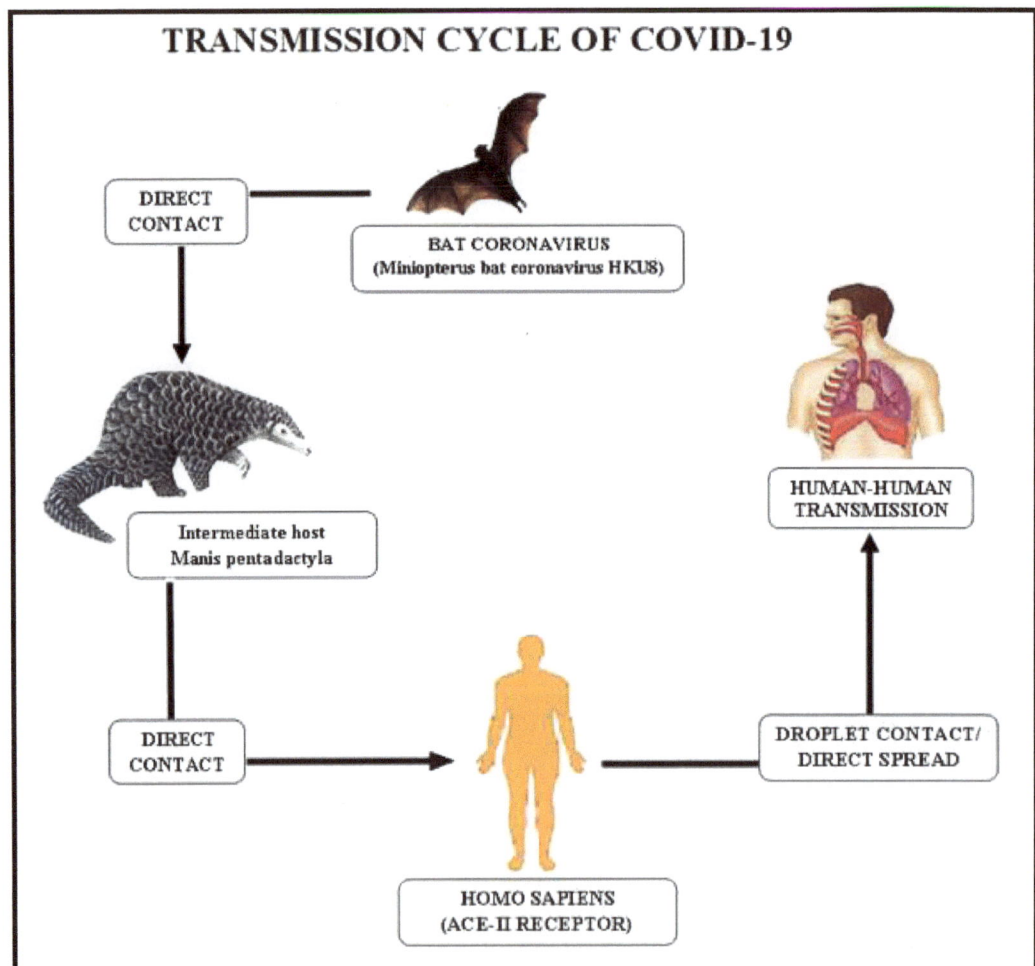

Fig. (7). Transmission Cycle of COVID-19.

LIST OF ABBREVIATIONS

2019-nCoV   Coronavirus

ACE-II   Angiotensin-Converting Enzyme-II

ACE2R	Angiotensin Converting Enzyme-II Receptor
ADP	Adenine diphosphate
ARDS	Acute respiratory Distress Syndrome
Bcl	B-Cell Lymphoma
CCL	Chemokine Ligand
CD	Cluster of Differentiation
CDC	Chinese Center for Disease Control and Prevention
CNS	Central nervous system
CoV	Coronavirus
COVID-19	Coronavirus disease 2019
FeCoV	Feline Enteric Coronavirus
FIPV	Feline infectious peritonitis Virus
HCoV-229E	Human Coronavirus 229E
HCoV-KHU1	Human Coronavirus KHU1
HCoV-NL63	Human Coronavirus NL63
HCoV-OC43	Human Coronavirus OC43
IBV	Infectious bronchitis virus
IgG	Immunoglobulin gamma
IgM	Immunoglobulin mu
IFN	Interferon
IL	Interleukins
kDa	Kilo Dalton
MCP	Monocyte chemoattractant protein
MERS	Middle East Respiratory Virus
MHV	Murine Hepatitis Virus
MIP	Macrophage inflammatory protein
ORF	Open Reading Frame
PEDV	Porcine Epidemic Disease Virus
pp	Polyproteins
PRCoV	Porcine respiratory virus
RANTES	Regulated upon Activation, Normal T cell Expressed, and Secreted
RBD	Receptor Binding Domain
RNA	Ribonucleic acid
SARS-CoV	Subacute Respiratory Syndrome Coronavirus
TGEV	Transmissible Gastroenteritis Virus

TNF	Tumor Necrosis Factor
WHO	World Health Organization

CONSENT FOR PUBLICATION

Not applicable.

CONFLICT OF INTEREST

The author declares no conflict of interest, financial or otherwise.

ACKNOWLEDGEMENTS

Declared none.

REFERENCES

Addie, DD (2004) Feline coronavirus--that enigmatic little critter. *Vet J,* 167, 5-6.
[http://dx.doi.org/10.1016/S1090-0233(03)00083-2] [PMID: 14623144]

Armstrong, J, Niemann, H, Smeekens, S, Rottier, P & Warren, G (1984) Sequence and topology of a model intracellular membrane protein, E1 glycoprotein, from a coronavirus. *Nature,* 308, 751-2.
[http://dx.doi.org/10.1038/308751a0] [PMID: 6325918]

Barthold, SW, Beck, DS & Smith, AL (1993) Enterotropic coronavirus (mouse hepatitis virus) in mice: influence of host age and strain on infection and disease. *Lab Anim Sci,* 43, 276-84.
[PMID: 8231082]

Bogoch, Watts (2020) Pneumonia of unknown etiology in Wuhan, China: potential for international spread *via* commercial air travel. *J Travel Med,* 27, 1-3.

Bond, CW, Leibowitz, JL & Robb, JA (1979) Pathogenic murine coronaviruses. II. Characterization of virus-specific proteins of murine coronaviruses JHMV and A59V. *Virology,* 94, 371-84.
[http://dx.doi.org/10.1016/0042-6822(79)90468-9] [PMID: 572113]

Boscarino, JA, Logan, HL, Lacny, JJ & Gallagher, TM (2008) Envelope protein palmitoylations are crucial for murine coronavirus assembly. *J Virol,* 82, 2989-99.
[http://dx.doi.org/10.1128/JVI.01906-07] [PMID: 18184706]

Bredenbeek, PJ, Pachuk, CJ, Noten, AF, Charité, J, Luytjes, W, Weiss, SR & Spaan, WJ (1990) The primary structure and expression of the second open reading frame of the polymerase gene of the coronavirus MHV-A59; a highly conserved polymerase is expressed by an efficient ribosomal frameshifting mechanism. *Nucleic Acids Res,* 18, 1825-32.
[http://dx.doi.org/10.1093/nar/18.7.1825] [PMID: 2159623]

Brian, DA, Hogue, BG & Kienzle, TE (1995) The coronavirus hemagglutinin esterase glycoprotein. In: Siddell, S.G., (Ed.), *The Coronaviridae.* Plenum Press, New York, N.Y.
[http://dx.doi.org/10.1007/978-1-4899-1531-3_8]

Brian, DA & Baric, RS (2005) Coronavirus genome structure and replication. *Curr Top Microbiol Immunol,* 287, 1-30.
[PMID: 15609507]

Cavanagh, D, Mawditt, K, Welchman, DdeB, Britton, P & Gough, RE (2002) Coronaviruses from pheasants (*Phasianus colchicus*) are genetically closely related to coronaviruses of domestic fowl (infectious bronchitis virus) and turkeys. *Avian Pathol,* 31, 81-93.

[http://dx.doi.org/10.1080/03079450120106651] [PMID: 12425795]

Cohen, JR, Lin, LD & Machamer, CE (2011) Identification of a Golgi complex-targeting signal in the cytoplasmic tail of the severe acute respiratory syndrome coronavirus envelope protein. *J Virol,* 85, 5794-803.
[http://dx.doi.org/10.1128/JVI.00060-11] [PMID: 21450821]

Coleman, CM & Frieman, MB (2014) Coronaviruses: important emerging human pathogens. *J Virol,* 88, 5209-12.
[http://dx.doi.org/10.1128/JVI.03488-13] [PMID: 24600003]

Du Toit, A (2020) Outbreak of a novel coronavirus. *Nat Rev Microbiol, no 18,* 123.
[http://dx.doi.org/10.1038/s41579-020-0332-0]

Enjuanes, L, Cavanagh, D, Holmes, K, Lai, MMC, Laude, H, Masters, P, Rottier, P, Sidell, SG, Spaan, WJM, Taguchi, F & Talbot, P (2000) *'Coronaviridae, Virus Taxonomy'* Classification and Nomemclature of Viruses.Accademic Press, San Diego, Calif.

Frana, MF, Behnke, JN, Sturman, LS & Holmes, KV (1985) Proteolytic cleavage of the E2 glycoprotein of murine coronavirus: host-dependent differences in proteolytic cleavage and cell fusion. *J Virol,* 56, 912-20.
[http://dx.doi.org/10.1128/JVI.56.3.912-920.1985] [PMID: 2999444]

Glass, WG, Chen, BP, Liu, MT & Lane, TE (2002) Mouse hepatitis virus infection of the central nervous system: chemokine-mediated regulation of host defense and disease. *Viral Immunol,* 15, 261-72.
[http://dx.doi.org/10.1089/08828240260066215] [PMID: 12081011]

Holshue, ML, DeBolt, C, Lindquist, S, Lofy, KH, Wiesman, J, Bruce, H, Spitters, C, Ericson, K, Wilkerson, S, Tural, A, Diaz, G, Cohn, A, Fox, L, Patel, A, Gerber, SI, Kim, L, Tong, S, Lu, X, Lindstrom, S, Pallansch, MA, Weldon, WC, Biggs, HM, Uyeki, TM & Pillai, SK Washington State 2019-nCoV Case Investigation Team (2020) 'First case of 2019 novel coronavirus in the United States'. *N Engl J Med,* 382, 929-36.
[http://dx.doi.org/10.1056/NEJMoa2001191] [PMID: 32004427]

Lee, HJ, Shieh, CK, Gorbalenya, AE, Koonin, EV, La Monica, N, Tuler, J, Bagdzhadzhyan, A & Lai, MM (1991) The complete sequence (22 kilobases) of murine coronavirus gene 1 encoding the putative proteases and RNA polymerase. *Virology,* 180, 567-82.
[http://dx.doi.org/10.1016/0042-6822(91)90071-I] [PMID: 1846489]

Li, W, Wong, SK, Li, F, Kuhn, JH, Huang, IC, Choe, H & Farzan, M (2006) Animal origins of the severe acute respiratory syndrome coronavirus: insight from ACE2-S-protein interactions. *J Virol,* 80, 4211-9.
[http://dx.doi.org/10.1128/JVI.80.9.4211-4219.2006] [PMID: 16611880]

Lu, H (2020) Drug treatment options for the 2019-new coronavirus (2019-nCoV). *Bioscience Trends,* 14, 69-71.
[http://dx.doi.org/10.5582/bst.2020.01020]

McIntosh, K (1974) 'Coronaviruses: a comparative review'. *Curr Top Microbiol Immunol,* 85-129.

Nie, QH, Luo, XD, Zhang, JZ & Su, Q (2003) Current status of severe acute respiratory syndrome in China. *World J Gastroenterol,* 9, 1635-45.
[http://dx.doi.org/10.3748/wjg.v9.i8.1635] [PMID: 12918094]

Perlman, S (1998) Pathogenesis of coronavirus-induced infections. Review of pathological and immunological aspects. *Adv Exp Med Biol,* 440, 503-13.
[http://dx.doi.org/10.1007/978-1-4615-5331-1_65] [PMID: 9782322]

Pyrc, K, Berkhout, B & van der Hoek, L (2007) The novel human coronaviruses NL63 and HKU1. *J Virol,* 81, 3051-7.
[http://dx.doi.org/10.1128/JVI.01466-06] [PMID: 17079323]

Ren, LL, Wang, YM, Wu, ZQ, Xiang, ZC, Guo, L, Xu, T, Jiang, YZ, Xiong, Y & Li, YJ (2020) Identification of a novel coronavirus causing severe pneumonia in human: a descriptive study. *Chin Med J (Engl),* 133, 1015-24.

Rothana, HA & Byrareddy, SN (2020) 'The epidemiology and pathogenesis of coronavirus disease (COVID-19) outbreak'. *J Autoimmun,* 1-5.
[http://dx.doi.org/10.1016/j.jaut.2020.102433]

Rottier, P, Brandenburg, D, Armstrong, J, van der Zeijst, B & Warren, G (1984) Assembly *in vitro* of a spanning membrane protein of the endoplasmic reticulum: The E1 glycoprotein of coronavirus mouse hepatitis virus A59. *Proc Natl Acad Sci USA,* 1421-5.
[http://dx.doi.org/10.1073/pnas.81.5.1421]

Saif, LJ (2004) 'Animal coronavirus vaccines: lessons for SARS'. *Dev Biol,* 129-40.

Saif, LJ (2004) Animal coronaviruses: what can they teach us about the severe acute respiratory syndrome? *Rev Sci Technol,* 643-60.
[http://dx.doi.org/10.20506/rst.23.2.1513]

Sturman, LS, Holmes, KV & Behnke, J (1980) Isolation of coronavirus envelope glycoproteins and interaction with the viral nucleocapsid. *J Virol,* 33, 449-62.
[http://dx.doi.org/10.1128/JVI.33.1.449-462.1980] [PMID: 6245243]

The WHO MERS-CoV Research Group (2013) State of Knowledge and Data Gaps of Middle East Respiratory Syndrome Coronavirus (MERS-CoV) in Humans, Edition 1. *PLOS Currents Outbreaks.*

Tsui, PT, Kwok, ML, Yuen, H & Lai, ST (2003) Severe acute respiratory syndrome: clinical outcome and prognostic correlates. *Emerg Infect Dis,* 9, 1064-9.
[http://dx.doi.org/10.3201/eid0909.030362] [PMID: 14519241]

Tyrrel, DAJ, Almedia, JD, Berry, DM, Cunningham, CH, Hamre, D, Hofstad, MS, Malluci, L & McIntosh, K (1968) 'Coronavirus'. *Nature,* 650.

Van der Hoek, L, Sure, K, Ihorst, G, Stang, A, Pyrc, K, Jebbink, MF, Petersen, G, Forster, J, Berkhout, B & Uberla, K (2005) Croup is associated with the novel coronavirus NL63. *PLoS Med,* 2, e240.
[http://dx.doi.org/10.1371/journal.pmed.0020240] [PMID: 16104827]

Verheije, MH, Hagemeijer, MC, Ulasli, M, Reggiori, F, Rottier, PJ, Masters, PS & de Haan, CA (2010) The coronavirus nucleocapsid protein is dynamically associated with the replication-transcription complexes. *J Virol,* 84, 11575-9.
[http://dx.doi.org/10.1128/JVI.00569-10] [PMID: 20739524]

World Health Organization (2003) *Severe Acute Respiratory Syndrome (SARS): Multi-country Outbreak.* World Health Organization, Geneva, Switzerland.

Zhao, S, Lin, Q, Ran, J, Musa, SS, Yang, G, Wang, W, Lou, Y, Gao, D, Yang, L, He, D & Wang, MH (2020) Preliminary estimation of the basic reproduction number of novel coronavirus (2019-nCoV) in China, from 2019 to 2020: A data-driven analysis in the early phase of the outbreak. *Int J Infect Dis,* 92, 214-7.
[http://dx.doi.org/10.1016/j.ijid.2020.01.050] [PMID: 32007643]

Zhong, NS, Zheng, BJ, Li, YM, Poon, , Xie, ZH, Chan, KH, Li, PH, Tan, SY, Chang, Q, Xie, JP, Liu, XQ, Xu, J, Li, DX, Yuen, KY, Peiris, & Guan, Y (2003) Epidemiology and cause of severe acute respiratory syndrome (SARS) in guangdong, people's republic of china, in february, 2003. *Lancet,* 362, 1353-8.
[http://dx.doi.org/10.1016/S0140-6736(03)14630-2] [PMID: 14585636]

Zhu, MS, Pan, Y, Chen, HQ, Shen, Y, Wang, XC, Sun, YJ & Tao, KH (2004) Induction of SARS-nucleoprotein-specific immune response by use of DNA vaccine. *Immunol Lett,* 92, 237-43.
[http://dx.doi.org/10.1016/j.imlet.2004.01.001] [PMID: 15081618]

CHAPTER 3

COVID-19: Epidemiology

Kamya Goyal[1,2,#], Shammy Jindal[1,#], Tarun Kumar[3], Jugnu Goyal[4], Reena Sharma[5], Ravinder Singh[6] and Samir Mehndiratta[7,8,*]

[1] *Laureate Institute of Pharmacy, Kathog, Distt- Kangra, H.P., India*

[2] *Chitkara College of Pharmacy, Chitkara University, Chandigarh-Patiala National Highway, Rajpura, Patiala, Punjab, India*

[3] *Department of ECE, Deenbandhu Chhotu Ram University of Science and Technology, Murthal, Haryana, India*

[4] *Swami Dayanand Institute of Pharmaceutical Sciences, UHS, Rohtak, Haryana, India*

[5] *Agricultural Biotechnology Research Center, Academia Sinica, Taipei, Taiwan*

[6] *Department of Chemistry, National Taiwan University, Taipei, Taiwan*

[7] *School of Pharmacy, University of Southern California, Los Angeles, USA*

[8] *School of Pharmacy, Taipei Medical University, Taipei, Taiwan*

Abstract: In the history, the year 2019 will be remembered as the year that has witnessed the beginning of a pandemic, primarily affecting the respiratory tract and then, spreading from human to human. A total of 25.18 million reported cases and 0.84 million deaths, as of 30th August 2020, and still counting, were caused by a novel coronavirus named COVID-19 that originated in Wuhan, China. By the beginning of the year 2020, this virus spread to several countries like Singapore, South Korea, Japan, Italy, Spain, Germany, the United Kingdom, and the United States of America. Between January 2020 and March 2020, the disease took a paradigm shift and started to affect the majority of European countries like Italy, Spain, France, Germany and UK. In the majority of the patients with a competent immune system, this disease goes unnoticed or without symptoms, thus making them highly susceptible to spread this disease to whoever comes in their contact. Aged patients (>60 years) or patients with chronic health issues like heart diseases, cancer, diabetes, and weak immunity are at greater risk of developing the symptoms. In severe conditions, patients need hospitalization and respiratory support (respirators/ventilators), thus causing an overload on the health system of the world. This initiated the movement of "flattening the curve" by social distancing and isolation to decrease the burden on the health system and to decrease the spread of the disease.

---

[*] **Corresponding author Samir Mehndiratta:** School of Pharmacy, University of Southern California, Los Angeles, California, USA; School of Pharmacy, Taipei Medical University, Taipei, Taiwan; E-mail: d301100006@tmu.edu.tw
[#] These authors contributed equally

Neeraj Mittal, Sanjay Kumar Bhadada, O. P. Katare and Varun Garg (Eds.)
All rights reserved-© 2021 Bentham Science Publishers

Keywords: China, Confirmed Cases, *Cordon sanitaire*, Coronavirus, COVID-19, Curfews, Epidemiology, Geographical distribution, Global Epidemiology, Hotspots, Lockdown, National Responses, Non-essential, Outbreak, Pandemic, Person-to-person Transmission, Quarantines, SARS-CoV-2, WHO Region, Wuhan.

INTRODUCTION

The year 2019 has witnessed the beginning of a pandemic majorly affecting the respiratory tract; however, effects on the other body organs have also been reported (Singh *et al.*, 2020a). The pandemic has affected 25,182,329 people across the globe, with a total death toll of 846,936 registered up to 30th August 2020. The total recovered cases from the COVID-19 pandemic are 17,515,059 and the active cases till 30th August 2020 are 6,820,334. Half of the total affected population of the world resides in the USA, Brazil, and India. This disease spreads from human to human *via* air-borne droplets. This pandemic is not the first pandemic world has ever seen; however, it is one of the biggest of our times and the most vulnerable after World War II. The severity of this can be estimated from the fact that it is as destructive as the influenza pandemic in 1918, which emerged after World War I and caused deaths of tens of millions of people due to lack of antibiotics. Similarly, Acquired Immune Deficiency Syndrome caused by a retrovirus was equally lethal before it was controlled by using antiretroviral drugs (DiMaio *et al.*, 2020).

Broadly, pandemics are the epidemics that spread worldwide and thus are not confined to any particular geographical region. This current world epidemic originated in Wuhan, China is caused by a novel coronavirus and has been named coronavirus disease 2019 or COVID-19. Due to its similarity with SARS (Severe Acute Respiratory Syndrome), ICTV (International Committee on Taxonomy of Viruses) coined it as SARS-CoV-2 virus. COVID-19 was officially proclaimed as PHEIC Public Health Emergency of International Concern by WHO on 30th January 2020 with various countries starting to impose travel restrictions, issuing traveling warnings, and also exercising travel bans (Malviya *et al.*, 2020; Tang *et al.*, 2020). However, the lag between identification of the first case of COVID-19 infection to realizing its person to person transmission and to declare it as a world pandemic led it to spread to various countries and as of now at least 208 countries are infected with this infection (Hamid *et al.*, 2020).

Fortunately, due to previous exposure and understanding of coronavirus infections, such as SARS (Severe Acute Respiratory Syndrome) and Middle Eastern Respiratory Syndrome (MERS), this causative agent of SARS-CoV2 was quickly identified and its genome was rapidly sequenced to help researchers around the globe to develop potential drugs and/or vaccines. Fig. (**1**) shows various events and developments happened so far related to SARS-CoV-2.

Report of Unspecified pneumonia in Wuhan	Chinese CDC identified virus as Novel Coronavirus	Genomic Sequence disclosed by Chinese CDC	Virus titled as 2019-nCoV by WHO	1st Confirmed case of Covid-19 outside China	Declared as public health emergency by WHO & 1st Case of Covid-19 reported by USA	Renamed as SARS CoV-2	67 territories outside china reported 8565 cases	Declared as pandemic by WHO
Late Dec. 2019	07-Jan-2020	11-Jan-2020	12-Jan-2020	13-Jan-2020	30-Jan-2020	11-Feb-2020	02-Mar-2020	11-Mar-2020

Fig. (1). Timeline of various developments in SARS-CoV-2 (Gennaro *et al.*, 2020; Park, 2020; Sun *et al.*, 2020; Srivastava *et al.*, 2020; Hamid *et al.*, 2020; Tang *et al.*, 2020).

In this chapter, we shall discuss the epidemiology of the COVID-19 pandemic. Basically, epidemiology is the study of various determinant factors of health and disease-related conditions or events in a sample population or globally, and the purpose of this study is to control the various factors related to disease and to control the spread of the disease. Therefore, from studying the epidemiology of COVID-19, one can conclude the frequency and pattern of this disease. In this chapter, the data has been collected and reported up to 12th June 2020. We shall discuss various determinants and factors like geographical distribution of the disease, patterns in the global spread of the pandemic, *etc*. Further, we shall discuss the comparison of the number of cases of COVID-19 in different WHO regions along with the effect of lockdown on the spread of the pandemic. Besides, the condition of the COVID-19 pandemic in India along with some published reports by clinicians/researchers will be discussed in the latter part of the chapter.

GEOGRAPHICAL DISTRIBUTION

On 13th January 2020, the first confirmed case of COVID-19 outside China was reported in Thailand. It made the situation clear that this virus is no longer confined to China or the provenances nearby Wuhan. Soon after, reports of confirmed cases started to emerge from different countries in Asia. In January 2020, this virus spread to many Asian countries like Thailand, South Korea, and Japan and also cases of patients affected by COVID-19 started to appear in the western part of the world, including Italy, Spain, Germany, the UK, and the USA. In early February, WHO realized that the occurrence of COVID-19 is very high and ranges between 2.24 to 3.38. From the end of January 2020 to March 2020, it took a paradigm shift and disease started to affect the majority of European countries like Italy, Spain, France and, Germany, and to UK and USA, surpassing China in the number of affected patients. As of 12th June 2020, the five countries with the most number of cases worldwide were: US, Brazil, Russia, India, and the UK. The majority of the patients with competent immune systems act as carriers of the COVID-19 as it goes un-noticed/without any symptoms in these patients thus making them highly susceptible to spread this disease far and near. Elderly patients (>60 years) or patients with underlying chronic health problems, like heart diseases, cancer, diabetes, and weak immune system, *etc.*, are at higher risk of developing severe symptoms of this novel coronavirus. Development of silent hypoxia in severely affected patients demanded hospitalization with respiratory support (respirators/ventilators), thus causing an overload on the health system. This initiated the movement of "flattening the curve" and effective parameters like social distancing and isolation were enforced to decrease the burden on the health care system and to decrease the person-to-person spread of the diseases. For more details, refer to the 'national responses of COVID-19' part mentioned later in this chapter. Fig. (**2**) enlists series of events during the initial spread and geographical distribution of the COVID-19 pandemic.

Event	Date
1 Patient passed away from 5 hospitalized reported with Acute respiratory distress syndrome	18-Dec-2019 to 29-Dec-2019
Number of confirmed cases rose to 41 in China	02-Jan-2020
571 cases reported in 25 provinces of China with COVID-19	22-Jan-2020
First two confirmed cases of Covid-19 in Italy	23-Jan-2020
Covid-19 cases rose to 1975 & 26 deaths in China	25-Jan-2020
India reported 1st confirmed case of Covid-19	30-Jan-2020
31,160 Covid-19 cases and more than 630 deaths in China	07-Feb-2020
From 1st case of Covid-19 in US, reported cases rose to 311,635	30-Jan-2020 to 05-April-2020
India reported 1st death due to Covid-19	12-Mar-2020

Fig. (2). Epidemiological events and geographical distribution of novel coronavirus (Giovanetti *et al.*, 2020; Hamid *et al.*, 2020).

GLOBAL EPIDEMIOLOGY OF COVID-19

Since the 1st confirmed case of Coronavirus (COVID-19) in Wuhan, China, the virus has widely and rapidly spread in various countries across the globe despite the efforts done by various counties to stop the spread (Guan *et al.*, 2020; Lai *et al.*, 2020). According to a WHO report, COVID-19 has affected 7,724,615 people in more than 210 countries and caused 427,675 mortalities till 12th of June 2020. The incidences of COVID-19 and number of affected cases globally explained are explained in Fig. (**3**).

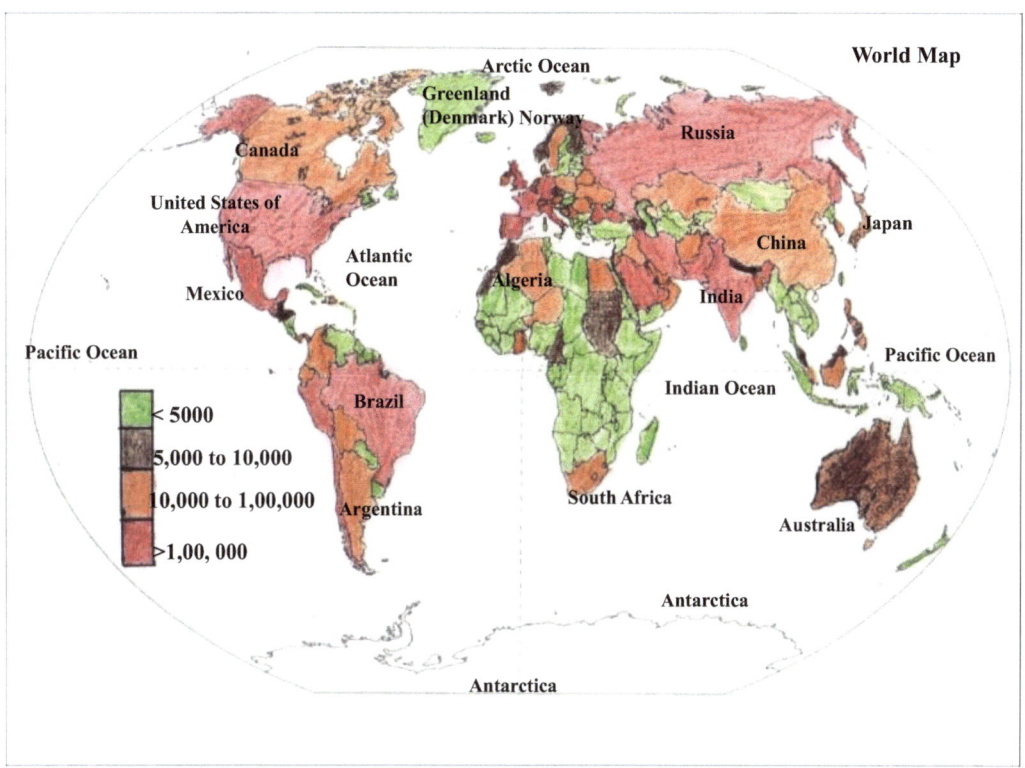

Fig. (3). World map showing COVID-19 cases as of 12th June 2020.

According to the data given in Table **1**, the countries with most cases of COVID-19 up to 12th June 2020 are:

1. USA, with total number of 2,116,211 patients and 116,814 total deaths along with 839,781 recovered cases and 1,159,616 active cases.
2. Brazil, with total number of 829,902 patients and 41,901 total deaths along with 396,692 recovered cases and 391,309 active cases.
3. Russia, with total number of 511,423 patients and 6,715 total deaths along with 269,370 recovered cases and 235,338 active cases.
4. India, with total number of 309,603 patients and 8,890 total deaths along with 154,231 recovered cases and 146,482 active cases.
5. Italy, with total number of 236,305 patients and with 34,223 total deaths along with 173,085 recovered cases and 28,997 active cases.
6. Peru, with total number of 220,749 patients and with 6,308 total deaths along with 107,133 recovered cases and 107,308 active cases.
7. Germany, with total number of 187,251 patients and with 8,863 total deaths

along with 171,600 recovered cases and 6,788 active cases.
8. Mainland China, with total number of 83,064 patients and with 4,634 total deaths along with 78,365 recovered cases and 65 active cases.

Table 1 enlists the global data of COVID-19 until 12th June 2020 indicating total number of COVID-19 cases worldwide & country-wise along with the total number of mortalities, recoveries and active cases. However, according to WHO these statistics will change in coming months as the spread of COVID-19 is expected to increase. The resurgence of corona cases in China has also supported this claim.

Table 1. Global Data of COVID-19 until 12th of June 2020 (Worldometer 2020).

S. No.	Country/ Other	Total Cases	Total Deaths	Total id="c3t Recovered	Active Cases	Population	1 Case Every X ppl
-	World	7,724,615	427,675	3,916,489	3,380,451	-	-
1	USA	2,116,211	116,814	839,781	1,159,616	330,901,704	156
2	Brazil	829,902	41,901	396,692	391,309	212,479,860	256
3	Russia	511,423	6,715	269,370	235,338	145,931,382	285
4	India	309,603	8,890	154,231	146,482	1,379,270,740	4,455
5	UK	292,950	41,481	N/A	N/A	67,867,577	232
6	Spain	290,289	27,136	N/A	N/A	46,753,887	161
7	Italy	236,305	34,223	173,085	28,997	60,466,117	256
8	Peru	220,749	6,308	107,133	107,308	32,946,025	149
9	Germany	187,251	8,863	171,600	6,788	83,770,376	447
10	Iran	182,525	8,659	144,649	29,217	83,933,136	460
11	Turkey	175,218	4,778	149,102	21,338	84,289,552	481
12	Chile	160,846	2,870	131,358	26,618	19,107,435	119
13	France	156,287	29,374	72,572	54,341	65,266,270	418
14	Mexico	133,974	15,944	98,064	19,966	128,859,025	962
15	Pakistan	125,933	2,463	40,247	83,223	220,638,507	1,752
16	Saudi Arabia	119,942	893	81,029	38,020	34,782,906	290
17	Canada	97,943	8,049	58,523	31,371	37,724,444	385
18	China	83,064	4,634	78,365	65	1,439,323,776	17,328
19	Bangladesh	81,523	1,095	17,249	63,179	164,600,549	2,019
20	Qatar	76,588	70	53,296	23,222	2,807,805	37
21	South Africa	61,927	1,354	35,006	25,567	59,267,163	957

(Table 1) cont.....

S. No.	Country/ Other	Total Cases	Total Deaths	Total Recovered	Active Cases	Population	1 Case Every X ppl
22	Belgium	59,819	9,646	16,498	33,675	11,587,039	194
23	Belarus	52,520	298	27,760	24,462	9,449,475	180
24	Sweden	49,684	4,854	N/A	N/A	10,095,978	203
25	Netherlands	48,461	6,053	N/A	N/A	17,132,971	354
26	Colombia	46,858	1,545	18,715	26,598	50,853,330	1,085
27	Ecuador	45,778	3,828	22,679	19,271	17,627,809	385
28	UAE	41,499	287	25,946	15,266	9,883,799	238
29	Egypt	41,303	1,422	11,108	28,773	102,220,760	2,475
30	Singapore	39,850	25	28,040	11,785	5,847,901	147
31	Indonesia	36,406	2,048	13,213	21,145	273,366,090	7,509
32	Portugal	36,180	1,505	22,200	12,475	10,198,122	282
33	Kuwait	34,952	285	25,048	9,619	4,266,990	122
34	Switzerland	31,063	1,938	28,800	325	8,651,283	279
35	Ukraine	29,753	870	13,567	15,316	43,745,847	1,470
36	Argentina	28,764	785	8,743	19,236	45,173,491	1,570
37	Poland	28,577	1,222	13,805	13,550	37,848,619	1,324
38	Ireland	25,250	1,705	22,698	847	4,934,765	195
39	Philippines	24,787	1,052	5,454	18,281	109,499,539	4,418
40	Afghanistan	23,546	446	3,928	19,172	38,874,978	1,651
41	Dominican Republic	22,008	568	12,754	8,686	10,842,017	493
42	Romania	21,404	1,380	15,445	4,579	19,243,552	899
43	Oman	21,071	96	7,489	13,486	5,098,511	242
44	Israel	18,795	300	15,288	3,207	9,197,590	489
45	Panama	18,586	418	10,977	7,191	4,310,882	232
46	Iraq	17,770	496	6,868	10,406	40,167,590	2,260
47	Japan	17,332	922	15,493	917	126,494,838	7,298
48	Bahrain	17,269	36	11,903	5,330	1,697,568	98
49	Austria	17,064	675	15,985	404	9,003,730	528
50	Bolivia	16,165	533	2,372	13,260	11,664,091	722
51	Armenia	15,281	258	5,639	9,384	2,962,966	194
52	Nigeria	15,181	399	4,891	9,891	205,822,203	13,558
53	Kazakhstan	13,872	70	8,829	4,973	18,764,311	1,353
54	Serbia	12,175	252	11,348	575	8,739,024	718

(Table 1) cont.....

S. No.	Country/ Other	Total Cases	Total Deaths	Total Recovered	Active Cases	Population	1 Case Every X ppl
55	Denmark	12,099	594	10,993	512	5,791,166	479
56	S. Korea	12,003	277	10,669	1,057	51,267,003	4,271
57	Moldova	11,093	385	6,229	4,479	4,034,411	364
58	Ghana	10,856	48	3,921	6,887	31,034,041	2,859
59	Algeria	10,698	751	7,322	2,625	43,804,765	4,095
60	Czechia	9,938	329	7,215	2,394	10,707,989	1,077
61	Azerbaijan	9,218	113	5,116	3,989	10,134,274	1,099
62	Cameroon	8,681	212	4,836	3,633	26,504,775	3,053
63	Norway	8,620	242	8,138	240	5,418,993	629
64	Morocco	8,610	212	7,618	780	36,886,438	4,284
65	Guatemala	8,561	334	1,567	6,660	17,896,120	2,090
66	Malaysia	8,402	119	7,168	1,115	32,342,925	3,849
67	Honduras	7,669	294	837	6,538	9,895,582	1,290
68	Australia	7,290	102	6,783	405	25,483,610	3,496
69	Finland	7,073	325	6,200	548	5,540,291	783
70	Sudan	6,879	433	2,416	4,030	43,786,472	6,365
71	Nepal	5,062	16	877	4,169	29,106,200	5,750
72	Tajikistan	4,902	49	3,158	1,695	9,524,612	1,943
73	Uzbekistan	4,869	19	3,758	1,092	33,441,780	6,868
74	Senegal	4,851	56	3,100	1,695	16,716,133	3,446
75	Ivory Coast	4,684	45	2,263	2,376	26,337,705	5,623
76	DRC	4,637	101	580	3,956	89,383,696	19,276
77	Djibouti	4,441	38	2,730	1,673	987,187	222
78	Guinea	4,426	24	3,106	1,296	13,110,203	2,962
79	Luxembourg	4,055	110	3,918	27	625,393	154
80	Hungary	4,053	555	2,447	1,051	9,661,522	2,384
81	Haiti	3,941	64	24	3,853	11,394,839	2,891
82	North Macedonia	3,701	171	1,694	1,836	2,083,378	563
83	El Salvador	3,481	68	1,587	1,826	6,484,517	1,863
84	Gabon	3,463	23	1,024	2,416	2,222,506	642
85	Kenya	3,305	96	1,164	2,045	53,699,517	16,248
86	Bulgaria	3,191	172	1,716	1,303	6,950,812	2,178
87	Thailand	3,129	58	2,987	84	69,791,171	22,305

(Table 1) cont.....

S. No.	Country/ Other	Total Cases	Total Deaths	Total Recovered	Active Cases	Population	1 Case Every X ppl
88	Greece	3,108	183	1,374	1,551	10,425,424	3,354
89	Ethiopia	2,915	47	451	2,417	114,786,713	39,378
90	Bosnia and Herzegovina	2,893	163	2,119	611	3,281,756	1,134
91	Venezuela	2,814	23	487	2,304	28,439,773	10,107
92	Somalia	2,513	85	532	1,896	15,864,908	6,313
93	Mayotte	2,268	28	1,790	450	272,408	120
94	Croatia	2,249	107	2,133	9	4,106,429	1,826
95	Cuba	2,233	84	1,902	247	11,326,953	5,073
96	Kyrgyzstan	2,166	26	1,668	472	6,517,994	3,009
97	CAR	2,044	7	360	1,677	4,824,890	2,361
98	Maldives	2,003	8	1,193	802	539,990	270
99	Estonia	1,970	69	1,703	198	1,326,491	673
100	Sri Lanka	1,880	11	1,196	673	21,408,657	11,388
101	Iceland	1,807	10	1,794	3	341,127	189
102	Lithuania	1,756	74	1,400	282	2,723,889	1,551
103	Mali	1,752	101	1,023	628	20,213,291	11,537
104	South Sudan	1,670	24	48	1,598	11,186,498	6,699
105	Costa Rica	1,612	12	731	869	5,091,620	3,159
106	Mauritania	1,572	81	278	1,213	4,641,964	2,953
107	Slovakia	1,542	28	1,409	105	5,459,512	3,541
108	New Zealand	1,504	22	1,482	0	5,002,100	3,326
109	Slovenia	1,490	109	1,359	22	2,078,924	1,395
110	Nicaragua	1,464	55	953	456	6,620,207	4,522
111	Guinea-Bissau	1,460	15	153	1,292	1,965,141	1,346
112	Lebanon	1,422	31	853	538	6,826,874	4,801
113	Albania	1,416	36	1,034	346	2,877,949	2,032
114	Zambia	1,321	10	1,104	207	18,351,048	13,892
115	Equatorial Guinea	1,306	12	200	1,094	1,399,912	1,072
116	Paraguay	1,254	11	633	610	7,127,687	5,684
117	Madagascar	1,240	10	344	886	27,646,431	22,296
118	Hong Kong	1,109	4	1,060	45	7,493,747	6,757
119	Sierra Leone	1,103	51	648	404	7,967,302	7,223

(Table 1) cont.....

S. No.	Country/ Other	Total Cases	Total Deaths	Total Recovered	Active Cases	Population	1 Case Every X ppl
120	Latvia	1,096	27	818	251	1,887,105	1,722
121	Tunisia	1,093	49	995	49	11,811,891	10,807
122	French Guiana	1,043	2	489	552	298,196	286
123	Cyprus	980	18	807	155	1,206,895	1,232
124	Niger	978	65	881	32	24,146,544	24,690
125	Jordan	915	9	671	235	10,197,652	11,145
126	Burkina Faso	892	53	791	48	20,866,826	23,393
127	Andorra	853	51	781	21	77,259	91
128	Chad	848	72	711	65	16,395,556	19,334
129	Uruguay	847	23	780	44	3,473,119	4,100
130	Georgia	843	13	697	133	3,989,535	4,733
131	Congo	728	24	221	483	5,509,663	7,568
132	*Diamond Princess*	712	13	651	48	-	-
133	Cabo Verde	697	6	294	397	555,657	797
134	San Marino	694	42	520	132	33,927	49
135	Uganda	686	-	161	525	45,645,761	66,539
136	Malta	645	9	600	36	441,484	684
137	Sao Tome and Principe	639	12	156	471	218,920	343
138	Yemen	632	139	28	465	29,786,156	47,130
139	Jamaica	611	10	408	193	2,960,505	4,845
140	Channel Islands	565	48	512	5	173,777	308
141	Togo	525	13	279	233	8,266,815	15,746
142	Rwanda	510	2	321	187	12,932,272	25,357
143	Tanzania	509	21	183	305	59,625,015	117,141
144	Mozambique	509	2	145	362	31,199,461	61,296
145	Palestine	489	3	414	72	5,094,148	10,417
146	Réunion	488	1	460	27	894,975	1,834
147	Malawi	481	4	65	412	19,098,955	39,707
148	Eswatini	472	3	246	223	1,159,511	2,457
149	Taiwan	443	7	431	5	23,814,623	53,758
150	Liberia	421	32	210	179	5,050,381	11,996
151	Libya	409	6	59	344	6,866,054	16,787

(Table 1) cont.....

S. No.	Country/ Other	Total Cases	Total Deaths	Total Recovered	Active Cases	Population	1 Case Every X ppl
152	Benin	388	5	217	166	12,103,226	31,194
153	Zimbabwe	343	4	51	288	14,850,685	43,296
154	Mauritius	337	10	325	2	1,271,663	3,773
155	Isle of Man	336	24	312	0	85,010	253
156	Vietnam	333	-	323	10	97,291,603	292,167
157	Montenegro	324	9	315	0	628,062	1,938
158	Myanmar	261	6	165	90	54,390,671	208,393
159	Martinique	202	14	98	90	375,279	1,858
160	Mongolia	197	-	95	102	3,275,260	16,626
161	Suriname	187	3	9	175	586,350	3,136
162	Cayman Islands	187	1	115	71	65,679	351
163	Faeroe Islands	187	-	187	0	48,854	261
164	Gibraltar	176	-	172	4	33,691	191
165	Guadeloupe	171	14	157	0	400,121	2,340
166	Syria	164	6	68	90	17,474,364	106,551
167	Comoros	163	2	97	64	868,486	5,328
168	Guyana	159	12	95	52	786,357	4,946
169	Bermuda	141	9	127	5	62,289	442
170	Brunei	141	2	138	1	437,253	3,101
171	Angola	130	5	42	83	32,799,138	252,301
172	Cambodia	126	-	125	1	16,705,964	132,587
173	Trinidad and Tobago	117	8	109	0	1,399,258	11,959
174	Bahamas	103	11	68	24	393,041	3,816
175	Aruba	101	3	98	0	106,743	1,057
176	Monaco	99	4	93	2	39,227	396
177	Barbados	96	7	83	6	287,358	2,993
178	Burundi	85	1	45	39	11,867,795	139,621
179	Liechtenstein	82	1	55	26	38,122	465
180	Sint Maarten	77	15	61	1	42,849	556
181	Bhutan	62	-	19	43	771,143	12,438
182	French Polynesia	60	-	60	0	280,824	4,680
183	Botswana	48	1	24	23	2,348,797	48,933

S. No.	Country/Other	Total Cases	Total Deaths	Total Recovered	Active Cases	Population	1 Case Every X ppl
184	Macao	45	-	45	0	648,839	14,419
185	Saint Martin	42	3	36	3	38,628	920
186	Eritrea	41	-	39	2	3,543,663	86,431
187	Namibia	31	-	17	14	2,538,214	81,878
188	Gambia	28	1	22	5	2,412,325	86,154
189	St. Vincent Grenadines	27	-	25	2	110,922	4,108
190	Antigua and Barbuda	26	3	20	3	97,886	3,765
191	Timor-Leste	24	-	24	0	1,316,964	54,874
192	Grenada	23	-	22	1	112,496	4,891
193	Curaçao	22	1	15	6	164,059	7,457
194	New Caledonia	21	-	20	1	285,350	13,588
195	Belize	20	2	16	2	397,206	19,860
196	Laos	19	-	19	0	7,269,590	382,610
197	Saint Lucia	19	-	18	1	183,584	9,662
198	Dominica	18	-	16	2	71,977	3,999
199	Fiji	18	-	18	0	896,103	49,784
200	Saint Kitts and Nevis	15	-	15	0	53,179	3,545
201	Falkland Islands	13	-	13	0	3,473	267
202	Greenland	13	-	13	0	56,765	4,367
203	Turks and Caicos	12	1	11	0	38,688	3,224
204	Vatican City	12	-	12	0	801	67
205	Montserrat	11	1	10	0	4,992	454
206	Seychelles	11	-	11	0	98,315	8,938
207	*MS Zaandam*	9	2	-	7	-	-
208	Western Sahara	9	1	6	2	596,428	66,270
209	British Virgin Islands	8	1	7	0	30,220	3,778
210	Papua New Guinea	8	-	8	0	8,937,038	1,117,130
211	Caribbean Netherlands	7	-	7	0	26,210	3,744
212	St. Barth	6	-	6	0	9,875	1,646

(Table 1) cont.....

S. No.	Country/ Other	Total Cases	Total Deaths	Total Recovered	Active Cases	Population	1 Case Every X ppl
213	Lesotho	4	-	2	2	2,141,348	535,337
214	Anguilla	3	-	3	0	14,996	4,999
215	Saint Pierre Miquelon	1	-	1	0	5,795	5,795
	Total:	7,724,615	427,675	3,916,489	3,380,451	-	-

X: Population Number.

As given in Table **1**, as of 12th June 2020 according to population density, Qatar has become the most affected country globally as it has one COVID-19 positive patient per every 37 people. San Marino occupied the second place with one COVID-19 positive patient per every 49 people followed by Bahrain having one COVID-19 positive patient per every 98 people.

Similarly, according to population density, Lesotho is the least affected country in the world as it has one COVID-19 positive patient per every 535,337 people followed by Vietnam, which has one COVID-19 positive patient per every 292,167 people. Myanmar stood third in this having one COVID-19 positive patient per every 208,393 people.

Effect of Age, Sex and other Factors on Covid-19-Related Deaths

Williamson *et al.* studied the various factors associated with COVID-19-death by creating an OpenSAFELY analytical platform in the field of health sciences. This study, which is related to the factors associated with COVID-19 mortality up to 6th May 2020, was carried on the behalf of NHS, England. The study included a total of 17,278,392 adults and reported that age and gender were entrenched risk factors for dreadful COVID-19 outcomes. The study revealed that about 90% of COVID-19-related deaths in the UK have been reported in the population over the age of 60 years with the majority of them being males (60%). The Chinese Center for Disease Control and Prevention revealed in an investigation including 44,672 individuals (1,023 deaths) that other diseases like hypertension, cardiovascular disease, respiratory disease, diabetes, and cancers were associated with an elevated risk of mortality; whereas, the establishment of a relationship with age was not possible. A UK cross-sectional survey including hospitalized 16,749 patients revealed that the death risk was greater for patients with pulmonary, cardiac, and renal disease, dementia, cancer, and obesity. In a recent communication, Sharma *et al.,* reported severity and risk factors of COVID-19 in cancer patients-based on various clinical evidence (Sharma *et al.*, 2020). Clinical evidence indicated that the patients with ophthalmic manifestations are also at high risk of COVID-19 infection (Singh *et al.*, 2020b). According to this study, the death rate increased with age as shown in Fig. (**4**). Among different sexes, males were more prone to COVID-19 as compared to females. (Williamson *et al.*, 2020).

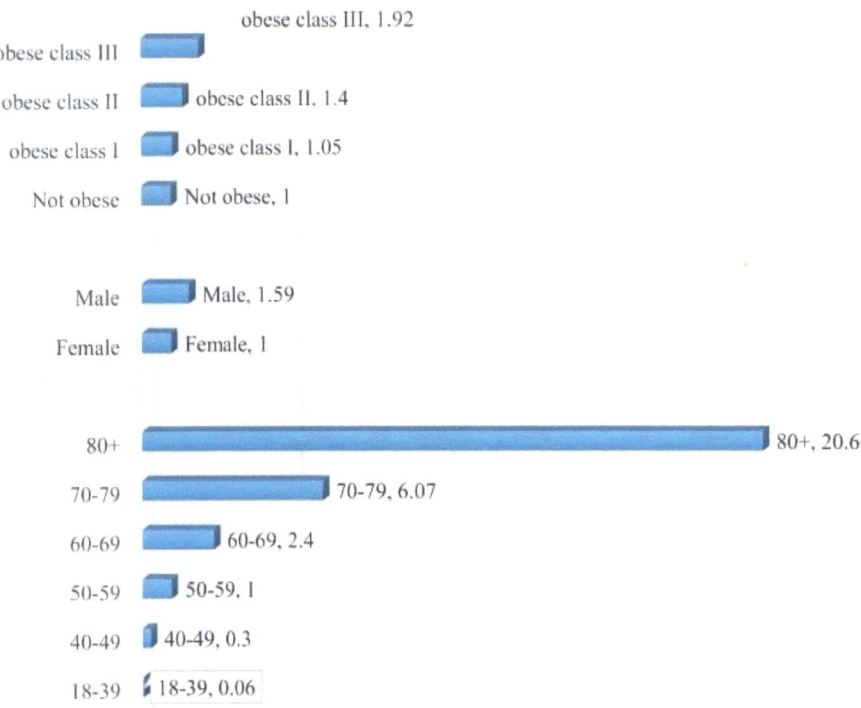

Fig. (4). Effect of Age, Sex and BMI on death related to COVID-19 (data represents hazard ratios in percentage for COVID-19).

COVID-19 CASE COMPARISONS IN DIFFERENT REGION OF WORLD (WORLD HEALTH ORGANIZATION, 2020)

WHO has divided the world into six regions, first being, Americas, which include various countries like Barbuda and Argentina, Barbados, Colombia, Grenada, Antigua, Costa Rica, Bahamas, Brazil, Jamaica, Bolivia, Canada, Chile, Cuba, Dominica, Dominican Republic, El Salvador, Saint Vincent, Guyana, Mexico, Nicaragua, United States, Paraguay, Ecuador, Guatemala, Haiti, The Grenadines, Honduras, Panama, Saint Kitts and Nevis, Saint Lucia, Belize, Suriname, Peru, Trinidad and Tobago, Uruguay, Venezuela, and Azerbaijan.

2nd region is European Region having Albania, Hungary, Armenia, Iceland, Austria, Belarus, Belgium, Bosnia, Herzegovina, Estonia, Bulgaria, Croatia, Andorra, Cyprus, Czech Republic, Denmark, Slovenia, Spain, Kyrgyzstan, San Marino, North Macedonia, Poland, Latvia, Finland, France, Germany, Georgia, Greece, Israel, Turkmenistan, Ukraine, United Kingdom, Slovakia, Netherlands, Ireland, Kazakhstan, Lithuania, Luxembourg, Italy, Malta Montenegro, Monaco, Norway, Portugal, Moldova, Romania, Russia, Serbia, Sweden, Switzerland, Tajikistan, Turkey, and Uzbekistan.

3rd region is Eastern Mediterranean Region having Afghanistan, Libya, Qatar, Jordan, Djibouti, Egypt, Somalia, Iran, Kuwait, United Arab Emirates, Saudi Arabia, Lebanon, Morocco, Sudan, Oman, Pakistan, Bahrain, Palestine, Syria, Tunisia, and Yemen.

4th region is South East Asia Region having North Korea, Maldives, Sri Lanka, Myanmar, Bhutan, Indonesia, Bangladesh, India, Nepal, Thailand, and Timor-Leste.

5th region is Western Pacific Region which includes South Korea, Australia, China, Laos, Cambodia, Marshall Islands, Nauru, Cook Islands, Fiji, Japan, Kiribati, Malaysia, Brunei, Micronesia, Mongolia, Niue, Papua, Taiwan, New Zealand, Palau, Vanuatu, New Guinea, Samoa Tonga, Solomon Islands, Singapore, Tuvalu, Philippines, and Vietnam.

6th region in the African Region which includes South Africa, Central African Republic, Ethiopia, Algeria, Botswana, Nigeria, Burundi, Madagascar, Burkina Faso, Cameroon, Equatorial Guinea, Cape Verde, Chad, Angola, Uganda, Comoros, Benin, Ivory Coast, Democratic Republic of Congo, Eritrea, Gabon, Gambia, Ghana, Guinea, Guinea- Bissau, Kenya, Lesotho, Liberia, Malawi, Mali, Mozambique, Mauritius, Niger, Namibia, Republic of Congo, Somalia, Rwanda, Mauritania, Tanzania, São Tomé and Príncipe, Senegal, Seychelles, Sierra Leone, Swaziland, Togo, Zambia, and Zimbabwe countries.

All the regions of the WHO have active COVID-19 cases. The most affected region is the Americas with 3,638,525 cases as of 12th June 2020. Whereas Europe stood 2nd with 2,378,958 cases and least affected is Africa with 161,254 cases as of 12th June 2020. In the Americas, the most affected countries are the USA, Brazil, and Canada. In Europe, the most affected countries are the United Kingdom, Germany, and Italy. Eastern Mediterranean is a third most affected region with 737,641 cases and Iran being the most affected country in this region. Southeast Asia is having 4,393,348 cases with India being the most affected country in the region. Western Pacific and Africa are also the affected regions as shown in Table **2** and Fig. (**5**).

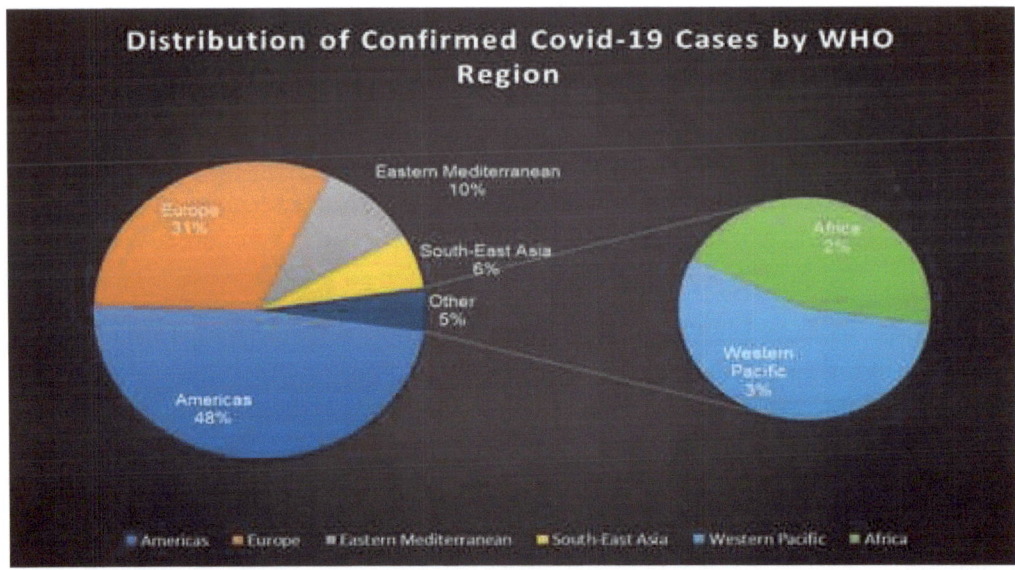

Fig. (5). Region-wise distribution of corona cases (as of 12 th June 2020).

Table 2. Total number of COVID-19 confirmed cases as per WHO regions.

WHO Region	No. of Confirmed Cases
Americas	3,638,525
Europe	2,378,958
Eastern Mediterranean	737,641
South-East Asia	439,348
Western Pacific	196,715
Africa	161,254

On comparing COVID-19 cases among the WHO regions, it is found that the Americas, South East Asia, Africa, and Eastern Mediterranean are still growing wrt number of patients, whereas, there is a steady decrease in corona cases in Europe and Western Pacific as shown in Table **3** and Fig. (**6**).

Table 3. Date wise comparison of COVID-19 cases in different WHO region.

Region	31st Dec. 2019	10th Jan. 2020	30th Jan	9th Feb.	29th Feb.	10th Mar.	30th Mar.	9th April	29th April	9th May	29th May	8th June
Americas	0	0	8	11	62	826	146,850	331,997	385,273	437,293	563,221	668,199
Europe	0	0	10	27	1,104	15,215	292,038	360,199	285,400	268,728	193,655	184,276

(Table 3) cont.....

Region	31st Dec. 2019	10th Jan. 2020	30th Jan	9th Feb.	29th Feb.	10th Mar.	30th Mar.	9th April	29th April	9th May	29th May	8th June
Eastern Mediterranean	0	0	4	3	500	7,069	24,983	39,355	52,344	69,353	125,770	166,580
South-East Asia	0	0	15	20	7	10	3,240	7,628	24,055	39,354	89,310	126,128
Western Pacific	27	32	7,547	29,604	8,194	6,628	10,475	11,314	15,327	12,064	9,321	12,746
Africa	0	0	0	0	2	7	2,833	4,547	9,156	16,611	28,363	42,216

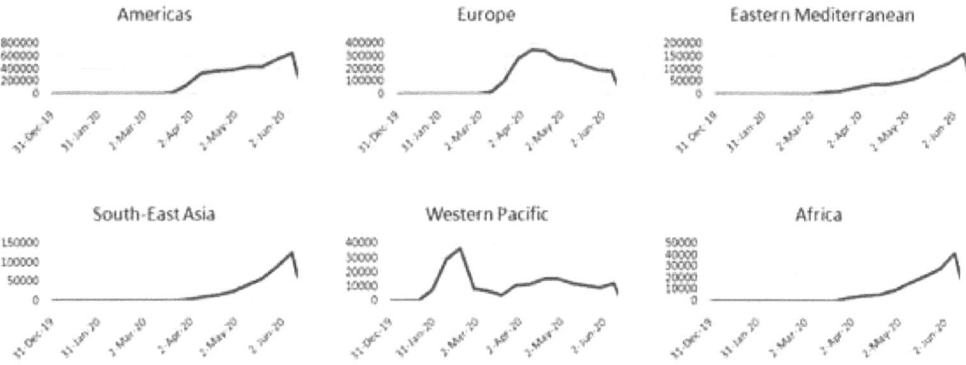

Fig. (6). Date-wise comparison of COVID-19 cases in different WHO regions.

The data shown in Table **3** and Fig. **(6)** indicates that some countries have witnessed a decline in the number of COVID-19 positive cases after strict lockdown restrictions (for more details regarding lockdown effects, refer to the next part of this chapter).

COVID-19 IN INDIA

India registered its first COVID-19 confirmed case at the end of January 2020. As of 12th June 2020, a total of 309,603 confirmed cases and 8,890 mortalities have been reported in India. The prevalence of confirmed COVID-19 cases with the number of cases in various states of India is shown in Fig. **(7)** (Worldometer, 2020). The figure represents states with more than 25,000 cases such as Maharashtra, Tamilnadu, and Gujrat. Various states had confirmed cases in the range of 10,000 to 25,000.

There were only three epidemiological surveys done in India till 12th June 2020:

- Twenty-one COVID-19 confirmed cases from the hospital of New Delhi.
- By Government of Maharashtra, with 12,296 cases data of the state.
- 41 sentinel sites of the country: data were taken and analyzed for Severe Acute Respiratory Infection (SARI) cases.

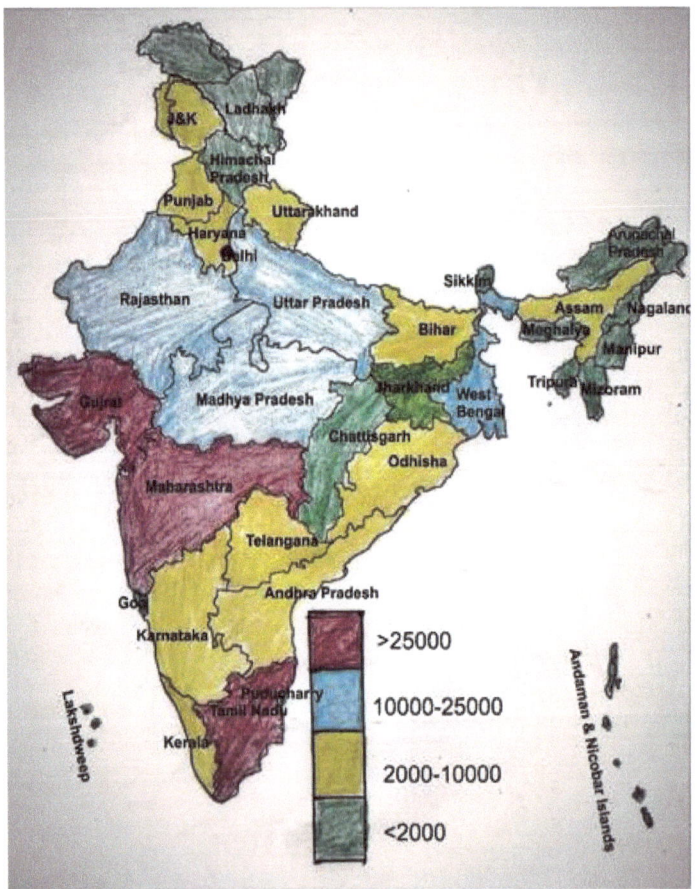

Fig. (7). Confirmed cases of COVID-19 in India as of 12th June 2020.

As of 3rd May 2020, 168,374 tests were completed in 41 sentry sites of Maharashtra for COVID-19. About 7.3%, approximately 12,300 patients were found positive in contrast with approximately 100 patients for SARI infections. Among the tested individuals, 84% were males and higher cases of infection also represented the poor unhygienic habits of the sanitary population. (Government of Maharashtra, 2020; Gupta *et al.*, 2020).

In another study conducted in Delhi, clinical data of the sample population showed that in all the tested individuals for COVID-19, 43% of patients were found to have cough and fever like symptoms, 24% patients with a sore throat, 14% with headache, and 5% were having breathlessness symptoms. This study revealed that symptomatic patients have a cough and fever-like symptoms (Gandhi *et al.*, 2020).

According to the government of Maharashtra, the case fatality rate was found to be 4.8% in males as compared to 4% in females and there was no correlation between gender and the death rate (p>0.05). This study further reported that the death rate is higher, *i.e.* 19.2% in the age group of 61-70 years as compared to 18 years old individuals who showed a 14% death rate. This study can be related to the clinical and physical conditions of the patients with their age (Government of Maharashtra, 2020; Gupta *et al.*, 2020).

Gupta *et al.*, studied 102 COVID-19 patients and found that the positive patients from sentinel sites having SARI infection had no abroad travel history or any kind of history of close contact with COVID-19 patients, and the source of infection was not known (Gupta *et al.*, 2020). Another study revealed that in India, community transmission had occurred very early in Pune and other cities, which is why the sources of infection were not traceable (Pulla, 2020).

All of these studies reported and concluded the basic demography of COVID-19 positive cases in India. These studies did not interpret the exact clinical outcomes; therefore, further studies were required to properly understand the epidemiology of corona cases in India.

More epidemiological information of the infection like co-morbidities, risk factors, mode of transmission and socio-demography, and their dynamics is needed in India. All these factors and their details are required to access the exact epidemiology of the COVID-19 pandemic in India.

REPORT BY ICMR ON COVID-19 ABOUT CONTAINMENT ZONE IN INDIA

Indian Council of Medical Research (ICMR) conducted a population-based survey on COVID-19 in India and found that 15-30 percent of the people living in the containment zones *i.e.* in main affected or hotspot cities were infected by the COVID-19 and were already recovered. These findings of ICMR have been shared with the union cabinet secretary and the Prime Minister's Office.

For this survey, ICMR collected the blood samples with the help of the National Centre for Disease Control, the World Health Organization's India office, and the state governments. Around 24,000 samples were collected from the 70 districts of Pune, Delhi, Indore, Kolkata, Chennai, Surat, Mumbai, and Jaipur where there is 70 percent of total COVID-19 cases of India. As many as 500 samples were collected from 10 randomly chosen containment areas in each of these cities. 400 samples each from the other 60 districts across 21 states, categorized based on the low, medium, and high caseloads, were also collected.

The report suggested that all the containment areas, except Surat and Kolkata, are the worst hit and have 100 to 200 times higher number of cases than the reported cases in the cities like Mumbai, Pune, Delhi, Ahmadabad, and Indore.

NATIONAL RESPONSES ON COVID-19 WORLDWIDE

Almost every country or territory in the world has reported at least one COVID-19 positive case. Different countries have taken different measures to contain viral infections. For instance, Schengen Area countries (Europe) have restricted any kind of movement and control the setup of borders (Schengen Visa Information, 2020). National responses include containment actions like curfews and quarantines, shelter-in-place, and stay-at-home orders.

In the last week of March 2020, globally 1.7 billion persons were under lockdown which got elevated to 3.9 billion people on the first week of April, which represents half of the world's population (Kaplan, 2020).

At the end of April, about 300 million people were under lockdown in different countries of Europe whereas about 200 million people were under lockdown in Latin America. Almost 90 percent of the United States population, around 100 million people in the Philippines (Buchholz, 2020), around 1.3 billion people in India, and 59 million people in South Africa (Nair, 2020) have been under lockdown. Ever since the beginning of the pandemic, over 100,000 new infections were reported on one single day worldwide on 21st May. Below are some detailed examples of corona-related developments in various countries and various measures taken to contain the COVID-19 virus.

Asia

All the countries present in the Asia continent reported COVID-19 positive cases by 19th May 2020 except North Korea and Turkmenistan.

Asia was the first in the world which got hit by the outbreak; however, South Korea, Vietnam, and Taiwan responded to the pandemic very well and were able to control the spread of the pandemic in their respective countries in the beginning, except Taiwan, which maintained to have very low infection rate.

China

As we discussed earlier, the first confirmed case of COVID-19 was reported in China in December 2019 (Chen *et al.*, 2020; Lu *et al.*, 2020) yet one unconfirmed report suggests that the cases were started to appear as early as 17th November 2019 (Ma, 2020). On 27th December 2019, patient samples reported the existence of a SARS-like coronavirus in original genetic testing. Wuhan Municipal Health Commission issued a public notice on 31st December 2019, confirmed 27 cases, and advised to wear masks (Zhu *et al.*, 2020), and on the very same day, WHO was also informed. The Chinese National Health Commission initially stated that there was no clear proof of person-to-person transmission; however, in a conference held on 14th January 2020, Chinese officials confidentially stated that there was a possibility of person-to-person transmission and preparations for the pandemic situation where required.

On 20th January, the Chinese National Health Commission confirmed person-to-person transmission of the virus. A lockdown in the city of Wuhan was enforced during Chinese New Year 2020 (Kuo, 2020). On 10th February, the Chinese government instigated a radical campaign called a "people's war" to contain the viral spread. On 23rd January, the "largest quarantine in human history", a *cordon sanitaire*, was declared with travel restrictions inside and outside of the city of Wuhan which was then extended to 15 cities of Hubei province affecting about 57 million people. Temporary hospitals were established including Huoshenshan Hospital (completed in ten days). Another hospital named Leishenshan Hospital was created to handle the load of additional patients. Facilities in Wuhan, like convention centers and stadiums, were converted into temporary hospitals (Ni *et al.*, 2020; Cai *et al.*, 2020).

On 26th January, the Chinese government instituted further measures as well as mandatory health declarations by travelers and postponing the Spring Festival season holidays. Institutes, schools, museums, universities, and other crowded places throughout China were temporarily closed and work from home was initiated in several regions. Controlled movement of the public was initiated in many cities and around 760 million people had restricted all kinds of outdoor activities. During the peak of the epidemic in Wuhan, in January-February 2020, about 5 million people lost their jobs. Almost 300 million migrants, belonging to rural areas, got trapped at their respective places during travel restrictions (Cai *et al.*, 2020; Ni *et al.*, 2020).

By the time pandemic reached its global phase in February-March 2020, it came under control in China, and therefore, strict measures were taken to prevent the re-entering of the virus in China from other countries. A 14-day compulsory quarantine was imposed for all international travelers entering China as enforced by Beijing. Regretfully, a strong anti-foreigner fury quickly took hold, and discrimination against foreigners such as forced evictions from hotels; lodges, and apartments were reported (Li et al., 2020).

On 24th March, the official announcement was made by Chinese Premier Li Keqiang that the outbreak has been contained in China. Except for Wuhan, travel restrictions were eased in Hubei from 24-26th March, after two months of lockdown. The Chinese Ministry of Foreign Affairs announced the suspension of visas or residence permits from 28th March onwards, with no specifications regarding its resumption. Re-application for visas in Chinese embassies or consulates had become mandatory for people who wish to enter China. Monetary stimulus packages for firms and factories were given to boost the local economy and to re-open businesses by the Chinese government on 30th March (Lau et al., 2020).

Coinciding with the Qingming Festival, a day of grief with a countrywide three-minute silence moment on 4th April was observed by the State Council. However, to avoid a transformed virus outbreak, the Chinese government suggested families pay their admirations online by observing physical distancing (Zhang, 2020). On 25th April, the last patients got discharged from hospitals in Wuhan; however, on 13th May, the city of Jilin was put on partial lockdown, by considering the fear of the second wave of COVID-19 infection (The Hindu, 2020).

South Korea

On 20th January 2020, COVID-19 was confirmed to have spread in South Korea as observed by the nation's health agency due to a substantial increase in the number of confirmed positive cases majorly attributed to an assembly of the Shincheonji Church of Jesus in Daegu. Shincheonji devotees who visited Daegu from Wuhan were supposed to be infected with the virus before entering S. Korea; and therefore, they were the carriers of the infection. By 22nd February, 1,261 supporters of the church (approx. 13%) amongst 9,336 in total reported viral symptoms following which, South Korea stated the highest level of alert on 23rd February 2020.

The number of confirmed cases in South Korea reached more than 2,000 on 28th February to 3,150 on 29th February. Furthermore, after examinations, three soldiers came positive for the COVID-19 virus and all of the South Korean military bases were sent for quarantine. Timetables of airline carriers were also changed.

A national-level drive to contain the virus was put into force by S. Korea which included screening the S. Korean population for the virus, isolating sick people, if any, and trace and quarantine people who had direct or indirect contact with the infected individuals. This drive is considered the largest and best-organized program in the world. Effective screening methods included were:

1. Compulsory self-reporting of symptoms through a mobile application by all new international arrivals.
2. Rapid testing for the virus was done through Drive-through testing resulting in next day.
3. 20,000 people were tested every day.

South Korea's program was successful in controlling the outbreak without imposing lockdown among all the cities of South Korea (Shim *et al.*, 2020).

On 23rd March, South Korea reported to had reported the lowest one-day case toll over the last four weeks. On 29th March, two weeks quarantine for all new overseas arrivals was announced to be implemented from the beginning of April. As per some reports, by early April, 121 different countries were reported to reach out to South Korea for assistance in virus testing. On 15th May, after a group of a hundred infected individuals was discovered, almost two thousand businesses were again closed briefly (Inocencio, 2020).

Middle Eastern

Iran

Iran recorded its first confirmed case of COVID-19 on 19th February in Qom. However, on the same day, two people had died due to COVID-19 as reported by the Ministry of Health and Medical Education. Primary actions were taken by the government involved:

1. Termination of cultural events, sports events, concerts, Friday prayers, and other similar actions.
2. Closings of schools, universities, and other higher education institutions.
3. Allocation of 5 trillion Rials to combat the virus.

However, on 26th February, President Hassan Rouhani declared that only infected individuals would be quarantined and that there were no plans to quarantine the affected areas. Despite travel restrictions announced in March, heavy traffic between cities was observed ahead of 'Nowruz'. Shrines were continually open to Shia pilgrims until 16th March in Qom.

After China, Iran became the center of the virus outbreak in February 2020 and over ten countries had outlined their cases related to Iran. On 3rd March, the Iranian Parliament had a blackout because twenty-three parliamentary members had tested positive out of 290 parliamentarians. Twelve government officials and various Iranian politicians succumbed to death due to the COVID-19 infection. On 15th March, over one hundred deaths were reported in one single day, the most recorded in Iran since the beginning of the outbreak. (Takian *et al.*, 2020). By 23rd March, there were fifty new cases per hour of corona infection, and one new death per ten minutes was also reported due to COVID-19. However, according to an official working with WHO, cases in Iran may be at least five times more than what is been reported. Furthermore, it was inferred that U.S. sanctions on Iran might be creating a financial crisis and affecting its ability to respond to the viral outbreak. Ease in economic sanctions was demanded by The UN High Commissioner for Human Rights, including Iran. On 20th April, Iran reopened various shopping malls and other areas with a high number of gatherings across the country; however, it sparked the risk of a second wave of infection. A new peak of the COVID-19 case was reported on 4th June, raising suspicions of the second wave (BBC, 2020).

Europe

The number of corona infected people in Europe increased very quickly and when on 13th March 2020, the number of infected people in Europe crossed China, WHO announced Europe as a new dynamic area of the pandemic. Infection cases in various countries in Europe started to double within 3 to 4 days, with some countries showing replication every 2 days.

By 17th March, there was at least one confirmed case of COVID-19 in all countries within Europe except Vatican City. Till 18th March, approximately 250 million people were restricted through lockdown in Europe (Henley, 2020).

Spain

After having the first confirmed positive case at the end of January 2020, Spain experienced community transmission starting from mid-February. Genetic examination of the samples from infected individuals revealed at least 15 strains of the virus indicating the adaptive nature of coronavirus. COVID-19 positive cases were confirmed in all of the 50 provinces of the country by 13th March (Ansede, 2020).

Lockdown was imposed on 14th March 2020. It was reported that all healthcare professionals and those living in old age homes were having greater rates of infection. Madrid recorded the greatest number of cases and deaths connected to

COVID-19 in the country by late March. On 25th March, the total number of death in Spain crossed 9,000 people approximately. On 2nd April, it was recorded that 950 people in a single day died due to corona infection (the highest number in any country within 24 hours) (Regencia, 2020).

There have been approximately 245,000 confirmed cases with COVID-19 infection and more than 27,000 deaths were reported till 14th June 2020. On 4th June, results of the nation-wide seroprevalence study directed by the Spanish Government showed that around 5.2% (roughly 2 million people) were infected during the pandemic and this figure was ten times more than the number of confirmed cases on that date. This study was based on a sample size of greater than 63,000 people and revealed that several provinces of Castilla–La Mancha, Castilla y León, and Madrid were amongst the most affected areas. (Andrino, 2020).

France

Originally, it was found that the first case of the COVID-19 pandemic in France was on 24th January 2020, with a confirmed case in Bordeaux. Christian Open Door annual assembly Church was organized during 17-24th February. This assembly was attended by about 2,500 people in Mulhouse and was suspected to be the main reason for the spread of the disease in the country. It was predicted that at least half of the attendees to have contracted the virus during this assembly (Point, 2020).

As of 16th March, the government of France announced a mandatory lockdown which was extended until 11th May. As of 23rd April, France reported more than 21,856 deaths, 42,088 recoveries, and 120,804 confirmed cases ranking fourth highest in the number of confirmed positive cases in Europe. Amidst the corona pandemic, when the situation appeared to be under control, the government decided to re-open schools; however, they were soon shut down due to COVID-19 cases flared up amongst children (CBS News, 2020).

North America

The cases of viral infection started to appear in the United States of the North American continent in January 2020. All North American countries had at least one COVID-19 positive case as of 25th March. With Bonaire confirming a case on 16th April, all North American territories had at least one positive case (Davis, 2020).

With over 82,000 cases on 26th March 2020, U.S. became the highest COVID-19 infected country surpassing China, and is still the country with the highest number of cases as of 12th June 2020. On 11th April 2020, U.S. reported the highest, more than 20,000 deaths, due to COVID-19 infection. As of 12th June 2020, the US confirmed 2,116,211 with 116,814 total deaths.

Canada reported 97,943 confirmed cases and 8,049 deaths on 12th June. Mexico has reported 133,974 COVID-19 cases and 15,944 mortalities till 12th June. Cuba, Dominican Republic, and Haiti are the only Caribbean countries that reported more than 1,000 confirmed cases; while Honduras and Panama led Central America with 7,669 and 18,586 cases respectively (Worldometer, 2020).

United States

As of 20th January, the first known confirmed case of COVID-19 was found in Washington in a man who had returned from China in January mid (Holshue *et al.*, 2020). On 31st January, government officials announced a public health emergency, limiting the entry of tourists and travelers, especially from China.

With a slow start in the testing of samples, the United States on 28th January developed its testing kit as announced by the Centers for Disease Control and Prevention (CDC). However, testing was impaired due to defective test kits; moreover, there was a lack of federal approval for the test kits approved by non-government bodies. Restrictive criteria for the inclusion of people for a test further impaired the effective testing. (Selsky, 2020).

By 2nd March, 80 confirmed cases were reported in the US with, a maximum of cases (almost half) in California. By that time, New York and Florida also stated their first two cases with Washington reporting many suspected cases along with the first death; however, Vice President stressed a small chance of the virus spreading all over the US (Heeb, 2020).

To deal with the rising number of cases in the States, on 6th March, Coronavirus Preparedness and Response Supplemental Appropriations Act were signed by President Trump, enabling federal agencies with $8.3 billion as emergency funding for the pandemic. Work from home was put into practice by various corporations and various sports events and related activities got cancelled (Heeb, 2020).

Despite ongoing efforts, the numbers of infected cases keep on increasing which led President Trump to declare a national emergency on 13th March. Beginning from 15th March, many businesses, schools, universities, stores, *etc.* across the country were either closed or had reduced working hours. By 17th March, all fifty states of the US had confirmed cases. In a survey of 323 hospitals across the U.S in late March, federal health inspectors reported severe shortages of test supplies, widespread shortages of Personal Protective Equipment (PPE), and other standard healthcare facilities due to the high load of patients.

On 22nd April, two Californians who were previously thought to have died (on 6th and 17th February respectively) from the influenza were reported to be dead because of the COVID-19 virus; however, it was three weeks later when first COVID-19 death officially occurred in U.S. New York Times database revealed over 1,474,600 patients had infected with COVID-19 in the US with at least 88,600 had died as of 17th May.

South America

South America reported its first case on 26th February with a confirmed case in São Paulo, Brazil. Soon after, by 3rd April, all the countries and territories of South America had reported at least one confirmed case.

As of April 17th, the highest number of COVID-19 infections and COVID-19 related mortalities were reported in Brazil followed by Chile and Peru.

On May 13th, Latin America and the Caribbean described over 400,000 COVID-19 positive cases with 23,091 deaths. With the rapid increase of patients having COVID-19 infection in Brazil, WHO stated South America as the new center of the coronavirus pandemic on May 22nd. Due to the lack of proper testing kits and medical facilities, it is considered that the actual numbers of affected people were far more than those reported.

Africa

Africa is of one particular concern by the experts as indicated by Michael Yao, Head of Emergency Operations of WHO in Africa. According to him, early detection would be vital in tackling the COVID-19 situation in Africa as the island's health systems are already overloaded due to other ongoing disease outbursts. To minimize lockdowns in African countries, an approach based on effective testing could be of particular use thus enabling those who depend on daily wages to be able to feed themselves and their families. However, as per a report of the United Nations, even in the best scenario, at least 74 million test kits and at least 30,000 ventilators will be needed for 1.3 billion people of African countries.

Maximum COVID-19 infected cases are reported from the six African countries, which are: South Africa, Ghana, Nigeria, Egypt, Morocco, and Algeria. Though, it is supposed that in African countries with poorer health care systems there is widespread under-reporting. As of 13th May 2020, all African countries reported

COVID-19 confirmed cases and Lesotho was the last country to report its 1st confirmed case on the same date.

Oceania

1st case of COVID-19 in Oceania was reported by the end of January 2020 with the first confirmed case reported in Melbourne, Australia. However, several small Pacific island countries had so far restricted the outbreak by closing their international borders.

On 19th May 2020, for an inquiry into the origins of the virus and the response of governments and the UN, Australia filed a motion in the UN. With the support from over 100 countries motion was passed unanimously in the UN.

EFFECT OF LOCKDOWN ON COVID-19 CASES IN TOP TEN MOST AFFECTED COUNTRIES OF WORLD

As discussed earlier, the most affected countries with the highest COVID-19 positive cases in the world include; USA, Russia, Brazil, Spain, India, UK, Peru, Germany, Italy, and Iran. All of these countries have imposed lockdowns in their respective areas. There is a huge influence of lockdown on the spread of this disease as shown in Table **4** (Worldometer 2020). During the lockdown, the numbers of corona cases were less as compared to cases before the lockdown. The possible reason behind this is the control of the movement of people, which is the main reason for the spread of the infection and thus preventing community spread of the infection.

Table 4. Corona cases from pre- to post lockdown (as of 12th June 2020).

Country	Pre-Lockdown				During Lockdown				Post-Lockdown			
	Period	No. of Confirmed Cases	Death	Average Confirmed Cases per Day	Period	No. of Confirmed Cases	Death	Average Confirmed Cases per Day	Period	No. of Confirmed Cases	Death	Average Confirmed Cases per Day
Brazil	25th Feb. to 23rd Mar.'20	45,775	25	1,635	24th Mar. to 20th Apr.'20	37,108	2,437	1,325	20th Apr. to till now	798,964	38,457	4,796
Russia	31st Jan. to 27th Mar.'20	840	02	15	28th Mar. to 15th May	251,405	2,303	5,130	15th May to till now	250,191	4,227	8,936
India	30th Jan. to 22nd Mar.'20	439	07	09	23rd Mar. to 31st May	181,704	5,157	2,634	31st May to till now	215,392	3,334	6,568

(Table 4) cont.....

Country	Pre-Lockdown				During Lockdown				Post-Lockdown			
	Period	No. of Confirmed Cases	Death	Average Confirmed Cases per Day	Period	No. of Confirmed Cases	Death	Average Confirmed Cases per Day	Period	No. of Confirmed Cases	Death	Average Confirmed Cases per Day
UK	22nd Jan. to 22nd Mar.'20	5,018	250	84	23rd Mar. to 10th May	210,242	31,337	4,280	11th May to till Now	76,149	9,692	2,380
Spain	31st Jan. to 13th Mar.'20	5,958	84	139	14th Mar. to 02nd May'20	211,846	25,016	4,237	3rd May to till now	25,405	2,036	620
Italy	30th Jan. to 21st Feb.	59,138	5,476	1,115	21st Feb. (partially) and 23rd Mar.'20 to 3rd May'20	150,198	23,234	3,664	3rd May to till now	26,804	5,457	682
Peru	6th Mar. to 14th Mar.'20	38	--	5	15th Mar. to till now	214,750	6,109	2,413	---	---	---	---
Germany	27th Jan. to 22nd Mar.'20	21,463	67	358	22nd Mar. to 19th Apr.'20	118,434	4,469	4,084	20th April to till now	45,777	4,469	848
Iran	19th Feb. to 12th Mar.'20	9,000	354	360	13th Mar. to 10th Apr.'20	57,220	3,756	1,974	11th April to till now	113,956	4,474	1,808

In the USA, there was lockdown executed only in some areas thus the infection throughout the period is the same. Moreover, the USA was dealing with a gigantic number of COVID-19 cases. New York reported 4,000 on 7th April, the highest number of cases in a day, and thus topped the country ever since the pandemic started to affect the country. Various states of the USA forced the restrictions; however, it was impossible to lock down the whole nation due to the federalist state system of the country and the independent nature of the states. In the mid of March'20, California imposed restrictions to avoid the non-essential outdoor movement & stay at home orders were also issued. Chicago executed the lockdown on 21st March 2020 being the 3rd most populated area of the country. There was no national strategy on lockdown; therefore, many US citizens are free to go anywhere throughout the country (Holshue et al., 2020).

Besides, many states of the USA had workplaces, educational institutes, and businesses to shut their services and imposed social distancing. Amongst them West Virginia, Washington, California, Indiana, Illinois, Wisconsin Michigan, and Ohio, adopted the policies of state-wide quarantine (Train, 2020). States such as Oklahoma and Mississippi, which were less-affected, had shut their educational institutes; however, other restrictions were not imposed as can be seen from the fact that, they permitted public gatherings of up to 10 people.

On 25th February 2020 Brazil reported the first positive case of COVID-19 in Sao Paulo. Until 12th June 2020, 802,828 cases were reported in the country and 40,919 deaths were reported. Globally, Brazil stood 2nd in the terms of highest number of confirmed cases of COVID-19. Brazilian government imposed lockdown from 24th March 2020 till 20th April 2020. Statistical data as given in Table **4** revealed that during the lockdown period the average number of confirmed cases was 1,325/day as compared to 14,796/day after lockdown indicating the effectiveness of restricted movement and home quarantine during the lockdown in tackling the spread of coronavirus (Schwartz, 2020; Painel Coronavírus, 2020; Shailesh, 2020).

In Peru, the first case was reported on 6th March 2020. A 25 years old man with a history of travel to France, the Czech Republic, and Spain tested positive. As of 15th of March, President Martín Vizcarra broadcast country-wide lockdown, limiting domestic travel, closing borders, and forbidding non-essential businesses except pharmacies, food vendors, health facilities, and institutions related to financial activities. With an extended state of emergency and a national lockdown until the end of June, Peru witnessed one of the world's longest compulsory isolation periods aimed at containing the coronavirus outbreak. Peru's confirmed COVID-19 positive cases were 111,698 the second-highest total in the American continent with total death of 3,244 as of 12th June'20.

In terms of Covid cases across the globe, Russia was on the 3rd spot as of 12th June 2020. According to official data, Russia had 511,423 confirmed cases till 12th June 2020. During treatment 269,370 cases recovered while 6,715 died. Pandemic started in country on 31st January 2020, when two citizens from China were found positive. Russia immediately imposed preventive measures and started testing every person crossing the Russia-China border. However, new cases of the infection were found on 2nd March 2020, with a history of travel to Italy, which led to an imposition of additional preventive actions such as cancelation of various events, closing theatres, educational institutes, and museums. Lockdown lasted until 11th May in most parts of the federal; including Moscow which was under lockdown until the end of March 2020. On 27th April, the total number of COVID-19 confirmed cases in Russia surpassed the number of cases in China. A similar trend in pre-and post-lockdown periods, like that of Brazil, was also observed in Russia with an average number of 8,936 cases per day after the lockdown was lifted compared to 5,130/day during the lockdown period (Table **4**) (Elsevier, 2020; Rainsford, 2020).

The first case of COVID-19 in India was reported on 30th January 2020. The Ministry of Health and Family Welfare (MoHFW) confirmed 309,603 numbers of cases, 154,231 recoveries, and 8,890 deaths in the country as of 12th June 2020. As of 12th June'20, India had the highest number of confirmed cases in Asia and was in the fourth number amongst the countries with the highest number of corona cases worldwide. However, India's fatality rate, 2.80%, was relatively lower than the global fatality rate of 6.13%. On 22nd March, India imposed 14 hours of Janta Curfew, which was followed by mandatory lockdown in all the major cities and states of India. On 24th March, a nationwide lockdown for 21 days was imposed, followed by extensions. From 1st June onwards, the government started unlocking the country with restrictions at places of containment zones. A similar trend, like that of Brazil and Russia, in the pre-and post- lockdown period, was observed in India.

In the UK, as of 12th June 2020, there were 292,950 confirmed cases and 41,481 confirmed deaths. This was the second-highest mortality rate per capita in the World. In the UK, among all the cities, London topped the country with cases of infections; but the rate of infection was found to be highest in North-East England.

In March, the UK government imposed a lockdown and barred all "non-essential" travel. The government also banned making contact with people outside one's domicile (including family and partners), closed businesses, schools, and other places of public gatherings. People with symptoms were asked to self-isolate, while the high-risk people (those over the 60s and with other diseases) were told to isolate and protect themselves. Social distancing was put into practice. Government efforts to contain the virus by lockdown resulted in a decrease in the rate at which people were getting infected before lockdown.

The first case of SARS-CoV-2 infection in Spain was reported on 31st January 2020, with COVID-19 positive tourists in La Gomera, Canary Islands, who came from Germany. Soon after, different provinces started to report corona cases and by 13th March, all 50 provinces of the country had COVID-19 positive cases. The lockdown was imposed on 14th March 2020. At the end of March, all government authorities ordered non-essential workers to stay at home for two weeks. In late March, Madrid recorded the highest number of infected persons and deaths in the whole country. Healthcare professionals and people living in old age homes were found to have higher rates of infection. As of 12th June 2020, there were 290,289 confirmed positive cases and 27,136 mortalities.

In Italy, the government implemented a nationwide quarantine on 9th March 2020, thus restricting the movement of the people except when required in case of work and health circumstances, to contain the mounting COVID-19 pandemic in the country. The temporary closure of unimportant shops and businesses was authorized by additional lockdown restrictions. Although approved by the public, these lockdown measures were the largest destruction of constitutional rights in the history of the republic. Nonetheless, lockdown effectively reduced the frequency and spread of the infection in the country. After the lockdown, the average per day corona cases were lowered to 682 as compared to the highest 3,664/day before lockdown.

The first case of the COVID-19 pandemic in Germany was a worker working in an automobile-parts producer and was confirmed on 27th January 2020. By the end of February 2020, multiple cases related to the coronavirus infection were detected in Baden-Württemberg named as 'Italian Outbreak'. Germany imposed a lockdown which lasted until 19th April 2020 with a decrease in the rate of infection transmission after lockdown. (Amante and Pollina, 2020; Seckin, 2020).

The coronavirus infection started in Iran on 19th February 2020. Iran reported its first confirmed case of infections in Qom. It was suspected that the virus may have entered the country from a merchant in Qom with travel history to China. Lockdown in Iran was started on 13th March 2020. To contain the infection, the government cancelled Friday prayers, public events, closed all educational institutes, markets, shopping centers, and holy shrines, and banned festival celebrations. Lockdown which ended on 10th April 2020 had successfully brought down the number of infected cases (Amante and Pollina, 2020; Seckin, 2020).

As can be seen, lockdown had a reasonable effect on containing the spread of the disease. Also, various countries have taken various other measures along with lockdown which was discussed in earlier parts of this chapter.

THE ROLE OF WHO AND INGOS FOR PROVIDING DATA IN COVID-19

To facilitate the wellbeing of public health worldwide, in 1948 World Health Organization (WHO) was established by United Nations with the main objective of obtaining reliable information and pieces of advice in the field of human health through publication. WHO supports national health strategies of various nations and addresses the alarming public health concerns by its publications. In the current pandemic situation, WHO is working actively in providing funding, information regarding disease progress, and giving statistical analysis on the COVID-19 to help control the spread of the disease in various part of the world and to help the researchers to find out the possible treatments of this disease; thus, helping to promote and protect health worldwide and to limit the spread of the disease throughout the world. Information provided by WHO contributes to achieving the organization's principal objective – the attainment by all people of the highest possible level of health. Similarly, various other International Non-Government Organizations (INGOs) are working day and night in parallel to various national agencies in and around their working area to keep updated information about COVID-19 by collecting samples, conducting studies, applying statistics, and publishing high impact papers on the spread, control, and management of the disease.

OUTCOMES FROM SOME PUBLISHED REPORTS ON COVID-19 EPIDEMIOLOGY

- Hamid *et al*. reported that the persons with age group 35-55 years got less infections as compared to children and infants. The study found that the median age of patients was 59 years and the majority were males (59%). Furthermore, the study reported that old age people with various problems were a high-risk group. They also found that transmissibility and pandemic risk of SARS-CoV-2 was at high rates as compared to that of SARS-CoV. The COVID-19 average incubation duration was estimated to be 4.8 ± 2.6 ranging from 2-11 days (Hamid *et al.*, 2020).
- Chen *et al.*, studied and analyzed the cases for demographic, epidemiological, radiological, and clinical features and laboratory data. The study reported that 49% of cases had exposure to the seafood market. They observed that the patients had clinical illustrations of fever (83%), cough (82%), breath shortness (31%), muscle ache (11%), confusion (9%), headache (8%), sore throat (5%), rhinorrhoea (4%), chest pain (2%), diarrhoea (2%) and nausea and vomiting (1%). They illustrated that according to imaging examination, 75% of patients manifested bilateral pneumonia, 14% patients showed multiple mottling and ground-glass opacity, and 1% of patients had observed pneumothorax. 17% of patients developed acute respiratory distress syndrome and 11% of patients had their conditions exacerbated in a short period of time and died of multiple organ failure (Chen *et al.*, 2020).
- Gandhi *et al.*, reported the epidemiological study on India which was based on literature from PubMed, WHO, GoI, and Google Scholar. They evaluated the study based on a test performed in various metro cities of India till 2nd April 2020 and found out that 1.8% cases were found positive with a corona in Maharashtra of which 39.7% were males with a mean age of 40.3. The median age of the patients in sentinel Delhi areas was 54. Furthermore, in the report, they revealed that 43.8% of cases had a travel history, and 31.3% of cases had direct contact with COVID-19 cases (Gandhi *et al.*, 2020).
- Ahn *et al*. reported epidemiology on COVID-19. They found that the death rate of SARS-CoV-2 (3.8%) is lesser as compared to SARS-CoV (10%) or MERS-

CoV (37.1%), but infection rates are 10 times more as compared to the other two. Reports suggested that SARS CoV-2 can be transmitted from patients which are having mild infections or are asymptomatic. The unexpected and immediate epidemic outspreading of the virus could be explained by these findings (Ahn et al., 2020).

- Zhai et al., reported in their study that the incubation period of COVID-19 was 5.2 days to 6.4 days. Authors also reported that the reproduction number in the majority of studies was found to be 2.24 to 3.58 which is higher than that of SARS (Zhai et al., 2020).
- Bulut, C et al., reported that the COVID-19 pandemic has R0 value of 2.3, which can be as high as up to 5.7, and the case fatality rate was found to be 6.3 which was different in various age groups amongst different countries. The study also suggested that 10-12 weeks are required for the control of pandemics in the community (Bulut et al., 2020).
- Sun et al. reported that the spread of the virus in the 2nd phase occurred in the hospitals and within the family starting from 13th January in Wuhan to other areas. The third phase was started on 26th January 2020. 1,716 staff members from 422 medical institutions were infected in February 2020 in China. In the initial evaluation, it was found that the reproductive number of COVID-19 was 1.4 to 3.9 (Sun et al., 2020).
- Lai et al., reported that there is a difference in the epidemiological data among the different countries whereas China registered a high number of deaths and illnesses than other sites of the world. The Daily Cumulative Index was calculated for COVID-19 as cumulative cases/no. of days between the first reported case and this number was highest in China (1,320.85) on 29th February 2020 followed by the Republic of Korea (78.78) and further followed by Iran (43.11) and Italy (30.62). In other countries/territories, the Daily Cumulative Index was not more than 10 per day (Lai et al., 2020).
- She et al., reported the epidemiology study on children infected with COVID-19. They found that around 56% (34/61) of children infected with COVID-19 were infected from their families. They reported that in China 17 days old baby was found COVID-19 positive. After that, a neonatal, 5 days old infant, was infected with corona as his mother was found corona positive. The report further revealed that the incubation period in the children was approximately 6.5 days as compared to 5.4 days in adults (She et al., 2020).
- Yoo et al. examined the epidemiological reports on the Republic of Korea and reported that as of March 2nd, 2020, the Republic of Korea had the second-highest number of confirmed cases (n = 4,212) after China (n = 80,026). The main cause of augmented elevation in CoV-2 patients in Korea appeared by the exposure between the Daegu Church gathering attending members with additional hospital and community transmission. Mainly, the detonation of

transmission occurs in Daegu and adjoining areas (Yoo *et al.*, 2020).
- In a hypothesis Singh *et al.*, reported the scope of lung biofabrication tool, 3D bio-printing technology in reducing the chances of clinical trial failures in COVID-19 treatments. However, this area needs to explore further to establish the hypothesis (Singh *et al.*, 2020c).

Herd Immunity-COVID-19

Immunity can be attained by recovering from a pre-infection or vaccination. Not every individual can attain immunity due to the medical affliction *i.e.* immunosuppression, immunodeficiency, hence for such a group, herd immunity is a crucial way of protection (Coughlin *et al.*, 2017). Herd immunity happens when the herd *i.e.* large portion of a community achieves immunity to a disease which results in an unlikely spread of disease from person to person. Hence, the whole community can be protected, not just those who are immune.

If the population proportion which is immune to the disease is more than the threshold, the disease spread will decline. This is referred to as the herd immunity threshold (Kwok *et al.*, 2020).

There are two ways to get herd immunity for COVID-19 *i.e.* vaccines and infection. The vaccine against the COVID-19 virus would be an ideal approach to achieve herd immunity. Utilizing the herd immunity concept, many deadly contagious diseases such as diphtheria, smallpox, polio, have been successfully controlled (Fine *et al.*, 2011). Obtaining herd immunity down vaccination has downsides, though *i.e.* re-vaccination, skepticism, religious objections, *etc.*

Considering the current scenario, even if infection with the COVID-19 virus generates enduring immunity, a large percentage of the population would have to get infected to gain the herd immunity threshold. Recent update estimates that in the U.S.A, >70% of the population (200 million) would have to recover to stop the epidemic (Poland, 2020). Under such circumstances, the amount of infection could also lead to millions of deaths, serious complications. Until the vaccine is developed against the COVID-19 virus, its critical decelerates the viral spread. Hence, to lower down the risk of infection (Giubilini 2019, Kwok *et al.*, 2020):

- Avoid mass gatherings, close contact with people.
- Stay home if you are feeling sick and avoid public transportation and ride-sharing.
- Keep the distance between yourself and others in public transportations.
- Avoid public transportation, taxis, and ride-sharing if you're sick.
- Cover your mouth and nose, wear masks.

- Disinfect the most used surfaces.
- Eat and drink healthy to boost your immune system.

CONCLUSION

COVID-19 has emerged as one of the most infectious pandemics of recent times. It has changed the world once and for all. With no vaccine and no medicine in the market as of 30th Aug. 2020, measures like quarantine, isolation, and social distancing are the only choices humans had. With the number of corona positive patients increasing every day, it appears that we are still far away from getting rid of this problem. With already reported mutations of this virus, it might not be an easy task to develop vaccines, but efforts are underway. However, measures like lockdown, wearing masks, and social distancing have proved the effectiveness and should be practiced. High-risk group people should be extra cautious. COVID-19 is probably one of those diseases with which the human race might need to learn how to co-exist!' However, continuous efforts of the researchers in finding vaccines and treatment drugs, health care providers, various NGOs, awareness groups, *etc.* are commendable and are surely a silver lining in clouds of the COVID-19 pandemic.

LIST OF ABBREVIATIONS

WHO	World Health Organization
ICTV	International Committee on Taxonomy of Viruses
SARS	Severe Acute Respiratory Syndrome
MERS	Middle Eastern Respiratory Syndrome
MoHFW	The Ministry of Health and Family Welfare
SARI	Severe Acute Respiratory Infections
NGO	Non-Government Organization

CONSENT FOR PUBLICATION

Not applicable.

CONFLICT OF INTEREST

The authors declare no conflict of interest, financial or otherwise.

ACKNOWLEDGEMENTS

Declared none.

REFERENCES

Ahn, DG, Shin, HJ, Kim, MH, Lee, S, Kim, HS, Myoung, J, Kim, BT & Kim, SJ (2020) Current status of epidemiology, diagnosis, therapeutics, and vaccines for novel coronavirus disease 2019 (COVID-19). *J Microbiol Biotechnol,* 30, 313-24.
[http://dx.doi.org/10.4014/jmb.2003.03011] [PMID: 32238757]

Amante, A & Pollina, E Two first coronavirus cases confirmed in Italy: prime minister, January 30, 2020. Reuters (2020) Accessed on 12 June 2020. https://www.reuters.com/article/us-China-health-italy/two-frst-coronavirus-cases-confirmed-in-italy-prime-minister-idUSKBN1ZT31H

Andrino, B, Grasso, D & Llaneras, K The excess of deaths in the coronavirus crisis rises to 43,000 dead, June 17, 2020. El Pais (2020) Accessed on 19 June 2020. https://elpais.com/sociedad/2020/05/27/actualidad/1590570927_371193.html

Ansede, M (2020) *Genetic Analysis Suggests that the Coronavirus was already Circulating in Spain in mid-February.* Accessed on 14 June 2020. https://elpais.com/ciencia/2020-04-22/el-analisis-genetico-sugiee-que-el-coronavirus-ya-circulaba-por-espana-a-mediados-de-febrero.html

Buchholz, K (2020) *What Share of the World Population Is Already on COVID-19 Lockdown?.* Accessed on 12 June 2020. https://www.statista.com/chart/21240/enforced-COVID-19-lockdowns-by-people-affeced-per-country/

Bulut, C & Kato, Y (2020) Epidemiology of COVID-19. *Turk J Med Sci,* 50, 563-70.
[http://dx.doi.org/10.3906/sag-2004-172] [PMID: 32299206]

Cai, Y, Huang, T, Liu, X & Xu, G (2020) The effects of fangcang, huoshenshan, and leishenshan makeshift hospitals and temperature on the mortality of COVID-19. *medRxiv.*
[http://dx.doi.org/10.1101/2020.02.26.20028472]

CBS News (2020) *Coronavirus Flare-ups Force France to Re-close some Schools.* Accessed on 12 June 2020. https://www.cbsnews.com/news/coronavirus-france-close-some-reopened-schools-covid-cass-flare-up- today-2020-05-18/

Chen, N, Zhou, M, Dong, X, Qu, J, Gong, F, Han, Y, Qiu, Y, Wang, J, Liu, Y, Wei, Y, Xia, J, Yu, T, Zhang, X & Zhang, L (2020) Epidemiological and clinical characteristics of 99 cases of 2019 novel coronavirus pneumonia in Wuhan, China: a descriptive study. *Lancet,* 395, 507-13.
[http://dx.doi.org/10.1016/S0140-6736(20)30211-7] [PMID: 32007143]

Coronavirus, BBC (2020) *Iran Fears the Second Wave After a Surge in Cases.* Accessed on 12 June 2020. https://www.bbc.com/news/world-middle-east-52903443

Coughlin, MM, Beck, AS, Bankamp, B & Rota, PA (2017) Perspective on global measles epidemiology and control and the role of novel vaccination strategies. *Viruses,* 9, 11.
[http://dx.doi.org/10.3390/v9010011] [PMID: 28106841]

Davis, S (2020) Update on coronavirus (COVID-19) by Bonaire's Lt. Governor InfoBonaire, April 16, 2020. *The Bonaire Information Site* Accessed 14 June 2020. https://www.infobonaire.com/update-on-coronavirs-COVID-19-by-bonaires-lt-governor/

Di Gennaro, F, Pizzol, D, Marotta, C, Antunes, M, Racalbuto, V, Veronese, N & Smith, L (2020) Coronavirus diseases (COVID-19) current status and future perspectives: A narrative review. *Int J Environ Res Public Health,* 17, 2690.
[http://dx.doi.org/10.3390/ijerph17082690] [PMID: 32295188]

DiMaio, D, Enquist, LW & Dermody, TS (2020) Introduction: a new coronavirus emerges, this time causing a pandemic. *Annual Review of Virology,* 7, iii-v.Elsevier, Novel Coronavirus Information Center, Elsevier Connect. Accessed 12 June 2020. https://www.elsevier.com/connect/coronavirus-information-center

Fine, P, Eames, K & Heymann, DL (2011) "Herd immunity": a rough guide. *Clin Infect Dis,* 52, 911-6.
[http://dx.doi.org/10.1093/cid/cir007] [PMID: 21427399]

Gandhi, PA & Kathirvel, S (2020) Epidemiological studies on coronavirus disease 2019 pandemic in India:

Too little and too late? *Med J Armed Forces India,* 76, 364-5.
[http://dx.doi.org/10.1016/j.mjafi.2020.05.003] [PMID: 32398889]

Giovanetti, M, Benvenuto, D, Angeletti, S & Ciccozzi, M (2020) The first two cases of 2019-nCoV in Italy: Where they come from? *J Med Virol,* 92, 518-21.
[http://dx.doi.org/10.1002/jmv.25699] [PMID: 32022275]

Giubilini, A (2019) Vaccination and herd immunity: individual, collective, and institutional responsibilities. *The Ethics of Vaccination Palgrave Studies in Ethics and Public Policy Palgrave Pivot, Cham,* 29-58.
[http://dx.doi.org/10.1007/978-3-030-02068-2_2]

Government of Maharashtra (2020) *Report of COVID-19 cases.* https://www.mgims.ac.in/files/covid/meddrep/MEDD REPORT 04-05-2020 (1).pdf

Gupta, N, Agrawal, S, Ish, P, Mishra, S, Gaind, R, Usha, G, Singh, B & Sen, MK (2020) Clinical and epidemiologic profile of the initial COVID-19 patients at a tertiary care center in India. *Monaldi Arch Chest Dis,* 90, 193-6.
[http://dx.doi.org/10.4081/monaldi.2020.1294]

Gupta, N, Praharaj, I, Bhatnagar, T, Vivian Thangaraj, JW, Giri, S, Chauhan, H, Kulkarni, S, Murhekar, M, Singh, S, Gangakhedkar, RR & Bhargava, B ICMR COVID Team (2020) Severe acute respiratory illness surveillance for coronavirus disease 2019, India, 2020. *Indian J Med Res,* 151, 236-40.
[PMID: 32362647]

Hamid, S, Mir, MY & Rohela, GK (2020) Novel coronavirus disease (COVID-19): a pandemic (epidemiology, pathogenesis and potential therapeutics). *New Microbes New Infect,* 35, 100679.
[http://dx.doi.org/10.1016/j.nmni.2020.100679] [PMID: 32322401]

Heeb, G (2020) Trump signs emergency coronavirus package, injecting $8.3 billion into efforts to fight the outbreak, 6 March 2020. *Business Insider.* Accessed 14 June 2020. https://www.businessinsider.in/finance/news/trump-signs-emergency-coronavirus-package-injecting-8-3-billion-into-efforts-to-fight-the-outbreak/articleshow/74516153.cms

Henley, J & Oltermann, P (2020) More than 250m people now in lockdown in the EU as Germany and Belgium adopt measures, March 18, 2020. *The Guardian.* Accessed 14 June 2020. https://www.theguardian.com/world/2020/mar/18/coronavirus-lockdown-eu-belgium-ger many-adopt-measures

Holshue, ML, DeBolt, C, Lindquist, S, Lofy, KH, Wiesman, J, Bruce, H, Spitters, C, Ericson, K, Wilkerson, S, Tural, A, Diaz, G, Cohn, A, Fox, L, Patel, A, Gerber, SI, Kim, L, Tong, S, Lu, X, Lindstrom, S, Pallansch, MA, Weldon, WC, Biggs, HM, Uyeki, TM & Pillai, SK Washington State 2019-nCoV Case Investigation Team (2020) First case of 2019 novel coronavirus in the United States. *N Engl J Med,* 382, 929-36.
[http://dx.doi.org/10.1056/NEJMoa2001191] [PMID: 32004427]

Inocencio, R (2020) Coronavirus flare-ups in China and South Korea prompt new fears of a 2nd wave, May 15, 2020. *CBS News.* Accessed 14 June 2020. https://www.cbsnews.com/news/China-coronavirus-souh-korea-outbreaks-fears-second-wave-infections/

Kaplan, J, Frias, L & Johnsen, MM A third of the global population is on coronavirus lockdown- here's our constantly updated list of countries and restrictions, July 11, 2020. Business Insider (2020) Accessed on 13 July 2020. https://www.businessinsider.in/international/news/a-third-of-the-global-population-is-on -coronavirus-lockdown-x2014-hereaposs-our-constantly-updated-list-of-coutries-and-restrictions/slidelist/75208623.cms

Kim, S (2020) How South Korea lost control of its coronavirus outbreak. *The New Yorker.* Accessed 14 June 2020. https://www.newyorker.com/news/news-desk/how-south-korea-lost-control-of-its-coronavirus-outbreak

Kuo, L (2020) China confirms human-to-human transmission of coronavirus. *The Guardian.* Accessed 13 June 2020. https://www.theguardian.com/world/2020/jan/20/coronavirus-spreads-to-beijing-as-China confirms-new-cases

Kwok, KO, Lai, F, Wei, WI, Wong, SYS & Tang, JWT (2020) Herd immunity - estimating the level required

to halt the COVID-19 epidemics in affected countries. *J Infect,* 80, e32-3.
[http://dx.doi.org/10.1016/j.jinf.2020.03.027] [PMID: 32209383]

Lai, CC, Wang, CY, Wang, YH, Hsueh, SC, Ko, WC & Hsueh, PR (2020) Global epidemiology of coronavirus disease 2019 (COVID-19): disease incidence, daily cumulative index, mortality, and their association with country healthcare resources and economic status. *Int J Antimicrob Agents,* 55, 105946.
[http://dx.doi.org/10.1016/j.ijantimicag.2020.105946] [PMID: 32199877]

Lau, H, Khosrawipour, V, Kocbach, P, Mikolajczyk, A, Schubert, J, Bania, J & Khosrawipour, T (2020) The positive impact of lockdown in Wuhan on containing the COVID-19 outbreak in China. *J Travel Med,* 27, 1-7.
[http://dx.doi.org/10.1093/jtm/taaa037]

Li, X, Zhao, X & Sun, Y (2020) The lockdown of Hubei Province causing different transmission dynamics of the novel coronavirus (2019-nCoV) in Wuhan and Beijing *medRxiv.*

Lu, H, Stratton, CW & Tang, YW (2020) Outbreak of pneumonia of unknown etiology in Wuhan, China: The mystery and the miracle. *J Med Virol,* 92, 401-2.
[http://dx.doi.org/10.1002/jmv.25678] [PMID: 31950516]

Ma, J (2020) Coronavirus: China's first confirmed Covid- 19 case traced back to November 17. *South China Morning Post.* Accessed 13 June 2020. https://www.scmp.com/news/China/society/article/3074991/coronavirus-Chinas-first-confirmed-COVID-19-case-traced-back

Malviya, R, Sharma, A & Awasthi, R (2020) Treatment and prevention of osteoporosis during COVID-19 outbreak: management and adherence to treatment guidelines. *Open Public Health J,* 13, 791-3.
[http://dx.doi.org/10.2174/1874944502013010791]

Nair, S (2020) For a billion Indians, the lockdown has not prevented the tragedy. *The Guardian.* Accessed 13 June 2020. https://www.theguardian.com/world/commentisfree/2020/mar/29/india-lockdown-trage-y-healthcare-coronavirus-starvation-mumbai

Ni, MY, Yang, L, Leung, CMC, Li, N, Yao, XI, Wang, Y, Leung, GM, Cowling, BJ & Liao, Q (2020) Mental health, risk factors, and social media use during the COVID-19 epidemic and cordon sanitaire among the community and health professionals in Wuhan, China: Cross-sectional survey. *JMIR Ment Health,* 7, e19009.
[http://dx.doi.org/10.2196/19009] [PMID: 32365044]

Painel Coronavírus Accessed 12 June, 2020 https://covid.saude.gov.br/

Park, SE (2020) Epidemiology, virology, and clinical features of severe acute respiratory syndrome - coronavirus-2 (SARS-CoV-2; Coronavirus Disease-19). *Clin Exp Pediatr,* 63, 119-24.
[http://dx.doi.org/10.3345/cep.2020.00493] [PMID: 32252141]

The point, L (2020) Coronavirus: the "atomic bomb" of the evangelical gathering in Mulhouse. Accessed 12 June, 2020 https://www.lepoint.fr/sante/coronavirus-la-bombe-atomique-du-rassemblement-evangel-que-de-mulhouse-28-03-2020-2369173_40.php

Poland, GA (2020) SARS-CoV-2: a time for clear and immediate action. *Lancet Infect Dis,* 20, 531-2.
[http://dx.doi.org/10.1016/S1473-3099(20)30250-4] [PMID: 32243818]

Pulla, P (2020) Covid-19: India imposes lockdown for 21 days and cases rise. *BMJ,* 368, m1251.
[http://dx.doi.org/10.1136/bmj.m1251] [PMID: 32217534]

Rainsford, S (2020) Coronavirus: Is putin rushing Russia out of lockdown? *BBC News.* Accessed 13 June, 2020 https://www.bbc.com/news/world-europe-52659481

Regencia, T, Varshalomidze, T & Allahoum, R (2020) White House: CDC 'let the country down' on testing- COVID-19 updates. *Aljazeera.* Accessed 14 June, 2020 https://www.aljazeera.com/news/2020/05/brazil-surpasses-spain-coronavirus-cases-live-updates-200516231547355.html/

Schengen Visa Information. Schengen Area Crisis: EU States Close Borders as Coronavirus Outbreak Grips Bloc (2020) Accessed on 13 June 2020 https://www.schengenvisainfo.com/news/schengen-area-crisis-eu-states-close-borders-as-coronavirus-outbreak-grips-bloc/

Schwartz, L (2020) Brazil confirms the first case of the disease. *Medscape Medical News.* Accessed on 10 June 2020. https://www.medscape.com/viewarticle/925806

Selsky, A (2020) Washington governor declares state of emergency over the virus. https://abcnews.go.com/US/wireStory/coronavirus-cases-unknown-origin-found-west-coast-69301250

Seckin, B (2020) *Italy reports third confirmed case of coronavirus.*https://www.aa.com.tr/en/europe/italy-reports-third-confirmed-case-of-coronavirus/1726934

https://inshorts.com/en/news/brazil-reports-over-1000-daily-covid19-deaths-for-first-time-1589994600598

Sharma, A, Malviya, R, Kumar, V, Gupta, R & Awasthi, R (2020) Severity and risk of COVID-19 in cancer patients: An evidence-based learning. *Dermatol Ther (Heidelb),* 33, e13778.
[http://dx.doi.org/10.1111/dth.13778] [PMID: 32515033]

She, J, Liu, L & Liu, W (2020) COVID-19 epidemic: Disease characteristics in children. *J Med Virol,* 92, 747-54.
[http://dx.doi.org/10.1002/jmv.25807] [PMID: 32232980]

Singh, AK, Bhushan, B, Maurya, A, Mishra, G, Singh, SK & Awasthi, R (2020) Novel coronavirus disease 2019 (COVID-19) and neurodegenerative disorders. *Dermatol Ther (Heidelb),* 33, e13591. a
[http://dx.doi.org/10.1111/dth.13591] [PMID: 32412679]

Singh, G, Sharma, PK, Malviya, R & Awasthi, R (2020) Novel corona virus disease (COVID-19) and ophthalmic manifestations: Clinical evidences. *Dermatol Ther (Heidelb),* 33, e13814.
[http://dx.doi.org/10.1111/dth.13814] [PMID: 32526073]

Singh, AK, Mishra, G, Maurya, A, Kulkarni, GT & Awasthi, R (2020) Biofabrication: An interesting tool to create in vitro model for COVID-19 drug targets. *Med Hypotheses,* 144, 110059.
[http://dx.doi.org/10.1016/j.mehy.2020.110059] [PMID: 32758895]

Srivastava, N, Baxi, P, Ratho, RK & Saxena, SK (2020) Global Trends in Epidemiology of Coronavirus Disease 2019 (COVID-19). In: Saxena, S., (Ed.), *Coronavirus Disease 2019 (COVID-19), Medical Virology: From Pathogenesis to Disease Control* Springer, Singapore 9-21.
[http://dx.doi.org/10.1007/978-981-15-4814-7_2]

Sun, J, He, WT, Wang, L, Lai, A, Ji, X, Zhai, X, Li, G, Suchard, MA, Tian, J, Zhou, J, Veit, M & Su, S (2020) 'COVID-19: epidemiology, evolution, and cross-disciplinary perspectives. *Trends Mol Med,* 26, 483-95.
[http://dx.doi.org/10.1016/j.molmed.2020.02.008] [PMID: 32359479]

Takian, A, Raoofi, A & Kazempour-Ardebili, S (2020) COVID-19 battle during the toughest sanctions against Iran. *Lancet,* 395, 1035-6.
[http://dx.doi.org/10.1016/S0140-6736(20)30668-1] [PMID: 32199073]

Tang, X, Wu, C, Li, X, Song, Y, Yao, X, Wu, X, Duan, Y, Zhang, H, Wang, Y, Qian, Z & Cui, J (2020) On the origin and continuing evolution of SARS-CoV-2. *Natl Sci Rev,* 7, 1012-23.
[http://dx.doi.org/10.1093/nsr/nwaa036]

The Hindu (2020) https://www.thehindu.com/news/international/jilin-imposes-partial-lockdown/article 31577030.ece

Train, R (2020) *Coronavirus lockdown in the USA: which states and what measures have been applied?.*https://en.as.com/en/2020/04/07/other_sports/1586293073_218312.html

Williamson, EJ, Walker, AJ, Bhaskaran, K, Bacon, S, Bates, C, Morton, CE, Curtis, HJ, Mehrkar, A, Evans, D, Inglesby, P, Cockburn, J, McDonald, HI, MacKenna, B, Tomlinson, L, Douglas, IJ, Rentsch, CT, Mathur, R, Wong, AYS, Grieve, R, Harrison, D, Forbes, H, Schultze, A, Croker, R, Parry, J, Hester, F, Harper, S, Perera, R, Evans, SJW, Smeeth, L & Goldacre, B (2020) Factors associated with COVID-19-related death using OpenSAFELY. *Nature,* 584, 430-6.
[http://dx.doi.org/10.1038/s41586-020-2521-4] [PMID: 32640463]

Worldometer (2020) Accessed on 13 June 2020. https://www.worldometers.info/coronavirus/?utm_campaign=homeAdvegas1?%20

World Health Organisation (2020) https://www.who.int/healthinfo/global_burden_disease/definition_regions/en/

Yoo, JH, Chung, MS, Kim, JY, Ko, JH, Kim, Y, Kim, YJ, Kim, JM, Chung, YS, Kim, HM, Han, MG & Kim, SY Korean Society of Infectious Diseases; (2020) Korean Society of Pediatric Infectious Diseases; (2020) Korean Society of Epidemiology; (2020) Korean Society for Antimicrobial Therapy; (2020) Korean Society for Healthcare-associated Infection Control and Prevention; (2020) Korea Centers for Disease Control and Prevention (2020) Report on the epidemiological features of Coronavirus disease 2019 (COVID-19) outbreak in the Republic of Korea from January 19 to March 2, 2020. *J Korean Med Sci,* 35, e112. [http://dx.doi.org/10.3346/jkms.2020.35.e112] [PMID: 32174069]

Zhai, P, Ding, Y, Wu, X, Long, J, Zhong, Y & Li, Y (2020) The epidemiology, diagnosis and treatment of COVID-19. *Int J Antimicrob Agents,* 55, 105955. [http://dx.doi.org/10.1016/j.ijantimicag.2020.105955] [PMID: 32234468]

Zhang, C (2020) COVID-19 in China: From 'Chernobyl Moment' to Impetus for Nationalism. May 4, 2020. *Made in China Journal.* Accessed 13 June 2020 https://madeinChinajournal.com/2020/05/04/covid-19--n-China-from-chernobyl-moment-to-impetus-for-nationalism/

Zhu, N, Zhang, D, Wang, W, Li, X, Yang, B, Song, J, Zhao, X, Huang, B, Shi, W, Lu, R, Niu, P, Zhan, F, Ma, X, Wang, D, Xu, W, Wu, G, Gao, GF & Tan, W China Novel Coronavirus Investigating and Research Team (2020) A novel coronavirus from patients with pneumonia in China, 2019. *N Engl J Med,* 382, 727-33. [http://dx.doi.org/10.1056/NEJMoa2001017] [PMID: 31978945]

CHAPTER 4

Pathophysiology

Anirban Ghosh[1] and Shamsher Singh[1,*]

[1] *Neuroscience Division, Department of Pharmacology, ISF College of Pharmacy, Moga, Punjab, India*

Abstract: The severe acute respiratory syndrome coronavirus 2 (SARS-CoV-2) is the causal pathogen of the novel coronavirus disease 2019. This novel Covid-19 has created a serious public health crisis throughout the world. The primary symptoms of coronavirus infection are common cold and influenza-like illness and with time it causes pneumonia. Although various studies are going on throughout the world, its actual pathophysiology is not very well clear to date. The Coronavirus is a positively charged single-stranded RNA virus. This virus gets easily transmitted from human to human. Numerous investigations have been found that the virus enters into the human body *via* its spike (S) proteins. The S-protein binds to ACE2 receptors and silently comes in contact with alveoli *via* blood. This entry hypersensitizes various receptors, epithelial cells, macrophages, T-cells, dendritic cells and thus implants pro-inflammatory cytokines and chemokines, resulting in stressful conditions. Studies found that Hemagglutinin-Esterase protein, Spike protein, Nucleocapsid protein, small envelope protein, internal proteins, group-specific proteins take part in viral pathogenesis, whereas, replication proteins (eIF4A, Cyclophilin, 3CLpro, RdRp) participates in Coronaviruses (CoVs) replication and translation phases, influencing both pathogenesis and pathophysiological conditions. In this chapter, we elaborate on viral pathogenesis, the various functions of proteins, structural, enzymatic, and accessory that are linked with the pathological conditions and will also highlight the correlation causing physiological alteration associated with this infection.

Keywords: ACE2 receptors, Covid-19, Hemagglutinin-Esterase protein, Life cycle, Membrane protein, Nsp1 protein, Nsp3 protein, Nsp8 primase, Nsp12 polymerase, Nsp13 helicase, Nsp14 protein, Nsp15 protein, Nsp16 protein, Nucleocapsid protein, Orf3b, Orf6, Orf7a, Pathogenesis, Pathophysiology, Spike proteins, Thrombosis, Transmission.

INTRODUCTION

Coronavirus (CoV) is a member of the Coronavirinae subfamily, which comprises a single positive-stranded RNA virus. The various endogenous proteins present in

---

* **Corresponding author Shamsher Singh:** Neuroscience Division, Department of Pharmacology, ISF College of Pharmacy, Moga, Punjab, India; Tel: +91 9779 9805 88; E-mail:shamshersinghbajwa@gmail.com

Neeraj Mittal, Sanjay Kumar Bhadada, O. P. Katare and Varun Garg (Eds.)
All rights reserved-© 2021 Bentham Science Publishers

it are integral membrane (M), spike (S), nucleocapsid (N), envelope (E), and other accessory proteins, which not only facilitate its entry into the cells but also helps in replication (Fig. **1**) (Garoff *et al.*, 1998). There are 3 different categories of CoVs- category 1, which includes human coronavirus 229e and transmissible gastric enteritis virus; category 2 includes human CoV-OC43, murine hepatitis virus, and bovine CoVs; class 3 comprehends avian infectious bronchitis virus (Fehr and Perlman, 2015). On 31st Dec 2019, China alerted WHO of a huge number of pneumonia-like cases in Wuhan city. After continuous investigations, Chinese scientists and WHO claimed the presence of a new strand of CoVs causing this pneumonia-like problem. CoV symptoms include- dry cough, shortness of breath, and respiratory distress. This virus has spread to almost every part of the world and costs about 469,587 lives worldwide till 23rd June 2020. From various investigations, WHO had declared that these CoVs are spreading through contacts by infected persons or patients. The S-protein of CoVs binds with ACE2 receptors and silently comes in contact with alveoli *via* blood. Initially, at the time of infection, the CoVs contaminates the epithelial cells, macrophages, T-cells, dendritic cells and execute pro-inflammatory cytokines and chemokines takes place, initiating stressful condition. In this chapter, we are discussing the viral pathology associated with proteins, enzymes, and accessory along with their roles in pathogenesis.

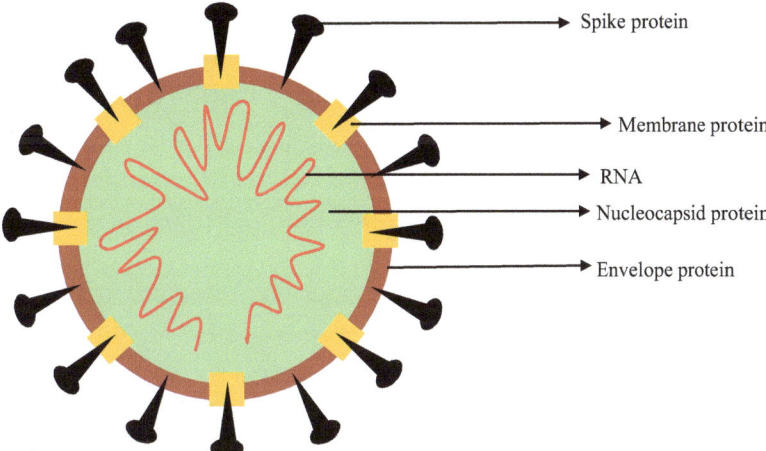

Fig. (1). Structure of CoV.

TRANSMISSION OF COV

Available reports have found that the CoVs are conveyed from animals to humans through close contact with animals like pigs, camels, and bats, are more susceptible to CoV infection, creating a reservoir (Mackay and Arden, 2015). At the early stage of CoV infection, the primary symptoms are not well expressed but as it gets matured and replication occurs CoVs slowly start to show their symptoms. The incubation time of CoV infection is 2 to 14 days. It has been found that Covid-19 gets transmitted from an individual to another *via* cough, sneezing, hands shaking and thus found to get settled themselves at the respiratory tract (Gunalan, 2011) (Fig. **2**).

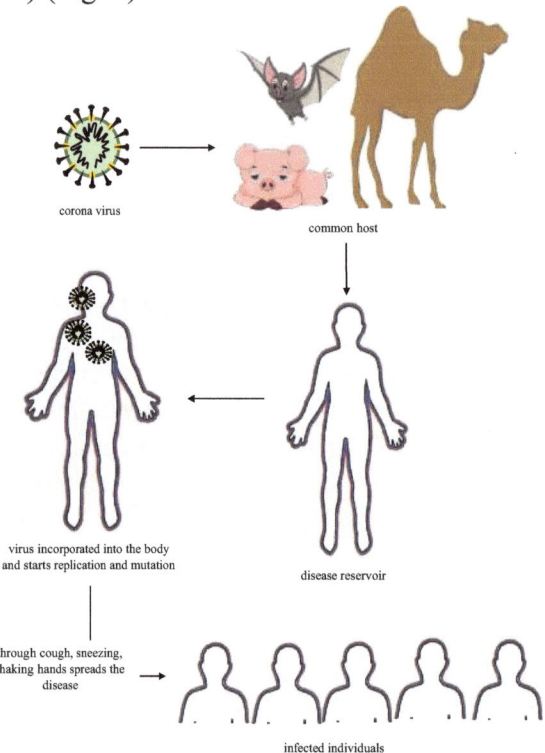

Fig. (2). Schematic representation of transmission of CoV.

Virus Life Cycle

The CoV life cycle has been summarized in this portion by discussing the various functions of viral proteins. It has been found that CoV with the help of the S-proteins gets attached with specific cellular receptors and thus initiates a conformational structural alteration of spike proteins, resulting in the liberation of the nucleocapsid into cells. After entering inside the cells, the 5' end of RNA, orf1a, and 1b gets translated to form pp1a and pp1ab. The orf1a represents the papain-like protease (PLpro) and a 3C-like protease (3CLpro), which acts to progress the pp1a and pp1ab to mature replicase protein (Lee *et al.*, 1991; Ziebuhr *et al.*, 2001). The orf1a X domain encodes the ADP-ribose1"-phosphatase activity (Ziebuhr, 2005; Snijder *et al.*, 2003), while the orf1b encodes a helicase and an RNA-dependent RNA polymerase (RdRp) which is processed by pp1ab (Gorbalenya, 2001). This orf1b also encodes various other enzymatic activities-

3'-to 5'- exonuclease (ExoN), poly (U)- specific endoribonuclease (XendoU), and S-adenosyl methionine- dependent ribose 2'-O- methyltransferase (Ziebuhr, 2005; Snijder *et al.*, 2003; Ivanov *et al.*, 2004). The downstream orf2a encodes the enzymatic activity of cyclic phosphodiesterase.

The infection of CoV involves replication and transcription of genomic mRNA. During replication, few long negative strands of RNA are being synthesized which acts as a template for genetic RNA. Several overlapping 3'- coterminal sub-genetic RNA acts as mRNA (75- to 78- nucleotide). These mRNA has a common initial sequence which is present at the 5' end (Lai *et al.*, 1984; Shieh *et al.*, 1987). With recent advancement and immense research, it has been found that interrupted transcription takes place during negative-stranded sub-genomic RNA synthesis, with an additional attachment of 3' end of negative RNA strands that acts as a template for mRNA synthesis (Enjuanes *et al.*, 2005). It has been found that the envelope (E) protein gets translated by a downstream or f5b of mRNA5. This translation of orf5b is intervened by the internal entry site of the ribosome (Jendrach *et al.*, 1999). The M and E protein gets immediately localized over the Golgi intracellular membrane just after translation. These M and E proteins are capable of producing virus-like particles without any viral protein and viral RNA (Corse and Machamer, 2003; Corse and Machamer, 2000; Klumperman *et al.*, 1994; Krijnse-Locker *et al.*, 1994). The distribution of spike (S) protein over intracellular membranes and also over the plasma membrane was found to take place. During assembly, this S-protein then interacts with M-protein's transmembrane region. The helical structure is found to occur due to interaction with genetic RNA and with nucleocapsid protein complexes. The interaction between N- and M-proteins (Kuo and Masters, 2002) leads to budding within the vesicles. Immediately, after budding, the viruses travel towards the cell surface and gradually leave the cell.

Role of Structural Proteins in The Pathogenesis

A. Spike Protein

The CoVs spike (S) are of type I glycoprotein which produces a peplomer-like structure on its envelope. During processing in the Golgi body, these spikes with the help of furin-like enzyme activities get cleaved into two distinct sub-units. The S1 subunits have an amino-terminal which forms the spherical head of the protein and also holds the receptor-binding domain (RBD) at its first 330 amino acids (Kubo *et al.*, 1994). The S2 subunits contain the carboxylic terminal which is supposed to form the stalk-like assembly which helps in anchorage over the membrane (Fig. **3A**). It comprehends two parts- 2 heptads repeat (HR) domains and a fusion peptide (La Monica *et al.*, 1991; Luo and Weiss, 1988; Parker *et al.*,

1989; Taguchi, 1995). A bridge-like connecting loop is formed by a cysteine enriched domain in between the anchor and the cytoplasmic tail which is essential for its fusion (Chang *et al.*, 2000). The RBD of CoVs is 192 amino acid regions reside over 319 to 510. The central part of CoV S-protein contains a loop which is also known as a receptor-binding motif (RBM); its role is to create direct connections with ACE2 receptors (Angiotensin-converting enzyme).

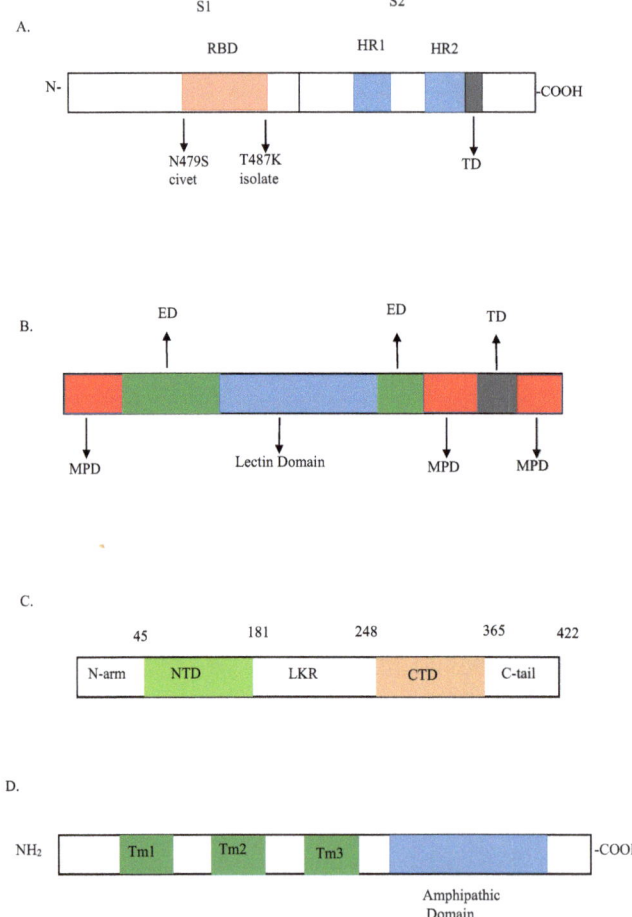

Fig. (3). Schematic representation of Spike Protein, Hemagglutinin-Esterase Protein, Nucleocapsid Protein, Membrane Protein structural proteins Where, RBD, Receptor binding domain; HR, Heptad repeats; TD, transmembrane domain; MPD, membrane-proximal domain; ED, Esterase domain.

Various researches have clarified that S-protein in addition to substitution of one or two amino acid groups interacts largely with human ACE-2 receptors. The S-RBM contains two residues – N479 and T487. These two residues are mostly preferred by human ACE-2 receptors and cause more pathogenicity. The CoVs S during synthesis does not get cleaved into S1 and S2 subunits. During viral entry, the cathepsin-L helps to facilitate the endosomal low pH requiring cleavage. In a study, it has been found that during viral entry, cathepsin facilitates the fusion, while for triggering the cell to cell fusion, the cellular protease facilitates the leupeptin-sensitive like cleavage (Simmons *et al.*, 2011). The S1/S1 boundary and in the S2 (R797) are the two cleavage events for mediating membrane fusion and for viral infection (Belouzard *et al.*, 2009; Belouzard *et al.*, 2010). It has been found that colocalization of ACE2 with transmembrane protease/subfamily of serine membrane 2 (TMPRSS2) increases the CoVs entry (Matsuyama *et al.*, 2010; Shulla *et al.*, 2011). This protease family TMPRSS2 is mainly found in the lungs and thus determines the viral pathogenesis. It has also been found that the virus after its entry regulates the renin-angiotensin system by downregulating the ACE2 in the plasma membrane and thus slowly initiates the CoVs infection (Haga *et al.*, 2008; Rockx *et al.*, 2009; Wang *et al.*, 2008). It is also known that the resin-angiotensin system maintains blood pressure and fluid balance. From various models of lung injury, it has been determined that ACE2 acts as a pneumo-protective agent and thus degrading the angiotensin II, proinflammatory mediators which are synthesized by ACE-1 (Kuba *et al.*, 2005; Hamming *et al.*, 2007; Wösten-van Asperen *et al.*, 2008). It has also been described that the S-protein activates the interleukin-8 (IL-8) by initiating MAPK and AP-1 in the lungs (Chang *et al.*, 2004).

B. Hemagglutinin-Esterase (HE) Protein

HE is a type of glycoprotein that forms a secondary type of S-protein, these types of S-proteins are smaller than the S-protein peplomer and are found on type 2 CoVs envelopes (Kienzle *et al.*, 1990; Yokomori *et al.*, 1989). This HE gets synthesized as an apoprotein of 42kDa which glycosylated to form 65kDa and homodimers are also formed due to disulfide links (Fig. **3B**). This HE is found to yield the activities hemagglutinating and esterase (Kienzle *et al.*, 1990; Brian *et al.*, 1995). It has also been noted that HE is found to acquire the group II CoVs homologous RNA recombination that contains no HE proteins (Snijder *et al.*, 2003). This HE protein was found to have sialic acid-binding and acetyl esterase activities, which activate the viral entry and its release from the cell surface by interconnecting the domains of sialic acid. It has been found that HE acts as a non-essential protein that gets activated by isolation of JHM (Yokomori *et al.*, 1991). It has been also found that HE acts as a binding molecule, where the spike acts by attaching to specified glycoprotein receptors over the cell. It has been notified to have a destructive activity towards the supplying receptors during virus removal from non-susceptible cells. After immense investigation, it has been found that the S-protein gets attached with sialic acid residues that produce the main role of HE for viruses that want to get released from glycans with the help of esterase activity (Wurzer *et al.*, 2002). It has also been noted that these S-protein increase its receptor specificity towards the residues of glycan (Langereis *et al.*, 2010).

Till now the proper role for pathogenesis of HE is not well clarified. From various investigations, it has been found that the A59 strain adapted from the genome of tissue culture shows not only a variety of HE mutations but also shows transcriptional regulatory sequences (TRS), which causes a negative impact over HE pseudogene and also over its lost expression on chimeric A59 during the *in-vitro* passage. HE also shows an immense impact in causing viral infection in CNS. When observed by comparing the isogenic recombinant viruses that express, HE wild type protein, the esterase activity of HE has been found eliminated whereas, short HE proteins were found to be synthesized by the virus (Kazi *et al.*, 2005).

In a mice study, it has been found that the virus having large polypeptides of HE shows more virulent activity and spreads vigorously in CNS. This result does not directly correlate the virulence with esterase activity but suggests the HE entertains the attachment or spread of the virus by forming bridges with molecules containing sialic acid. From various studies, it has been found that the communication of HE with molecules residing on the cellular surface increases the binding of neural cell types, whereas the isogenic recombinant JHM strains do not show any discrimination in the case of neurovirulence; cumulatively suggesting that HE does not always aim for neuropathogenesis. The esterase activity may not be an important event for neurons but is a vital event for the gastrointestinal tract which allows the virus to pass through mucous or may have the power to get detached from cells and are believed to cause neuraminidase. During the influenza neuraminidase, the sialic acids specified enzymatic activity which may cause cell subtype infection in the respiratory tract and cause pathogenic severity (Matrosovich *et al.*, 2004).

C. Membrane (M) Protein

Earlier the M-protein was known as envelop-1 (E1) protein. It is a several-layered bridge protein consisting of 221 to 262 amino acids and is found to be adequate in viral envelopes (Escors *et al.*, 2001). It is a short hydrophilic protein and its glycosylated N-terminal motif is present on the outer surface of the virion. The inner surface of the virus contains 3 transmembrane motifs, positioned at its long C-terminal end. The two motifs are present at the C-terminal ends, an amphipathic motif is also present just next to the third transmembrane motif which contains a small hydrophilic portion (Fig. **3D**). It has been found that both alpha and gamma CoVs contain an N-glycosylated N-terminal motif. This domain is very sensitive to protease and is in contact with the viral surface.

In an *in-vitro* study, it has also been found that this domain gets translocated into the lumen of ER during cDNA translation, containing the M-protein in the presence of microsome. It has also been found that the N-terminal domain is capable of neutralizing the viral infectivity by recognizing the monoclonal antibodies. The C-terminal end contains maximum amphipathic motifs which are linked through the viral envelop protein or by the vesicular part of the cytoplasmic region where viral assembly and budding takes place depending upon the sensitivity of protease during *in-vitro* translation of cDNA that encodes the M-protein in presence of microsome. It has been found that when the m-protein is expressed alone it gets localized on the Golgi apparatus (Nal *et al*., 2005). A fact has been found that the first transmembrane motif of M-protein possesses an indicator that can keep the membrane protein into cis-Golgi apparatus, but in some cases, it has been found that due to deletion of first two transmembrane, or the tail of cytoplasm may cause loss of membrane protein in the Golgi apparatus. The M-protein is present inside the intracellular region of the ER-Golgi intermediate compartment (ERGIC). In infected cells, it has been found that the position of ERGIC depends on the expression of E-protein (Lim and Liu, 2001). It has been found that this M-protein has a vital role in assembling and budding viral particles (de Haan and Rottier, 2005). This M-protein has been found to interconnect with themselves and also with N, E, S, HE proteins (Kuo and Masters, 2002; de Haan *et al*., 2000). Various reverse genetic, biochemical, and two-hybrid studies have been conducted using virus-like particles (VLP) or by other protein interactions to monitor the role of M-protein for CoVs assembly (Corse and Machamer, 2003; Arndt *et al*., 2010; Verma *et al*., 2007; Nakauchi *et al*., 2008; He *et al*., 2004; Hsieh *et al*., 2008; McBride and Machamer, 2010). The M-M protein interactions are mostly umpired by transmembrane motifs (de Haan *et al*., 2000) and also by SWWSFNPETNNL a classified protected belt of 12 amino acids that continues up to the third transmembrane motif (Arndt *et al*., 2010). The M-S protein interactions are controlled through the remnant of cytoplasmic tail whereas it can be proved that half of the N-terminal residues participate in this event (McBride and Machamer, 2010; Voß *et al*., 2009). It has been found that the M-N protein interactions are also umpired by the M-cytoplasmic motif (Kuo and Masters, 2002; Verma *et al*., 2007; Hsieh *et al*., 2008; Fang *et al*., 2005).

Besides, all these interactions it has also been found that the M-protein also interacts directly with the signal of RNA packaging in N-protein independent ways to process the genomic packing into the virions (Narayanan and Makino,

2001; Narayanan et al., 2003). It has been notified that for assembly and binding of the virus, the interaction between M-cytoplasmic domain protein and b-actin is important (Wang et al., 2009). With the initiation of interferon responses as a role of M-protein for CoV infection has been found, whereas, with the initiation of interferon-α in peripheral blood mononuclear cells (PBMCs) by the help of glutaraldehyde-fixed purified virus or the cells infected by viruses, that can be inhibited by monoclonal antibodies which are sensitive for N-terminal domains of M-protein. Various studies have claimed that the VLPs consisting of M-proteins of CoVs (α, β, γ) confirmed the interferogenic actions of M-protein are not restricted in only a few CoVs. Some genetic studies have been performed using recombinant A59 mutants, in which alteration of M-protein was done for stoppage of glycosylation or for altering N-glycosylation site in place of o-glycosylation site. In this case, this N-glycosylated M-protein modulates the interferogenic activity and can cause a better inducer than in O-glycosylated M-protein (de Haan et al., 2003). It has been found that the unglycosylated M-protein mutation does not cause any conformational induction of interferon. During *in-vivo* studies, it has been found that these viruses can replicate in hepatic surroundings but not in the brain which correlates their *in-vitro* interferogenic capacity (de Haan et al., 2003). This study can also explain the interaction of the virus with lectins, a mannose receptor, present in the liver, which induces interferon-α in dendritic cells. The overexpression of M-protein correlates with RIG-I, TBK-1, IKKe, and TRAF3 and can inhibit the IRF3 and IRF7, which results in inhibition of interferon-β, advocated by dsRNA (Siu et al., 2009).

D. Small Envelop (E) Protein

The envelope (E) proteins are endogenous membrane proteins (Yu et al., 1994). This E-protein along with M-proteins takes part in viral assembly (Vennema et al., 1996). The expression of E-protein in the presence or absence of M-protein is capable of producing viral particles. This E-protein has been found to play an important role in causing infection (Kuo and Masters, 2003). It has been found that disarrangement of the E gene in TGEV proteins causes lethal effects (Curtis et al., 2002; Ortego et al., 2002). It has been found that the E-protein has significant specific ion channel activity (Wilson et al., 2004), although this needs to be further excavated. This E-protein ion channel acts as a site for budding and increases the morphogenesis and assembly of viruses. During *in-vitro* studies, it has been found that E-protein induces apoptosis in A59 infected 17Cl-1 cells by modulating the caspase-dependent pathways which get suppressed by excessive Bcl-2 expression. It has also been found that inhibition of apoptosis may increase viral production during the terminal section of infection, which suggests that this apoptosis may be the host response that checks the expression of viral production

(An *et al.*, 1999), but this data needs to be verified for an *in-vivo* condition also. At the time of Jurkat-T cell, it has been found that the E-protein could result in apoptosis, but their activity can be suppressed by the expression of anti-apoptotic protein Bcl-xL (Yang *et al.*, 2005), thus suggesting that this T-cell apoptosis may lead to activation of lymphopenia, which is observed in most patients.

E. Nucleocapsid (N) Protein and Internal (I) Protein

The N-protein acts as a primary RNA binding protein, which is encoded in 30 portions of the CoV genome (Fig. **3C**). It has been found to act both as structural as well as non-structural roles during infection. This N-protein binds with genomic RNA, resulting in virus capsid and during assembly, it interacts with M-protein (Hurst *et al.*, 2005). In addition to all these, the N-protein binds to both genomic and sub-genomic mRNA and gets placed specifically over TRS (Grossoehme *et al.*, 2009) and thus preferentially increases the recovery rate of infectious virus from transfected genome length synthetic RNA (Yount *et al.*, 2002). From various studies, it has been found that the N-protein gets attached with replication transcription complexes in infected cells and thus causes the attachment of N-protein to them which requires the C-terminal N2b domain and thus helps to interact with other N-proteins (Verheije *et al.*, 2010). This N-protein is quite well distinguishable from other structural proteins and is present in the nucleus of the infectious cells (Wurm *et al.*, 2001).

Few available data have already claimed that N-protein has a prominent role in CNS pathogenesis and also for hepatitis. After observing the viruses that contain the N-genes have explained that the N-protein of A-59 causes increased neurovirulence and also increases the viral antigen spread within the brain (Cowley *et al.*, 2010). It has been found that this N-protein is linked with microtubules and thus takes part in axonal transport and trafficking in neurons, and does not participate in spreading viral infection in an artificially prepared primary hippocampal neuronal cell (Cowley *et al.*, 2010). It has been reported during investigation in 17Cl-1 cells, the N-protein acts as an antagonist of type-I interferon by inhibiting the activity of RNase L. In these 17Cl-1 cells, type-I INF does not get activated as the N-protein binds with RNA which causes hiding from deletion of recognized receptors and also induces type-I interferon (Ye *et al.*, 2007). In a study, it has been found that N-protein is also likely to induce the fibrinogen-link protein 2 (fgl2), which acts as a procoagulant and immunosuppressant and thus causes drastic liver damage during the infectious case. During *in-vitro* studies conducted upon 293J cells, the over-expressed N-protein causes inhibition of production of IFN by blocking IRF3 and suppresses the expression of NF-kB responsive promoter (Kopecky-Bromberg *et al.*, 2007).

The internal (I) protein is about 23kDa, containing hydrophobic structural protein of unknown functions that are not precise. This I-gene gets encoded inside the +1 N orf reading frame. During both *in-vivo* and *in-vitro* studies, no differences in replication have been found to take place in any of the systems-brain and liver, when compared between the negative recombinant I-gene of A59 virus with its isogenic control wild type. It has been found that loss of expression of I-protein leads to hepatitis, however, further investigations need to be done.

F. Replicase Proteins

The site of CoV replication has been demonstrated by pp1a and pp1ab that has been exercised into 16 non-structural proteins that can provide some essential functions- RNA-dependent RNA polymerases (RdRp). This RdRp acts as an enzyme that can alter the genomic 5' end with a methylated cap and also by some proteases for processing precursor proteins. There is another replicase protein that shows non-essential functions during the interaction between virus and host. These proteins are expressed as below:

1. **Nsp12 polymerase and Nsp8 primase:** Nsp12 is embedded within orf1b, featuring the translational frameshift domain orf1a/1b. It comprises the central action of RdRp, which is liable for amplification of the viral genome through a negative intermediate strand. It also causes transcription of several sub-genomic mRNAs which contain 5' termini, originating from genomic 5' end even *via* intermediate negative segment. Depending on frameworks the RdRp character has been noted previously. It has been found that the catalytic domain forms a three-dimensional model and with located conserved motifs which get shared by all RdRps (Xu *et al.*, 2003). This behavior has been little defined as a consequence of protein expression difficulties. During the *in-vitro* study, the expression of nsp12 has been found in E. coli along with its ordinary N-terminus, showing primer-dependent activity on RNA substrates like poliovirus and Hepatitis C enzymes (TeVelthuis *et al.*, 2010). It has also been found that Nsp8 provides the operation of RdRp, which recommends internal 5'-(G/U) CC-3' sequences to induce oligonucleotide replications for not more than six residues. Consequently, the nsp8 C-terminal end has similarities with the RNA viral polymeric catalytic palm domain. These studies indicate that nsp8 may represent a primase for the production of nsp12-dependent coronavirus RNA synthesis primers (Imbert *et al.*, 2006).

2. **Nsp15 protein:** The CoV orf1b encodes the nsp15 protein which synthesizes the part of precursor polyprotein (pp1ab), it establishes 38kDa of nsp15 protein to get released by 3CLpro protease (Hegyi and Ziebuhr, 2002; Prentice *et al.*,

2004). This nsp15 has been found to contain a motif that suggests being familiar to Xenopus laevis U representing endonuclease, which helps the processing of small nucleolar RNA (Snijder *et al.*, 2003). Various studies claimed that true recombinant nsp15 contains an endo-ribosomal property which gets facilitated by the presence of divalent cations along with strong Mn^{2+} and thus focused over cleaving at uridine nucleotide in S or dsRNA substrates by cutting its 2'-3' cyclic phosphate end (Ivanov *et al.*, 2004; Bhardwaj *et al.*, 2004). It has been found that cleavage of enzyme takes place at 3' site of specified uridylate residues but it is well preferred by the U-site and has very little interaction towards the substrates containing C (Bhardwaj *et al.*, 2006). After conducting the mutagenic studies, it has been found that the structure of nsp15 towards the Xenopus sequence claims to have two histidines and a lysin component that helps to conduct various functions of enzymes (Guarino *et al.*, 2005). It has been found that the nsp15 structure containing catalytic residues of RNase A claims to conduct enzymatic-like mechanistic action (Bhardwaj *et al.*, 2008). After studying the nsp15 amino acid sequence of β-CoV it has been found to contain retinoblastoma (pRb)- binding domain which is present on the surface of protein near to the active site of Nendo U. During the *in-vitro* study when pRb gets attached with the recombinant nsp15, it has been found to stimulate the endonuclease activity, along with it the immunoprecipitated of two proteins has also been noted from cellular extracts. The nsp15 expression in cellular environments has been found to alter pRb cellular distribution from the cytoplasm and thus increases pRb ubiquitination with a decreased level of pRb. It has also been found to increase the cell fraction during the S-phase of the cell cycle and thereby increases the amount of 3T3 cell proliferation site. The growth phenotype has been found to get reduced by mutation of the LXCXE/D domain. From all this information, it has been clarified that nsp15 and pRb participate in cellular proliferation and affect CoV replication.

3. **Nsp13 protein:** The nsp13 is a 66kDa protein that comprises an N-terminal zinc finger configuration that is bound to a helicase motif of the C-terminal superfamily1. The α-CoV is of 229E protein containing a histidine-labeled version which gets expressed by vectors of baculovirus or by SARS-CoV nsp13 maltose-binding protein (MBP)- fusion (Ivanov and Ziebuhr, 2004). It has been found that the processed recombinant proteins contain unwinding functions of both RNA and DNA duplex 5' to 3'. This 5' to 3' direction is directly opposite to flaviviral helicase and may be found to cause the function of reflecting the multiple sub-genomic mRNAs synthesis and their templets of negative polarity. It has been found that glutathione S-transferase labeled CoV nsp13 (GST-nsp13) gets expressed with the help of recombinant baculovirus inside the cells and also clarifies the relaxes of nucleic acids 2 to 3 times more

frequently than other helicases (His tagged or MBP-fusion nsp13 protein). Many studies claimed that nsp13 complexes act more rapid relaxation of nucleic acid when it is with nsp12 than its alone state. Some studies claimed that the addition of triphosphatase activity along with helicase helps to process out the first step of genomic capping and for mRNAs.

4. **Nsp3 protein:** The orf1a of CoV encodes the nsp3 – multifunctional protein. The 18-200kDa of nsp3 contains multiple domains, two of which are the PLP domain and an ADP-ribosome 100 phosphate or ADRP (macrodomain) which are the cause of virulence factors. The mass spectroscopic, kinase-profiling studies, and bioinformatic analysis claimed that nsp3 contains a chaperone-like motif that encodes the PLP domain downstream and a cysteine-coordinated metal ion binding domain. These two domains are the RNA binding motif. It has been found that the PLP and its analogous (PLP2) have a deubiquitinating property along with protease activity and cause activation of type-I INF antagonism (Barretto *et al*., 2005; Zheng *et al*., 2008). It has been found that the PLP causes inhibition of IRF3 and NF-kB signaling pathways (Devaraj *et al*., 2007; Frieman *et al*., 2009).

The macrodomains are highly conserved and have been ubiquitous property. It has been found that histone-associated macro H2A which regulates the cell type sensitive regulation/ pathway for transcription (Changolkar *et al*., 2008). The CoV has ADRP which contains the activity of phosphatase and thus converts ADP-ribose 100 phosphate to inorganic phosphate and ADP-ribose (Puticset al., 2005; Putics *et al*., 2006). It has been found that the mutation of the conserved residues of the ADRP domain causes enzymatic loss and decreases the induction of inflammatory cytokines (Eriksson *et al*., 2008). It has also been found that the ADRP domain restricts the type-I IFN treatment (Kuri *et al*., 2011). It has also been found that these macrodomains having a binding activity of mono- and poly- ADP-ribose which indicates the participation of ribosylation of host protein causes mediation of apoptosis or necrosis and thus monitors various host body pathways (Egloff *et al*., 2006).

5. **Nsp1 Protein:** The nsp1, the N-terminal protein present in the orf1a polyprotein (pp1a) which has been found to get cleaned by papain-like protease (PLP) from pp1a, is also confined in orf1a (nsp3). From immunofluorescence studies, it has been found that nsp1 gets co-recruited with some proteins that facilitate replication complexes at early time infection; whereas, during late infection, this protein binds with M-protein at viral budding and assembly site (Brockway *et al*., 2004). It has been found from various studies that this nsp1 protein is RNA binding protein that may act as a regulator for viral genome translation or replication. Cell cycle gets arrested at G_0/G_1 phases due to

infection, which also found to reduce the G_1 cyclin-Cdk complexes, activates Cdk, and inadequate phosphorylation of pRb (Chen and Makino, 2004). The nsp1 has been found to get expressed from plasmid vectors in normal cells, resulting in comparable cell arrest of G_0/G_1 phases, along with inactivation of cell proliferation (Chen et al., 2004). During studying the cell cycle regulatory protein, it has been found that expression of p28 causes hyperphosphorylation of pRb and thereby enhances the tumor suppressor levels- p53 and Cdk inhibitor (p21Cip1). This study suggests that expression of p28 can stabilize p53 and can increase the p53 level which can activate the p21Cip1 by inhibiting Cyclin E/ Cdk2 activity and as a result of which pRb phosphorylation gets inhibited with cell cycle arrest at G0/G1 phase. The external expression of the nsp1 also has been found to decrease cell proliferation with an increased level of cell accumulation in G_0/G_1 phases (Wathelet et al., 2007). The pathological role of nsp1 has also been found as it causes inhibition of type-I interferon synthesis and activates the interferon-dependent antiviral protein- ISG15 and ISG56 (Frieman et al., 2007; Wathelet et al., 2007; Kamitani et al., 2006). It has also been found that expression of nsp1 can inhibit three translational factors- IRF3, NF-kB, and c-Jun, which are found to activate the interferon-b promoter (Wathelet et al., 2007). The biochemical studies have claimed that inhibition of recombinant nsp1 during in-vitro translation reaction are found to bound with 40S ribosomal subunit and inhibition of 80S ribosomal synthesis but allows the synthesis of 48S complex with mRNA (Kamitani et al., 2009).

6. **eIF4A:** Eukaryotic translation initiation factor 4 A (eIF4A) is an associate of the DEAD-box protein helices family, consisting of two recA-like domains separated by a flexible hinge region in the center lined by conserved motifs (Fig. 4). This preserved motif is called the DEAD-box which contains amino acid sequences like aspartic acid glutamic acid- alanine- aspartic acid. The motif of eIF4A possibly interact with nucleic acid and participates in ATP binding and ATPase activity. As a consequence, eIF4A has been demonstrated to have RNA-dependent ATPase activity, ATP-dependent duplex RNA unwinding activity, and involvement in the initiation of translation. The action of eIF4A is synchronized with other translation initiation factors, that initiate its all activities and mediate interaction with RNA for translation (Hilbert et al., 2011). Further, the main functions of eIF4A include removal of secondary complex structures from the 5'-untranslated region and also to displace proteins attachment to mRNA for protein synthesis (Andreou and Klostermeier, 2013; Cencic et al., 2011).

The eIF4A protein is a key factor involved in translation during viral infection. A study demonstrated that viral mRNA uses eIF4A for the synthesis of its protein (Nakagawa *et al.*, 2016). Genomic mRNAs of CoV have a 5-cap structure and undergo cap-dependent translation using eIF4F. The eIF4A is a part of the eIF4F protein complex which is associated with other two translation initiation factors such as eIF4E and eIF4G, in turn, connected with eIF4A which is further connected with eIF4E. In the cap-dependent mechanism of translation, the viral mRNA is engaged with the eIF4F protein complex, which is composed of three proteins: eIF4E, eIF4A, and eIF4G. The eIF4A and eIF4F are essential for the recruitment of ribosomes in protein synthesis during CoV infection. Consequently, eIF4A is important for controlling translation and for regulating gene expression at the translational level. Inhibition of eIF4A might play an important role in the treatment of CoV (Montero *et al.*, 2019).

7. **Cyclophilin:** Cyclophilins (Cyps) are a subgroup of immunophilins belong to the enzyme peptidyl-prolyl cis/trans isomerases family. Totally 80 iso-forms of dissimilar molecular masses have been illustrated in human tissues. Among these isoforms, seven are major Cyps present in humans such as CypA, CypB, CypC, CypD, CypE, Cyp40, and CypNK. Cyps are present in both extracellular and intracellular space of the cell and secreted in response to various stimuli having different nature and intensity (Rajiv and Davis, 2018). The extracellular cyclophilins CypA and CypB are concerned with cell-to-cell communication. Cyps are contemplation to be concerned in different signaling pathways such as mitochondrial apoptosis, inflammation, RNA splicing, and adaptive immunity. Cyps bind to the CD147 cell membrane receptor as well as heparins and then initiate several arrays of intracellular signaling cascades which are involved in inflammatory processes (Singh *et al.*, 2018). Besides, CypA is also competent in controlling human IFN-I reactions to viral infections (von Hahn and Ciesek, 2015).

Moreover, CypA and CypB have significant functions in the duplication of many viruses including coronavirus (CoV), human immunodeficiency virus (HIV), hepatitis C virus (HCV), measles virus, and influenza A virus (Dawar *et al.*, 2017). A study demonstrated that CypA is an essential cyclophilin that acts as binding factors for CoV proteins and is required for CoV replication (Tanaka *et al.*, 2017). Another study conducted using surface plasmon resonance biosensor technology reported the interaction of CypA with nucleocapsid (N) protein of SARS-CoV. This statement gets verified by another technique which observed CypA AS one of the cellular proteins integrated into purified SARS-CoV particles by using spectrometric profiling (Carbajo-Lozoya *et al.*, 2012; von Brunn *et al.*, 2015). Furthermore, research using nucleocapsid protein (NP) of SARS-CoV shown that segment Val235-Pro369 of SARS NP interacts with human CypA (hCypA) more accurately, and SARS NP loop Trp302-Pro310 lock into the active-site groove of hCypA through hydrogen bonding indicate human CypA (hCypA) binds NP of SARS-CoV with high affinity, resulting in CypA play important role in CoV replication and virus growth (Luo et al., 2004).

8. **3CLpro** : Genomes of CoVs comprise two exposed reading frames orf1a and orf1b, programmed by host ribosomes into two specific viral polyproteins-pp1a and pp1ab. The orf1a encrypts two cysteine proteases, a protease specific to papain (PLpro) and a protease specific to 3C (3CLpro). Although PLpro cuts the polyprotein's first three cleavage sites, 3CLpro is accountable for cleavage of the subsequent 11 positions culminating in a sum of 16 non-structural proteins (nsp) being released into CoVs. The viral key proteinase (Mpro, also known as 3CLpro) regulates the coronavirus duplication complex activities. 3CLpro is a homodimeric process effective in the company of substrates. Both 3CLpros crystal structures revealed that each monomer consists of three structural domains: domains I and II construct a chymotrypsin-like framework through a catalytic cysteine and are linked by a long loop to a third C-terminal domain (Needle et al., 2015). 3CLpro monomer contains three domains, domain I (residues 8–101), domain II (residues 102–184), and domain III (residues 201–303), and a large coil binds domain II and III (residues 185–200). The effective zone of 3CLpro seems to have a CysHis catalytic dyad (Cys145 and His41) found in the distance between domains I and II (Yang et al., 2003). At the proteolytic stage, both 3CLpros choose glutamine in positions P1 and leucine, simple residues, low hydrophobic residues in positions P2, P3, and P4 respectively (Chuck et al., 2011). Limited residues are expected at positions P1′ and P2′; however, position P3′ shows no clear preference. Recent studies report has reported that the structure of 3CLpro from SARS-CoV2 (Liu et al., 2020) (PDB code 6LU7) and the available structure of 3CLpro from CoV (Yang et al., 2003) (PDB code 1UK4), can only be able to differentiate through their two main proteases by only 12 amino acids, along with the α carbon atoms, which all are lying at least 1 nm away from the 3CLpro active site. The substrate-binding pockets of Covid-19 main proteases display an extraordinarily high level of alignment of the prime residues involved in substrate binding, including the CYS145···HIS41 dyad, and HIS163/HIS172/GLU166. The latter residues are supposed to offer the inaugural gate for the substrate in the active state of the protomer (Yang et al., 2003). The PLpro and 3CLpro process ORFs and concoct 16 non-structural proteins that are vital for membrane-associated duplication complex. The PLpro was detected to be multipurpose enzymes with deISGylating (deletion of ISG15 conjugates from host cell factors) and deubiquitinating (cleavage of ubiquitin from host cell factors) properties (Clasman et al., 2017). This subsidized to antagonization of the host antiviral immune response and the growth of viral duplication. PLpro can hamper the behavior of the IFN-β

reporter prompted by the mitochondrial antiviral signaling protein and dwindle the event of TNF-α-induced NF-kB reporter.

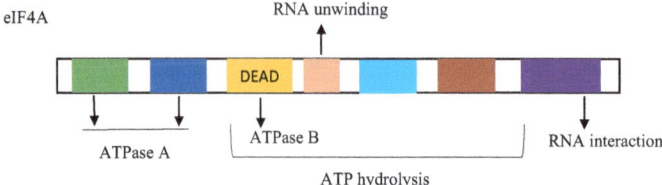

Fig. (4). Schematic representation of eIF4A.

G. CoV Associated Protein

The CoV genome is known to have encoded numerous associated proteins that have identified homologies with other host cell proteins. The CoVs associated proteins encodes within orf3a, 3b, 7a, 7b, 8a, 8b and 9b. It has been found that the encoded proteins of orf3b, 7b, and 8b are translational by the involvement of internal downstream initiation which encodes the same RNA for 3a, 7a, and 8a respectively. While investigating the viral particles, the proteins which encode in orf3a, 6, 7a, and 7b have been found (Narayanan *et al.*, 2008). From *in-vitro* studies, it has been found that deletion of combined or individual orf3a, 3b, 6, 7a, or 7b in the recombinant viruses does not influence the replication. However, with the deletion of orf3a, some loss in efficiency has been found in viral replication (Yount *et al.*, 2005). From various investigations, it has been found that the type-I interferon activation and signaling antagonizing capacity are influenced by orf3b and 6, whereas the orf3a and 7a also take place in apoptosis signaling pathways.

i. **Orf6:** From *in-vitro* studies and histological analysis of the patient's lungs and intestine, it has been found that orf6 contains 63-amino acid ER/Golgi membrane-associated protein (Narayanan *et al.*, 2008). The protein which is encoded in orf6 has been found to cause some virulence factors (Tangudu *et al.*, 2007). It has been found that this orf6 protein causes inhibition of nuclear imports and causes inactivation of interferon signaling by resisting the entry of ISGF3 (STAT1/STAT2/IRF-9). This ISGF3 is the transcriptional factor that umpires the illustration of the gene responsible for type-I interferon-stimulation or complexes of STAT1/STAT2. Near to the C-terminal end of orf6, it gets attached to karyopherin alpha2 (KPNA2) that places KPNB1, a nuclear importer complex, and thereby blocks the protein along with the help of import signals (Frieman *et al.*, 2007; Hussain *et al.*, 2008). It has been found that expression of this orf6 in absence of other viral proteins activates the construction of membranous structure which is very much alike to that of double-layered vesicles which takes part in viral replications and partially placed with non-structural protein3 (nsp3), confirming the presence of orf6 role in viral replication (Zhou *et al.*, 2010).

ii. **Orf3b:** During CoVs infection, it has been found that orf3b encoded proteins contain various functions (Chan *et al.*, 2005). In *in-vitro* studies, it has been found that highly expressed orf3b proteins get localized initially over the nucleus of A549 cells and it causes inhibition of both interferons signaling and its activation (Vennema *et al.*, 1996). From other studies, it has also been found that orf3b expression also activates cell growth arrest (Yuan *et al.*, 2005) or also promotes apoptosis and necrosis (Khan *et al.*, 2006).

iii. **Orf7a:** The orf7a is a 122 amino acid type-I transmembrane encoded protein, placed in the perinuclear part in SARS-infected cells (Nelson *et al.*, 2005) by connecting with M and E protein (Huang *et al.*, 2006). From various studies, various functions of orf7a have come into account which includes activation of apoptosis by caspase-dependent pathways (Tan *et al.*, 2004), it can cause negative impulse for cellular protein synthesis, it has also been found to cause activation of p38 mitogen-activated protein kinase (Kopecky-Bromberg *et al.*, 2006) and also arrests cell cycle at G_0/G_1 phases (Yuan *et al.*, 2006).

Pathophysiology from a Cell Biology Perspective

CoV is the major health concern of 2020 with the everyday devastating scenario. Various studies had performed to study mortality of clinical disease but their cellular responses towards the viral disease are not known. The pathophysiology of CoV has been described in Figs. (**5A** and **B**). The basis of cell response towards infected CoV can be divided into some different clinical stages (Wu and McGoogan, 2020).

Phase I. Asymptomatic Stage (First 1-2 Days of Infection)

When the virus gets inhaled, it gets binds to epithelial cells in the respiratory tract and initiates replication. From various investigations, it has been that ACE2 is the main receptor Covid-19 (Wan *et al.*, 2020; Hoffmann *et al.*, 2020). During *in-vitro* studies, it has been found that ciliated cells get infected first in conducting airways (*Sims et al.*, 2005). Again, it has also been found that scRNA points out the lowered expression of ACE2 in conducting airway cells (Reyfman *et al.*, 2019). In this situation, there causes native diffusion of the virus but does not show any huge intrinsic immune response. In this phase, the virus is well spotted or identified by using a nasal swab. From the data generated by RT-PCR for viral RNA, it can be easily predicted that the viral load and causes infection with clinical course.

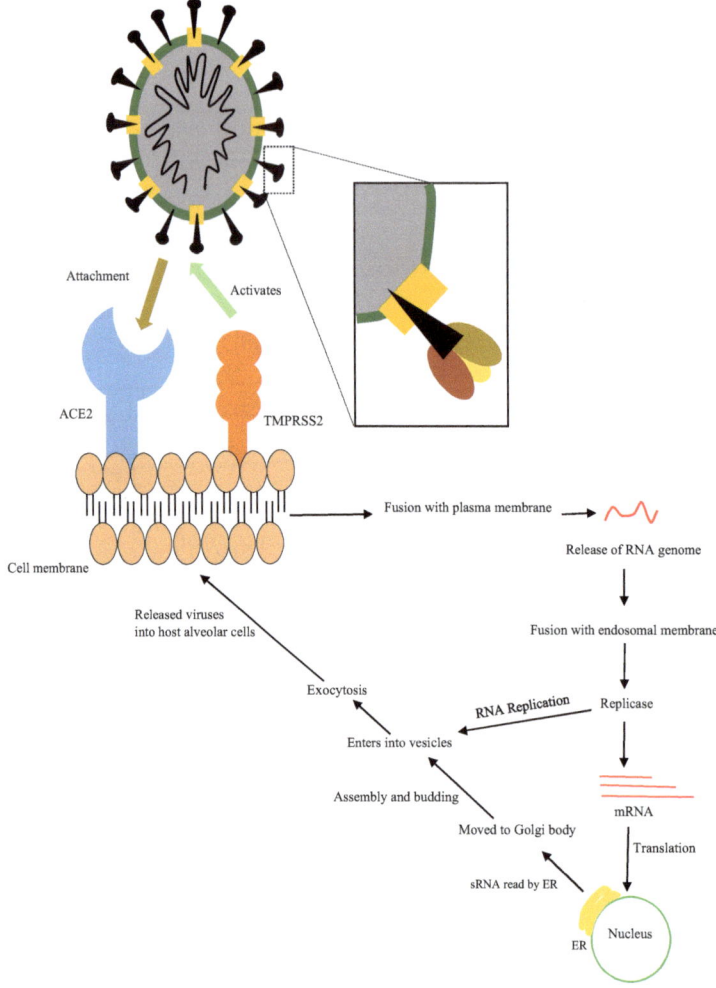

Fig. (5A). Transmission and Pathophysiology mechanism of Coronavirus inside the cell membrane.

Phase II. Upper Airway and Conducting Airway Response (Next Few Days)

In this stage, the virus grows and travels down into the respiratory tract along the conducting airways and thus triggers the initiation of immune responses. From nasal swab or sputum test can conclude the presence of the virus or by preliminary immune markers can be also used for its presence. It has been found that level of intrinsic cytokine response, CXCL-10 can cause clinical course (Tang *et al.*, 2005). The epithelial cells which get infected form the main source of beta and lambda interferons (Hancock *et al.*, 2018). It has also been found that the CXCL-10, an interferon responsive gene shows a strong signal towards the noise ratio that is formed in the alveolar type II cells during CoVs and influenza (Qian *et al.*, 2013; Wang *et al.*, 2011). It has been found that about 80% of infected patients show mild and upper and conducting airways infection (Wu and McGoogan, 2020). These individuals need to be home quarantine.

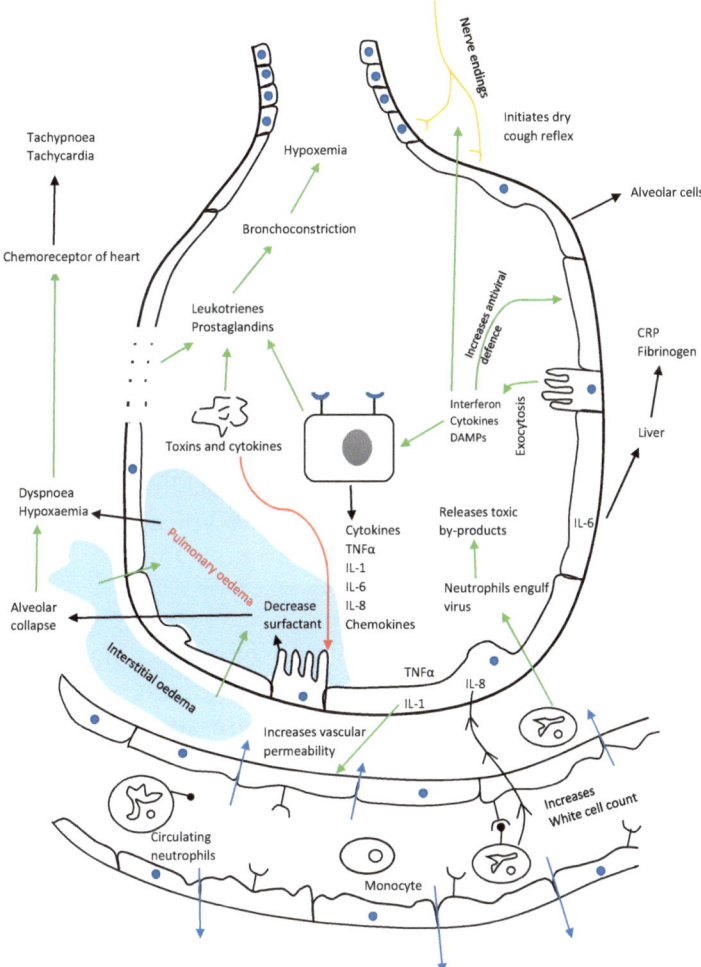

Fig. (5B). Pathophysiology of Coronavirus outside the cell membrane. The green arrow signifies activation/ enhancement and the red arrow signifies inhibition/ negative impact; the blue arrow shows permeability.

Phase III. Hypoxia, Ground-glass Infiltrates, Progression to ARDs

It has been noted that about 20% of the infected patients come to this phase and as a symptom, they show pulmonary infiltrates and sometimes develop severe illness. In this case, the virus reaches the lungs and infects the type-II alveolar cells. It has been noted that type II alveolar cells are more preferred than type I in case of CoV infection (Mossel *et al.*, 2008; Weinheimer *et al.*, 2012). The alveolar units which are infected are inclined to be peripheral and subpleural (Wu *et al.*, 2019; Zhang *et al.*, 2020). The CoVs gradually increase into the type II alveolar cells and the release of huge viral particles causes activation of apoptosis followed by cell death (Qian *et al.*, 2013). Near to the end, a self-replicating pulmonary toxin gets released as the type II cells get infected and gradually lose all these cells, initiating the secondary pathways for the regeneration of epithelial cells. It has been found that diffused alveolar damage favored by fibrin enriched hyaline membranes and the presence of few poly-nucleated giant cells are the pathological reason behind CoV (Gu and Korteweg 2007; Xu *et al.*, 2020). The abnormal healing of wounds causes more severity due to the formation of scaring and fibrosis; their recovery may employ inherent or acquired immune responses for the regeneration of epithelial cells. It is harmful to administrating the epithelial growth factors, KGF, and may also enhance the ACE2 expressing cells (Nikolaidis *et al.*, 2017). The lowering of immune response with an increase in age is the reason for mortality for elderly individuals and thereby decreases the capability of epithelial damage repair. As age increases the mucociliary clearance gets slowly diminished, allowing the virus to spread more vigorously into the lungs (Ho *et al.*, 2011). It has been found that CD209L acts as an alternative receptor for CoV (Jeffers *et al.*, 2004), and the apical cilia and microvilli on airway cells and type II cells, respectively are now found to have an important role in viral entry.

Various histopathological studies and from postmortem reports it has been found that death is mostly due to respiratory failures inpatients and at the same time it has been surprisingly found that early and progressive stages of blood clotting supply and gaseous exchange. Although the exact reason for blood clotting has not yet been excavated some mechanisms support this incidence. There are in total three debatable points for blood clotting which are as- in many patients of Covid-19 it has been found that there is an elevated level of d-dimer, a marker of thrombosis. Again, in some studies, evidence has been found that this extensive microvascular thrombosis has been observed during autopsy studies. In this study, extensive blood clotting has been observed in small lung vessels (microvascular thrombosis-MVT) which also suggests blood clotting with poor oxygenation and respiratory failure. Another point has also been found that the ACE2 receptor of the host facilitates the entry of the virus into the endothelial cells where the blood vessels lie. Autopsy studies suggest that specific contamination into cells can activate the clotting in the small blood vessels that form unresponsive respiratory failure. Various clinical reports suggest that many patients suffer from 'silent pneumonia' or 'silent hypoxia' which is due to low blood oxygen which can lead to extensive pulmonary thrombosis.

CONCLUSION

The CoVs infection is one of the major health risk factors of the current destructive outbreak worldwide. These CoVs are very well adapted human viruses in humans. The transmission of CoVs has caused a serious pandemic situation. The CoV is a single-stranded positive RNA virus that utilizes the host viral proteins and cellular components for completion of its replication cycle- viral entry, replication. Throughout the world, researchers are working day and night for the development of the vaccine. Several pathological, viral mechanisms of action, various biomarkers need to be excavated. Several series of small molecular CoVs endosomal proteins need to be discussed for a better understanding of the pathophysiology of CoV.

LIST OF ABBREVIATIONS

SARS-CoV-2	Severe acute respiratory syndrome coronavirus 2
CoV	Coronavirus
M	Membrane
S	Spike
N	Nucleocapsid
E	Envelope
PLpro	Papain-like protease
3CLpro	3C-like protease
RdRp	RNA-dependent RNA polymerase
ExoN	Exonuclease
poly U- XendoU	Specific endoribonuclease
RBD	Receptor binding domain
HR	Heptad repeat
RBM	Receptor-binding motif
ACE2	Angiotensin converting enzyme 2
TMPRSS2	Transmembrane protease/ subfamily of serine membrane 2
IL-8	interleukin-8
TRS	Transcriptional regulatory sequences
E1	Envelop-1
ERGIC	ER-Golgi intermediate compartment
VLP	Virus like particles
PBMCs	Peripheral blood mononuclear cells
I	Internal protein

pp1ab	Precursor polyprotein
MBP	Maltose binding protein
pp1a	Polyprotein
eIF4A	Eukaryotic translation initiation factor 4 A
Cyps	Cyclophilins
HIV	Human immunodeficiency virus
HCV	Hepatitis C virus
hCypA	Human CypA
nsp	Non-structural proteins
KPNA2	Karyopherin alpha2

CONSENT FOR PUBLICATION

Not applicable.

CONFLICT OF INTEREST

The author declares no conflict of interest, financial or otherwise.

ACKNOWLEDGEMENTS

The authors express their gratitude to Chairman, Mr. Parveen Garg, ISF College of Pharmacy, Moga (Punjab), India for their great vision and support.

REFERENCES

An, S, Chen, CJ, Yu, X, Leibowitz, JL & Makino, S (1999) Induction of apoptosis in murine coronavirus-infected cultured cells and demonstration of E protein as an apoptosis inducer. *J Virol,* 73, 7853.
[http://dx.doi.org/10.1128/JVI.73.9.7853-7859.1999]

Andreou, AZ & Klostermeier, D (2013) The DEAD-box helicase eIF4A: paradigm or the odd one out? *RNA Biology,* 10, 19.
[http://dx.doi.org/10.4161/rna.21966]

Arndt, AL, Larson, BJ & Hogue, BG (2010) A conserved domain in the coronavirus membrane protein tail is important for virus assembly. *J Virol,* 84, 11418.

Barretto, N, Jukneliene, D, Ratia, K, Chen, Z, Mesecar, AD & Baker, SC (2005) The papain-like protease of severe acute respiratory syndrome coronavirus has deubiquitinating activity. *J Virol,* 79, 15189.
[http://dx.doi.org/10.1128/JVI.79.24.15189-15198.2005]

Belouzard, S, Chu, VC & Whittaker, GR (2009) Activation of the SARS coronavirus spike protein *via* sequential proteolytic cleavage at two distinct sites. *Proc Natl Acad Sci USA,* 106, 5871.
[http://dx.doi.org/10.1073/pnas.0809524106]

Belouzard, S, Madu, I & Whittaker, GR (2010) Elastase-mediated activation of the severe acute respiratory syndrome coronavirus spike protein at discrete sites within the S2 domain. *J Biol Chem,* 285, 22758.
[http://dx.doi.org/10.1074/jbc.M110.103275]

Bhardwaj, K, Guarino, L & Kao, CC (2004) The severe acute respiratory syndrome coronavirus Nsp15

protein is an endoribonuclease that prefers manganese as a cofactor. *J Virol,* 78, 12218.
[http://dx.doi.org/10.1128/JVI.78.22.12218-12224.2004]

Bhardwaj, K, Palaninathan, S, Alcantara, JMO, Yi, LL, Guarino, L, Sacchettini, JC & Kao, CC (2008) Structural and functional analyses of the severe acute respiratory syndrome coronavirus endoribonuclease Nsp15. *J Biol Chem,* 283, 3655.
[http://dx.doi.org/10.1074/jbc.M708375200]

Bhardwaj, K, Sun, J, Holzenburg, A, Guarino, LA & Kao, CC (2006) RNA recognition and cleavage by the SARS coronavirus endoribonuclease. *J Mol Biol,* 361, 243.
[http://dx.doi.org/10.1016/j.jmb.2006.06.021]

Brian, D, Hogue, BG & Kienzle, TE (1995) The coronavirus hemagglutinin esterase glycoprotein. In: Siddell, S.G., (Ed.), *The Coronaviridae The Viruses,* Springer, Boston, MA 165-79.

Brockway, SM, Lu, XT, Peters, TR, Dermody, TS & Denison, MR (2004) Intracellular localization and protein interactions of the gene 1 protein p28 during mouse hepatitis virus replication. *J Virol,* 78, 11551.

Carbajo-Lozoya, J, Müller, MA, Kallies, S, Thiel, V, Drosten, C & von Brunn, A (2012) Replication of human coronaviruses SARS-CoV, HCoV-NL63 and HCoV-229E is inhibited by the drug FK506. *Virus Res,* 165, 112.
[http://dx.doi.org/10.1016/j.virusres.2012.02.002]

Cencic, R, Desforges, M, Hall, DR, Kozakov, D, Du, Y, Min, J, Dingledine, R, Fu, H, Vajda, S, Talbot, PJ & Pelletier, J (2011) Blocking eIF4E-eIF4G interaction as a strategy to impair coronavirus replication. *J Virol,* 85, 6381.

Chan, WS, Wu, C, Chow, SC, Cheung, T, To, KF, Leung, WK, Chan, PK, Lee, KC, Ng, HK, Au, DM & Lo, AW (2005) Coronaviral hypothetical and structural proteins were found in the intestinal surface enterocytes and pneumocytes of severe acute respiratory syndrome (SARS). *Mod Pathol,* 18, 1432.
[http://dx.doi.org/10.1038/modpathol.3800439]

Chang, KW, Sheng, Y & Gombold, JL (2000) Coronavirus-induced membrane fusion requires the cysteine-rich domain in the spike protein. *Virology,* 269, 212.
[http://dx.doi.org/10.1006/viro.2000.0219]

Chang, YJ, Liu, CYY, Chiang, BL, Chao, YC & Chen, CC (2004) Induction of IL-8 release in lung cells *via* activator protein-1 by recombinant baculovirus displaying severe acute respiratory syndrome-coronavirus spike proteins: identification of two functional regions. *J Immunol,* 173, 7602.
[http://dx.doi.org/10.4049/jimmunol.173.12.7602]

Changolkar, LN, Singh, G & Pehrson, JR (2008) macroH2A1-dependent silencing of endogenous murine leukemia viruses. *Mol Cell Biol,* 28, 2059.
[http://dx.doi.org/10.1128/MCB.01362-07]

Chen, CJ & Makino, S (2004) Murine coronavirus replication induces cell cycle arrest in G0/G1 phase. *J Virol,* 78, 5658.
[http://dx.doi.org/10.1128/JVI.78.11.5658-5669.2004]

Chen, CJ, Sugiyama, K, Kubo, H, Huang, C & Makino, S (2004) Murine coronavirus nonstructural protein p28 arrests cell cycle in G0/G1 phase. *J Virol,* 78, 10410.
[http://dx.doi.org/10.1128/JVI.78.19.10410-10419.2004]

Chuck, CP, Chow, HF, Wan, DCC & Wong, KB (2011) Profiling of substrate specificities of 3C-like proteases from group 1, 2a, 2b, and 3 coronaviruses. *PloS one,* 6.
[http://dx.doi.org/10.1371/journal.pone.0027228]

Clasman, JR, Báez-Santos, YM, Mettelman, RC, O'Brien, A, Baker, SC & Mesecar, AD (2017) X-ray Structure and Enzymatic Activity Profile of a Core Papain-like Protease of MERS Coronavirus with utility for structure-based drug design. *Sci Rep,* 7, 40292.
[http://dx.doi.org/10.1038/srep40292] [PMID: 28079137]

Corse, E & Machamer, CE (2000) Infectious bronchitis virus E protein is targeted to the Golgi complex and

directs release of virus-like particles. *J Virol,* 74, 4319.
[http://dx.doi.org/10.1128/JVI.74.9.4319-4326.2000]

Corse, E & Machamer, CE (2003) The cytoplasmic tails of infectious bronchitis virus E and M proteins mediate their interaction. *Virology,* 312, 25.
[http://dx.doi.org/10.1016/S0042-6822(03)00175-2]

Cowley, TJ, Long, SY & Weiss, SR (2010) The murine coronavirus nucleocapsid gene is a determinant of virulence. *J Virol,* 84, 1752.
[http://dx.doi.org/10.1128/JVI.01758-09]

Curtis, KM, Yount, B & Baric, RS (2002) Heterologous gene expression from transmissible gastroenteritis virus replicon particles. *J Virol,* 76, 1422.
[http://dx.doi.org/10.1128/JVI.76.3.1422-1434.2002]

Dawar, FU, Tu, J, Khattak, MN, Mei, J & Lin, L (2017) 'Cyclophilin A: a key factor in virus replication and a potential target for antiviral therapy. *Curr Issues Mol Biol,* 21, 1-20.
[PMID: 27033630]

de Haan, CA & Rottier, PJ (2005) Molecular interactions in the assembly of coronaviruses. *Adv Virus Res,* 64, 165-230.
[http://dx.doi.org/10.1016/S0065-3527(05)64006-7] [PMID: 16139595]

de Haan, CA, de Wit, M, Kuo, L, Montalto-Morrison, C, Haagmans, BL, Weiss, SR, Masters, PS & Rottier, PJ (2003) The glycosylation status of the murine hepatitis coronavirus M protein affects the interferogenic capacity of the virus *in vitro* and its ability to replicate in the liver but not the brain. *Virology,* 312, 395.
[http://dx.doi.org/10.1016/S0042-6822(03)00235-6]

De Haan, CA, Vennema, H & Rottier, PJ (2000) Assembly of the coronavirus envelope: homotypic interactions between the M proteins. *J Virol,* 74, 4967.
[http://dx.doi.org/10.1128/JVI.74.11.4967-4978.2000]

Devaraj, SG, Wang, N, Chen, Z, Chen, Z, Tseng, M, Barretto, N, Lin, R, Peters, CJ, Tseng, CTK, Baker, SC & Li, K (2007) Regulation of IRF-3-dependent innate immunity by the papain-like protease domain of the severe acute respiratory syndrome coronavirus. *J Biol Chem,* 282, 32208.
[http://dx.doi.org/10.1074/jbc.M704870200]

Egloff, MP, Malet, H, Putics, A, Heinonen, M, Dutartre, H, Frangeul, A, Gruez, A, Campanacci, V, Cambillau, C, Ziebuhr, J & Ahola, T (2006) Structural and functional basis for ADP-ribose and poly (ADP-ribose) binding by viral macro domains. *J Virol,* 80, 8493.
[http://dx.doi.org/10.1128/JVI.00713-06]

Enjuanes, L, Sola, I, Alonso, S, Escors, D & Zúñiga, S (2005) Coronavirus reverse genetics and development of vectors for gene expression. coronavirus replication and reverse genetics. In: Enjuanes, L., (Ed.), *Current Topics in Microbiology and Immunology* Springer, Berlin, Heidelberg 161.

Eriksson, KK, Cervantes-Barragán, L, Ludewig, B & Thiel, V (2008) Mouse hepatitis virus liver pathology is dependent on ADP-ribose-1 ″-phosphatase, a viral function conserved in the alpha-like supergroup. *J Virol,* 82, 12325.
[http://dx.doi.org/10.1128/JVI.02082-08]

Escors, D, Camafeita, E, Ortego, J, Laude, H & Enjuanes, L (2001) Organization of two transmissible gastroenteritis coronavirus membrane protein topologies within the virion and core. *J Virol,* 75, 12228.
[http://dx.doi.org/10.1128/JVI.75.24.12228-12240.2001]

Fang, X, Ye, L, Timani, KA, Li, S, Zen, Y, Zhao, M, Zheng, H & Wu, Z (2005) Peptide domain involved in the interaction between membrane protein and nucleocapsid protein of SARS-associated coronavirus. *BMB Reports,* 38, 381.
[http://dx.doi.org/10.5483/BMBRep.2005.38.4.381]

Fehr, AR & Perlman, S (2015) Coronaviruses: An Overview of Their Replication and Pathogenesis. In: Maier, H., Bickerton, E., Britton, P., (Eds.), *Coronaviruses Methods in Molecular Biology* Humana Press,

New York, NY 1282.
[http://dx.doi.org/10.1007/978-1-4939-2438-7_1]

Frieman, M, Ratia, K, Johnston, RE, Mesecar, AD & Baric, RS (2009) SARS Coronavirus Papain-Like Protease Ubiquitin-like domain and Catalytic domain regulate antagonism of IRF3 and NFkB signaling. *J Virol*, 83, 6689.

Frieman, M, Yount, B, Heise, M, Kopecky-Bromberg, SA, Palese, P & Baric, RS (2007) Severe acute respiratory syndrome coronavirus ORF6 antagonizes STAT1 function by sequestering nuclear import factors on the rough endoplasmic reticulum/Golgi membrane. *J Virol*, 81, 9812.
[http://dx.doi.org/10.1128/JVI.01012-07]

Garoff, H, Hewson, R & Opstelten, DJE (1998) Virus maturation by budding. *Microbiol Mol Biol Rev*, 62, 1171.
[http://dx.doi.org/10.1128/MMBR.62.4.1171-1190.1998]

Gorbalenya, AE (2001) Big Nidovirus Genome. The Nidoviruses. In: Lavi, E., Weiss, S.R., Hingley, S.T., (Eds.), *Advances in Experimental Medicine and Biology* Springer, Boston, MA.

Grossoehme, NE, Li, L, Keane, SC, Liu, P, Dann, CE, III, Leibowitz, JL & Giedroc, DP (2009) Coronavirus N protein N-terminal domain (NTD) specifically binds the transcriptional regulatory sequence (TRS) and melts TRS-cTRS RNA duplexes. *J Mol Biol*, 394, 544.
[http://dx.doi.org/10.1016/j.jmb.2009.09.040]

Gu, J & Korteweg, C (2007) Pathology and pathogenesis of severe acute respiratory syndrome. *Am J Pathol*, 170, 1136.
[http://dx.doi.org/10.2353/ajpath.2007.061088]

Guarino, LA, Bhardwaj, K, Dong, W, Sun, J, Holzenburg, A & Kao, C (2005) Mutational analysis of the SARS virus Nsp15 endoribonuclease: identification of residues affecting hexamer formation. *J Mol Biol*, 353, 1106.
[http://dx.doi.org/10.1016/j.jmb.2005.09.007]

Gunalan, V (2011) *Virus host interactions in SARS coronavirus infection Inst for microbiology, tumor-and cell biology/Department of Microbiology*.Tumor and Cell Biology. ISBN: 978-91-7457-510-1, http://hdl.handle.net/10616/40750

Haga, S, Yamamoto, N, Nakai-Murakami, C, Osawa, Y, Tokunaga, K & Sata, T (2008) Modulation of TNF--converting enzyme by the spike protein of SARS-CoV and ACE2 induces TNF- production and facilitates viral entry. *Proc Natl Acad Sci*, 105, 7809.

Hamming, I, Cooper, ME, Haagmans, BL, Hooper, NM, Korstanje, R, Osterhaus, AD, Timens, W, Turner, AJ, Navis, G & van Goor, H (2007) The emerging role of ACE2 in physiology and disease. *J Pathol*, 212, 1-11.
[http://dx.doi.org/10.1002/path.2162]

Hancock, AS, Stairiker, CJ, Boesteanu, AC, Monzón-Casanova, E, Lukasiak, S, Mueller, YM, Stubbs, AP, Garcia-Sastre, A, Turner, M & Katsikis, PD (2018) Transcriptome analysis of infected and bystander type 2 alveolar epithelial cells during influenza A virus infection reveals *in vivo* Wnt pathway downregulation', J. Virol. *J Virol*, 92, e01325.
[http://dx.doi.org/10.1128/JVI.01325-18]

He, R, Leeson, A, Ballantine, M, Andonov, A, Baker, L, Dobie, F, Li, Y, Bastien, N, Feldmann, H, Strocher, U & Theriault, S (2004) Characterization of protein-protein interactions between the nucleocapsid protein and membrane protein of the SARS coronavirus. *Virus Res*, 105, 121.
[http://dx.doi.org/10.1016/j.virusres.2004.05.002]

Hegyi, A & Ziebuhr, J (2002) Conservation of substrate specificities among coronavirus main proteases. *J Gen Virol*, 83, 595.
[http://dx.doi.org/10.1099/0022-1317-83-3-595]

Hilbert, M, Kebbel, F, Gubaev, A & Klostermeier, D (2011) eIF4G stimulates the activity of the DEAD-box

protein eIF4A by a conformational guidance mechanism. *Nucl Acids Res,* 39, 2260.
[http://dx.doi.org/10.1093/nar/gkq1127]

Ho, JC, Chan, KN, Hu, WH, Lam, WK, Zheng, L, Tipoe, GL, Sun, J, Leung, R & Tsang, KW (2001) The effect of aging on nasal mucociliary clearance, beat frequency, and ultrastructure of respiratory cilia. *Am J Resp Crit Care Med,* 163, 983.
[http://dx.doi.org/10.1164/ajrccm.163.4.9909121]

Hoffmann, M, Kleine-Weber, H, Schroeder, S, Krüger, N, Herrler, T, Erichsen, S, Schiergens, TS, Herrler, G, Wu, NH, Nitsche, A, Müller, MA, Drosten, C & Pöhlmann, S (2020) SARS-CoV-2 cell entry depends on ACE2 and TMPRSS2 and is blocked by a clinically proven protease inhibitor. *Cell,* 181, 271-280.e8.
[http://dx.doi.org/10.1016/j.cell.2020.02.052] [PMID: 32142651]

Hsieh, YC, Li, HC, Chen, SC & Lo, SY (2008) Interactions between M protein and other structural proteins of severe, acute respiratory syndrome-associated coronavirus. *J Biomed Sci,* 15, 707.

Huang, C, Ito, N, Tseng, CTK & Makino, S (2006) Severe acute respiratory syndrome coronavirus 7a accessory protein is a viral structural protein. *J Virol,* 80, 7287.
[http://dx.doi.org/10.1128/JVI.00414-06]

Hurst, KR, Kuo, L, Koetzner, CA, Ye, R, Hsue, B & Masters, PS (2005) A major determinant for membrane protein interaction localizes to the carboxy-terminal domain of the mouse coronavirus nucleocapsid protein. *J Virol,* 79, 13285.
[http://dx.doi.org/10.1128/JVI.79.21.13285-13297.2005]

Hussain, S, Perlman, S & Gallagher, TM (2008) Severe acute respiratory syndrome coronavirus protein 6 accelerates murine hepatitis virus infections by more than one mechanism. *J Virol,* 82, 7212.
[http://dx.doi.org/10.1128/JVI.02406-07]

Imbert, I, Guillemot, JC, Bourhis, JM, Bussetta, C, Coutard, B, Egloff, MP, Ferron, F, Gorbalenya, AE & Canard, B (2006) A second, non-canonical RNA-dependent RNA polymerase in SARS Coronavirus. *The EMBO J,* 25, 4933.
[http://dx.doi.org/10.1038/sj.emboj.7601368]

Ivanov, KA & Ziebuhr, J (2004) Human coronavirus 229E nonstructural protein 13: characterization of duplex-unwinding, nucleoside triphosphatase, and RNA 5'-triphosphatase activities. *J Virol,* 78, 7833.
[http://dx.doi.org/10.1128/JVI.78.14.7833-7838.2004]

Ivanov, KA, Hertzig, T, Rozanov, M, Bayer, S, Thiel, V, Gorbalenya, AE & Ziebuhr, J (2004) Major genetic marker of nidoviruses encodes a replicative endoribonuclease. *Proc Natl Acad Sci,* 101, 12694.
[http://dx.doi.org/10.1073/pnas.0403127101]

Jeffers, SA, Tusell, SM, Gillim-Ross, L, Hemmila, EM, Achenbach, JE, Babcock, GJ, Thomas, WD, Thackray, LB, Young, MD, Mason, RJ & Ambrosino, DM (2004) CD209L (L-SIGN) is a receptor for severe acute respiratory syndrome coronavirus. *Proc Natl Acad Sci,* 101, 15748.
[http://dx.doi.org/10.1073/pnas.0403812101]

Jendrach, M, Thiel, V & Siddell, S (1999) Characterization of an internal ribosome entry site within mRNA 5 of murine hepatitis virus. *Arch Virol,* 144, 921.
[http://dx.doi.org/10.1007/s007050050556]

Kamitani, W, Huang, C, Narayanan, K, Lokugamage, KG & Makino, S (2009) A two-pronged strategy to suppress host protein synthesis by SARS coronavirus Nsp1 protein. *Nat Struct Mol Biol,* 16, 1134.
[http://dx.doi.org/10.1038/nsmb.1680]

Kamitani, W, Narayanan, K, Huang, C, Lokugamage, K, Ikegami, T, Ito, N, Kubo, H & Makino, S (2006) Severe acute respiratory syndrome coronavirus nsp1 protein suppresses host gene expression by promoting host mRNA degradation. *Proc Natl Acad Sci,* 103, 12885.

Kazi, L, Lissenberg, A, Watson, R, de Groot, RJ & Weiss, SR (2005) Expression of hemagglutinin esterase protein from recombinant mouse hepatitis virus enhances neurovirulence. *J Virol,* 79, 15064.
[http://dx.doi.org/10.1128/JVI.79.24.15064-15073.2005]

Khan, S, Fielding, BC, Tan, TH, Chou, CF, Shen, S, Lim, SG, Hong, W & Tan, YJ (2006) Over-expression of severe acute respiratory syndrome coronavirus 3b protein induces both apoptosis and necrosis in Vero E6 cells. *Virus Res,* 122, 20.
[http://dx.doi.org/10.1016/j.virusres.2006.06.005]

Kienzle, TE, Abraham, S, Hogue, BG & Brian, DA (1990) Structure and orientation of expressed bovine coronavirus hemagglutinin-esterase protein. *J Virol,* 64, 1834.
[http://dx.doi.org/10.1128/JVI.64.4.1834-1838.1990]

Klumperman, J, Locker, JK, Meijer, A, Horzinek, MC, Geuze, HJ & Rottier, PJ (1994) Coronavirus M proteins accumulate in the Golgi complex beyond the site of virion budding. *J Virol,* 68, 6523.
[http://dx.doi.org/10.1128/JVI.68.10.6523-6534.1994]

Kopecky-Bromberg, SA, Martinez-Sobrido, L & Palese, P (2006) 7a protein of severe acute respiratory syndrome coronavirus inhibits cellular protein synthesis and activates p38 mitogen-activated protein kinase. *J Virol,* 80, 785.
[http://dx.doi.org/10.1128/JVI.80.2.785-793.2006]

Kopecky-Bromberg, SA, Martínez-Sobrido, L, Frieman, M, Baric, RA & Palese, P (2007) Severe acute respiratory syndrome coronavirus open reading frame (ORF) 3b, ORF 6, and nucleocapsid proteins function as interferon antagonists. *J Virol,* 81, 548.
[http://dx.doi.org/10.1128/JVI.01782-06]

Krijnse-Locker, J, Ericsson, M, Rottier, PJ & Griffiths, G (1994) Characterization of the budding compartment of mouse hepatitis virus: evidence that transport from the RER to the Golgi complex requires only one vesicular transport step. *J Cell Biol,* 124, 55.
[http://dx.doi.org/10.1083/jcb.124.1.55]

Kuba, K, Imai, Y, Rao, S, Gao, H, Guo, F, Guan, B, Huan, Y, Yang, P, Zhang, Y, Deng, W & Bao, L (2005) A crucial role of angiotensin-converting enzyme 2 (ACE2) in SARS coronavirus–induced lung injury. *Nat Med,* 11, 875.
[http://dx.doi.org/10.1038/nm1267]

Kubo, H, Yamada, YK & Taguchi, F (1994) Localization of neutralizing epitopes and the receptor-binding site within the amino-terminal 330 amino acids of the murine coronavirus spike protein. *J Virol,* 68, 5403.
[http://dx.doi.org/10.1128/JVI.68.9.5403-5410.1994]

Kuo, L & Masters, PS (2002) Genetic evidence for a structural interaction between the carboxy termini of the membrane and nucleocapsid proteins of mouse hepatitis virus. *J Virol,* 76, 4987.
[http://dx.doi.org/10.1128/JVI.76.10.4987-4999.2002]

Kuo, L & Masters, PS (2003) The small envelope protein E is not essential for murine coronavirus replication. *J Virology,* 77, 4597.

Kuri, T, Eriksson, KK, Putics, A, Züst, R, Snijder, EJ, Davidson, AD, Siddell, SG, Thiel, V, Ziebuhr, J & Weber, F (2011) The ADP-ribose-1″-monophosphatase domains of severe acute respiratory syndrome coronavirus and human coronavirus 229E mediate resistance to antiviral interferon responses. *J Gen Virol,* 92, 1899.
[http://dx.doi.org/10.1099/vir.0.031856-0]

La Monica, N, Banner, LR, Morris, VL & Lai, MM (1991) Localization of extensive deletions in the structural genes of two neurotropic variants of murine coronavirus JHM. *Virology,* 182, 883.
[http://dx.doi.org/10.1016/0042-6822(91)90635-O]

Lai, M, Baric, RS, Brayton, PR & Stohlman, SA (1984) Characterization of leader RNA sequences on the virion and mRNAs of mouse hepatitis virus, a cytoplasmic RNA virus. *Proc Natl Acad Sci,* 81, 3626.
[http://dx.doi.org/10.1073/pnas.81.12.3626]

Langereis, MA, van Vliet, AL, Boot, W & de Groot, RJ (2010) Attachment of mouse hepatitis virus to O-acetylated sialic acid is mediated by hemagglutinin-esterase and not by the spike protein. *J Virol,* 84, 8970.
[http://dx.doi.org/10.1128/JVI.00566-10]

Lee, HJ, Shieh, CK, Gorbalenya, AE, Koonin, EV, La Monica, N, Tuler, J, Bagdzhadzhyan, A & Lai, MM (1991) The complete sequence (22 kilobases) of murine coronavirus gene 1 encoding the putative proteases and RNA polymerase. *Virology,* 180, 567.
[http://dx.doi.org/10.1016/0042-6822(91)90071-I]

Lim, KP & Liu, DX (2001) The missing link in coronavirus assembly retention of the avian coronavirus infectious bronchitis virus envelope protein in the pre-Golgi compartments and physical interaction between the envelope and membrane proteins. *J Biol Chem,* 276, 17515.

Liu, C, Zhou, Q, Li, Y, Garner, LV, Watkins, SP, Carter, LJ, Smoot, J, Gregg, AC, Daniels, AD, Jervey, S & Albaiu, D (2020) Research and development on therapeutic agents and vaccines for COVID-19 and related human coronavirus diseases. *ACS Cent Sci,* 6, 315.
[http://dx.doi.org/10.1021/acscentsci.0c00272]

Luo, C, Luo, H, Zheng, S, Gui, C, Yue, L, Yu, C, Sun, T, He, P, Chen, J, Shen, J & Luo, X (2004) Nucleocapsid protein of SARS coronavirus tightly binds to human cyclophilin A. *Biochem Biophys Res Commun,* 321, 557.
[http://dx.doi.org/10.1016/j.bbrc.2004.07.003]

Luo, Z & Weiss, SR (1998) Roles in the cell-to-cell fusion of two conserved hydrophobic regions in the murine coronavirus spike protein. *Virology,* 244, 483.
[http://dx.doi.org/10.1006/viro.1998.9121]

Mackay, IM & Arden, KE (2015) MERS coronavirus: diagnostics, epidemiology, and transmission. *Virol J,* 12, 222.
[http://dx.doi.org/10.1186/s12985-015-0439-5]

Matrosovich, MN, Matrosovich, TY, Gray, T, Roberts, NA & Klenk, HD (2004) Human and avian influenza viruses target different cell types in cultures of human airway epithelium. *Proc Natl Acad Sci,* 101, 4620.
[http://dx.doi.org/10.1073/pnas.0308001101]

Matsuyama, S, Nagata, N, Shirato, K, Kawase, M, Takeda, M & Taguchi, F (2010) Efficient activation of the severe acute respiratory syndrome coronavirus spike protein by the transmembrane protease TMPRSS2. *J Virol,* 84, 12658.
[http://dx.doi.org/10.1128/JVI.01542-10]

McBride, CE & Machamer, CE (2010) A single tyrosine in the severe acute respiratory syndrome coronavirus membrane protein cytoplasmic tail is important for efficient interaction with spike protein. *J Virol,* 84, 1891.
[http://dx.doi.org/10.1128/JVI.02458-09]

Montero, H, Pérez-Gil, G & Sampieri, CL (2019) Eukaryotic initiation factor 4A (eIF4A) during viral infections. *Virus genes,* 55, 267.
[http://dx.doi.org/10.1007/s11262-019-01641-7]

Mossel, EC, Wang, J, Jeffers, S, Edeen, KE, Wang, S, Cosgrove, GP, Funk, CJ, Manzer, R, Miura, TA, Pearson, LD & Holmes, KV (2008) SARS-CoV replicates in primary human alveolar type II cell cultures but not in type I-like cells. *Virology,* 372, 127.
[http://dx.doi.org/10.1016/j.virol.2007.09.045]

Nakagawa, K, Lokugamage, KG & Makino, S (2016) Viral and cellular mRNA translation in coronavirus-infected cells. *Adv Virus Res* Academic Press Inc 165.

Nakauchi, M, Kariwa, H, Kon, Y, Yoshii, K, Maeda, A & Takashima, I (2008) Analysis of severe acute respiratory syndrome coronavirus structural proteins in virus-like particle assembly. *Microbiol Immunol,* 52, 625.
[http://dx.doi.org/10.1111/j.1348-0421.2008.00079.x]

Nal, B, Chan, C, Kien, F, Siu, L, Tse, J, Chu, K, Kam, J, Staropoli, I, Crescenzo-Chaigne, B, Escriou, N & van der Werf, S (2005) Differential maturation and subcellular localization of severe acute respiratory syndrome coronavirus surface proteins S, M and E. *J Gen Virol,* 86, 1423.

[http://dx.doi.org/10.1099/vir.0.80671-0]

Narayanan, K & Makino, S (2001) Cooperation of an RNA packaging signal and a viral envelope protein in coronavirus RNA packaging. *J Virol,* 75, 9059.
[http://dx.doi.org/10.1128/JVI.75.19.9059-9067.2001]

Narayanan, K, Chen, CJ, Maeda, J & Makino, S (2003) Nucleocapsid-independent specific viral RNA packaging *via* viral envelope protein and viral RNA signal. *J Virol,* 77, 2922.
[http://dx.doi.org/10.1128/JVI.77.5.2922-2927.2003]

Narayanan, K, Huang, C & Makino, S (2008) SARS coronavirus accessory proteins. *Virus Res,* 133, 113.
[http://dx.doi.org/10.1016/j.virusres.2007.10.009]

Needle, D, Lountos, GT & Waugh, DS (2015) Structures of the Middle East respiratory syndrome coronavirus 3C-like protease reveal insights into substrate specificity. *Acta Crystallogr D Biol Crystallogr,* 71, 1102.

Nelson, CA, Pekosz, A, Lee, CA, Diamond, MS & Fremont, DH (2005) Structure and intracellular targeting of the SARS-coronavirus Orf7a accessory protein. *Structure,* 13, 75.
[http://dx.doi.org/10.1016/j.str.2004.10.010]

Nikolaidis, NM, Noel, JG, Pitstick, LB, Gardner, JC, Uehara, Y, Wu, H, Saito, A, Lewnard, KE, Liu, H, White, MR & Hartshorn, KL (2017) Mitogenic stimulation accelerates influenza-induced mortality by increasing susceptibility of alveolar type II cells to infection. *Proc Natl Acad Sci,* 114, E6613.
[http://dx.doi.org/10.1073/pnas.1621172114]

Ortego, J, Escors, D, Laude, H & Enjuanes, L (2002) Generation of a replication-competent, propagation-deficient virus vector based on the transmissible gastroenteritis coronavirus genome. *J Virol,* 76, 11518.
[http://dx.doi.org/10.1128/JVI.76.22.11518-11529.2002]

Parker, S, Gallagher, T & Buchmeier, M (1989) Sequence analysis reveals extensive polymorphism and evidence of deletions within the E2 glycoprotein gene of several strains of murine hepatitis virus. *Virology,* 173
[http://dx.doi.org/10.1016/0042-6822(89)90579-5]

Prentice, E, McAuliffe, J, Lu, X, Subbarao, K & Denison, MR (2004) Identification and characterization of severe acute respiratory syndrome coronavirus replicase proteins. *J Virol,* 78, 9977.
[http://dx.doi.org/10.1128/JVI.78.18.9977-9986.2004]

Putics, A, Filipowicz, W, Hall, J, Gorbalenya, AE & Ziebuhr, J (2005) ADP-ribose-1"-monophosphatase: a conserved coronavirus enzyme that is dispensable for viral replication in tissue culture. *J Virol,* 79, 12721.

Putics, Á, Gorbalenya, AE & Ziebuhr, J (2006) Identification of protease and ADP-ribose 1"-monophosphatase activities associated with transmissible gastroenteritis virus non-structural protein 3. *J Virol,* 87, 651-.
[http://dx.doi.org/10.1099/vir.0.81596-0]

Qian, Z, Travanty, EA, Oko, L, Edeen, K, Berglund, A, Wang, J, Ito, Y, Holmes, KV & Mason, RJ (2013) Innate immune response of human alveolar type ii cells infected with the severe acute respiratory syndrome–coronavirus. *Am J Respir Cell Mol Biol,* 48, 742.
[http://dx.doi.org/10.1165/rcmb.2012-0339OC]

Rajiv, C & Davis, TL (2018) Structural and functional insights into human nuclear cyclophilins. *Biomolecules,* 8, 161.
[http://dx.doi.org/10.3390/biom8040161]

Reyfman, PA, Walter, JM, Joshi, N, Anekalla, KR, McQuattie-Pimentel, AC, Chiu, S, Fernandez, R, Akbarpour, M, Chen, CI, Ren, Z & Verma, R (2019) Single-cell transcriptomic analysis of human lung provides insights into the pathobiology of pulmonary fibrosis *Am J Respir Crit Care Med,* 199, 1517.
[http://dx.doi.org/10.1164/rccm.201712-2410OC]

Rockx, B, Baas, T, Zornetzer, GA, Haagmans, B, Sheahan, T, Frieman, M, Dyer, MD, Teal, TH, Proll, S, van den Brand, J & Baric, R (2009) Early upregulation of acute respiratory distress syndrome-associated cytokines promotes lethal disease in an aged-mouse model of severe acute respiratory syndrome coronavirus infection. *J Virol,* 83, 7062.

Shieh, CK, Soe, LH, Making, S, Chang, MF, Stohlman, SA & Lai, MM (1987) The 5′-end sequence of the murine coronavirus genome: implications for multiple fusion sites in leader-primed transcription *Virology,* 156, 321.
[http://dx.doi.org/10.1016/0042-6822(87)90412-0]

Shulla, A, Heald-Sargent, T, Subramanya, G, Zhao, J, Perlman, S & Gallagher, T (2011) A transmembrane serine protease is linked to the severe acute respiratory syndrome coronavirus receptor and activates virus entry. *J Virol,* 85, 873.
[http://dx.doi.org/10.1128/JVI.02062-10]

Simmons, G, Bertram, S, Glowacka, I, Steffen, I, Chaipan, C, Agudelo, J, Lu, K, Rennekamp, AJ, Hofmann, H, Bates, P & Pöhlmann, S (2011) Different host cell proteases activate the SARS-coronavirus spike-protein for cell–cell and virus–cell fusion. *Virology,* 413, 265.
[http://dx.doi.org/10.1016/j.virol.2011.02.020]

Sims, AC, Baric, RS, Yount, B, Burkett, SE, Collins, PL & Pickles, RJ (2005) Severe acute respiratory syndrome coronavirus infection of human ciliated airway epithelia: role of ciliated cells in the viral spread in the conducting airways of the lungs. *J Virol,* 79, 15511.
[http://dx.doi.org/10.1128/JVI.79.24.15511-15524.2005]

Singh, K, Winter, M, Zouhar, M & Ryšánek, P (2018) Cyclophilins: less studied proteins with critical roles in pathogenesis *Phytopathology,* 108, 6.
[http://dx.doi.org/10.1094/PHYTO-05-17-0167-RVW]

Siu, KL, Kok, KH, Ng, MHJ, Poon, VKM, Yuen, KY, Zheng, BJ & Jin, DY (2009) Severe acute respiratory syndrome coronavirus m protein inhibits type I interferon production by impeding the formation of TRAF3·TANK·TBK1/IKKε complex. *J Biol Chem,* 284, 16202.
[http://dx.doi.org/10.1074/jbc.M109.008227]

Snijder, EJ, Bredenbeek, PJ, Dobbe, JC, Thiel, V, Ziebuhr, J, Poon, LL, Guan, Y, Rozanov, M, Spaan, WJ & Gorbalenya, AE (2003) Unique and conserved features of genome and proteome of SARS-coronavirus, an early split-off from the coronavirus group 2 lineage *J Mol Biol,* 331, 991.
[http://dx.doi.org/10.1016/S0022-2836(03)00865-9]

Taguchi, F (1995) The S2 subunit of the murine coronavirus spike protein is not involved in receptor binding *J Virol,* 69, 7260.
[http://dx.doi.org/10.1128/JVI.69.11.7260-7263.1995]

Tan, YJ, Fielding, BC, Goh, PY, Shen, S, Tan, TH, Lim, SG & Hong, W (2004) Overexpression of 7a, a protein specifically encoded by the severe acute respiratory syndrome coronavirus, induces apoptosis *via* a caspase-dependent pathway. *J Virol,* 78, 14043.
[http://dx.doi.org/10.1128/JVI.78.24.14043-14047.2004]

Tanaka, Y, Sato, Y & Sasaki, T (2017) Feline coronavirus replication is affected by both cyclophilin A and cyclophilin B. *J Gen Virol,* 98, 190.
[http://dx.doi.org/10.1099/jgv.0.000663]

Tang, NLS, Chan, PKS, Wong, CK, To, KF, Wu, AKL, Sung, YM, Hui, DSC, Sung, JJY & Lam, CWK (2005) Early enhanced expression of interferon-inducible protein-10 (CXCL-10) and other chemokines predict adverse outcome in severe acute respiratory syndrome. *Clin Chem,* 51, 2333.
[http://dx.doi.org/10.1373/clinchem.2005.054460]

Tangudu, C, Olivares, H, Netland, J, Perlman, S & Gallagher, T (2007) Severe acute respiratory syndrome coronavirus protein 6 accelerates murine coronavirus infections. *J Virol,* 81, 1220.
[http://dx.doi.org/10.1128/JVI.01515-06]

TeVelthuis, AJ, Arnold, JJ, Cameron, CE, van den Worm, SH & Snijder, EJ (2010) The RNA polymerase activity of SARS-coronavirus nsp12 is primer dependent. *Nucleic Acids Res,* 38, 203.

Vennema, H, Godeke, GJ, Rossen, JW, Voorhout, WF, Horzinek, MC, Opstelten, DJ & Rottier, PJ (1996) Nucleocapsid-independent assembly of coronavirus-like particles by co-expression of viral envelope protein genes. *The EMBO J*, 15, 2020.
[http://dx.doi.org/10.1002/j.1460-2075.1996.tb00553.x]

Verheije, MH, Hagemeijer, MC, Ulasli, M, Reggiori, F, Rottier, PJ, Masters, PS & de Haan, CA (2010) The coronavirus nucleocapsid protein is dynamically associated with the replication-transcription complexes. *J Virol*, 84, 11575.
[http://dx.doi.org/10.1128/JVI.00569-10]

Verma, S, Lopez, LA, Bednar, V & Hogue, BG (2007) Importance of the penultimate positive charge in mouse hepatitis coronavirus A59 membrane protein *J Virology*, 81, 5339.
[http://dx.doi.org/10.1128/JVI.02427-06]

von Brunn, A, Ciesek, S, von Brunn, B & Carbajo-Lozoya, J (2015) Genetic deficiency and polymorphisms of cyclophilin A reveal its essential role for Human Coronavirus 229E replication. *Curr Opin Virol*, 14, 56-61.
[http://dx.doi.org/10.1016/j.coviro.2015.08.004] [PMID: 26318518]

von Hahn, T & Ciesek, S (2015) Cyclophilin polymorphism and virus infection. *Curr Opin Virol*, 14, 47-9.
[http://dx.doi.org/10.1016/j.coviro.2015.07.012] [PMID: 26281011]

Voß, D, Pfefferle, S, Drosten, C, Stevermann, L, Traggiai, E, Lanzavecchia, A & Becker, S (2009) Studies on membrane topology, N-glycosylation and functionality of SARS-CoV membrane protein. *J Virol*, 6, 1-13.

Wan, Y, Shang, J, Graham, R, Baric, RS & Li, F (2020) Receptor recognition by the novel coronavirus from Wuhan: an analysis based on decade-long structural studies of SARS coronavirus. *J Virol*, 94.
[http://dx.doi.org/10.1128/JVI.00127-20]

Wang, J, Fang, S, Xiao, H, Chen, B, Tam, JP & Liu, DX (2009) Interaction of the coronavirus infectious bronchitis virus membrane protein with β-actin and its implication in virion assembly and budding. *PLoS One*, 4.
[http://dx.doi.org/10.1371/journal.pone.0004908]

Wang, J, Nikrad, MP, Phang, T, Gao, B, Alford, T, Ito, Y, Edeen, K, Travanty, EA, Kosmider, B, Hartshorn, K & Mason, RJ (2011) Innate immune response to influenza A virus in differentiated human alveolar type II cells. *Am J Respir Cell Mol Biol*, 45, 582.
[http://dx.doi.org/10.1165/rcmb.2010-0108OC]

Wang, S, Guo, F, Liu, K, Wang, H, Rao, S, Yang, P & Jiang, C (2008) Endocytosis of the receptor-binding domain of SARS-CoV spike protein together with virus receptor ACE2. *Virus Res*, 136, p.8.
[http://dx.doi.org/10.1016/j.virusres.2008.03.004]

Wathelet, MG, Orr, M, Frieman, MB & Baric, RS (2007) Severe acute respiratory syndrome coronavirus evades antiviral signaling: role of nsp1 and rational design of an attenuated strain. *J Virol*, 81, 11620.
[http://dx.doi.org/10.1128/JVI.00702-07]

Weinheimer, VK, Becher, A, Tönnies, M, Holland, G, Knepper, J, Bauer, TT, Schneider, P, Neudecker, J, Rückert, JC, Szymanski, K & Temmesfeld-Wollbrueck, B (2012) Influenza A viruses target type II pneumocytes in the human lung. *J Infect Dis*, 206, 1685.
[http://dx.doi.org/10.1093/infdis/jis455]

Wilson, L, Mckinlay, C, Gage, P & Ewart, G (2004) SARS coronavirus E protein forms cation-selective ion channels. *Virology*, 330, 322.
[http://dx.doi.org/10.1016/j.virol.2004.09.033]

Wösten-van Asperen, RM, Lutter, R, Haitsma, JJ, Merkus, MP, van Woensel, JB, Van Der Loos, CM, Florquin, S, Lachmann, B & Bos, AP (2008) ACE mediates ventilator-induced lung injury in rats *via* angiotensin II but not bradykinin. *Eur Respir J*, 31, 363.
[http://dx.doi.org/10.1183/09031936.00060207]

Wu, J, Wu, X, Zeng, W, Guo, D, Fang, Z, Chen, L, Huang, H & Li, C (2020) Chest CT findings in patients

with coronavirus disease 2019 and its relationship with clinical features. *Invest Radiol*, 55, 257.
[http://dx.doi.org/10.1097/RLI.0000000000000670]

Wu, Z & McGoogan, JM (2020) Characteristics of and important lessons from the coronavirus disease 2019 (COVID-19) outbreak in China: summary of a report of 72314 cases from the chinese center for disease control and prevention. *JAMA*.
[http://dx.doi.org/10.1001/jama.2020.2648]

Wurm, T, Chen, H, Hodgson, T, Britton, P, Brooks, G & Hiscox, JA (2001) Localization to the nucleolus is a common feature of coronavirus nucleoproteins, and the protein may disrupt host cell division. *J Virol*, 75, 9345.
[http://dx.doi.org/10.1128/JVI.75.19.9345-9356.2001]

Wurzer, WJ, Obojes, K & Vlasak, R (2002) The sialate-4-O-acetyl esterase of coronaviruses related to mouse hepatitis virus: a proposal to reorganize group 2 Coronaviridae. *J Gen Virol*, 83, 395.

Xu, X, Liu, Y, Weiss, S, Arnold, E, Sarafianos, SG & Ding, J (2003) Molecular model of SARS coronavirus polymerase: implications for biochemical functions and drug design. *Nucleic Acids Res*, 31, 7117.
[http://dx.doi.org/10.1093/nar/gkg916]

Xu, Z, Shi, L, Wang, Y, Zhang, J, Huang, L, Zhang, C, Liu, S, Zhao, P, Liu, H, Zhu, L & Tai, Y (2020) Pathological findings of COVID-19 associated with acute respiratory distress syndrome. *Lancet Respir Med*, 8, 420.
[http://dx.doi.org/10.1016/S2213-2600(20)30076-X]

Yang, H, Yang, M, Ding, Y, Liu, Y, Lou, Z, Zhou, Z, Sun, L, Mo, L, Ye, S, Pang, H & Gao, GF (2003) The crystal structures of severe acute respiratory syndrome virus main protease and its complex with an inhibitor. *Proc Natl Acad Sci*, 100, 13190.
[http://dx.doi.org/10.1073/pnas.1835675100]

Yang, Y, Xiong, Z, Zhang, S, Yan, Y, Nguyen, J, Ng, B, Lu, H, Brendese, J, Yang, F, Wang, H & Yang, XF (2005) Bcl-xL inhibits T-cell apoptosis induced by expression of SARS coronavirus E protein in the absence of growth factors. *Biochem J*, 392, 135.
[http://dx.doi.org/10.1042/BJ20050698]

Ye, Y, Hauns, K, Langland, JO, Jacobs, BL & Hogue, BG (2007) Mouse hepatitis coronavirus A59 nucleocapsid protein is a type I interferon antagonist. *J Virol*, 81, 2554.
[http://dx.doi.org/10.1128/JVI.01634-06]

Yokomori, K, Banner, L & Lai, M (1991) Heterogeneity of gene expression of the hemagglutinin-esterase (HE) protein of murine coronaviruses. *Virology*, 183.
[http://dx.doi.org/10.1016/0042-6822(91)90994-M]

Yokomori, K, La Monica, N, Makino, S, Shieh, CK & Lai, MM (1989) Biosynthesis, structure, and biological activities of envelope protein gp65 of murine coronavirus. *Virology*, 173, 683.
[http://dx.doi.org/10.1016/0042-6822(89)90581-3]

Yount, B, Denison, MR, Weiss, SR & Baric, RS (2002) Systematic assembly of a full-length infectious cDNA of mouse hepatitis virus strain A59. *J Virol*, 76, 11065.
[http://dx.doi.org/10.1128/JVI.76.21.11065-11078.2002]

Yount, B, Roberts, RS, Sims, AC, Deming, D, Frieman, MB, Sparks, J, Denison, MR, Davis, N & Baric, RS (2005) Severe acute respiratory syndrome coronavirus group-specific open reading frames encode nonessential functions for replication in cell cultures and mice. *J Virol*, 79, 14909.
[http://dx.doi.org/10.1128/JVI.79.23.14909-14922.2005]

Yu, X, Bi, W, Weiss, SR & Leibowitz, JL (1994) Mouse hepatitis virus gene 5b protein is a new virion envelope protein. *Virology*, 202, 1018.
[http://dx.doi.org/10.1006/viro.1994.1430]

Yuan, X, Shan, Y, Zhao, Z, Chen, J & Cong, Y (2005) G0/G1 arrest and apoptosis induced by SARS-CoV 3b protein in transfected cells. *Virology*, 2, 66.

Yuan, X, Wu, J, Shan, Y, Yao, Z, Dong, B, Chen, B, Zhao, Z, Wang, S, Chen, J & Cong, Y (2006) SARS coronavirus 7a protein blocks cell cycle progression at G0/G1 phase *via* the cyclin D3/pRb pathway. *Virology,* 346, 74.
[http://dx.doi.org/10.1016/j.virol.2005.10.015]

Zhang, S, Li, H, Huang, S, You, W & Sun, H (2020) High-resolution computed tomography features of 17 cases of coronavirus disease 2019 in Sichuan province, China. *Eur Respir J,* 5, 2000334.

Zheng, D, Chen, G, Guo, B, Cheng, G & Tang, H (2008) PLP2, a potent deubiquitinase from murine hepatitis virus. strongly inhibits cellular type I interferon production. *Cell Res,* 18, 1105.

Zhou, H, Ferraro, D, Zhao, J, Hussain, S, Shao, J, Trujillo, J, Netland, J, Gallagher, T & Perlman, S (2010) The N-terminal region of severe acute respiratory syndrome coronavirus protein 6 induces membrane rearrangement and enhances virus replication. *J Virol,* 84, 3542.
[http://dx.doi.org/10.1128/JVI.02570-09]

Ziebuhr, J (2005) The coronavirus replicase. *Curr Top Microbiol Immunol* 287, 57.
[http://dx.doi.org/10.1007/3-540-26765-4_3]

Ziebuhr, J, Thiel, V & Gorbalenya, AE (2001) The autocatalytic release of a putative RNA virus transcription factor from its polyprotein precursor involves two paralogous papain-like proteases that cleave the same peptide bond. *J Biol Chem,* 276, 33220.
[http://dx.doi.org/10.1074/jbc.M104097200]

CHAPTER 5

Clinical Presentation and Comorbidities

Jasleen Kaur[1], Baljinder Singh[2], Bikash Medhi[3] and Gurpreet Kaur[1,*]

[1] *Department of Pharmaceutical Sciences and Drug Research, Punjabi University, Patiala, Punjab, India*

[2] *MM School of Pharmacy, MM University, Sadopur, Ambala, Haryana, India*

[3] *Department of Pharmacology, PGIMER, Chandigarh, India*

Abstract: Presently, the whole world is going through a historic yet a troublesome situation following COVID-19 outbreak. The clinicians have observed a wide variety of respiratory and non-respiratory clinical manifestations in COVID-19 patients. Accumulating reports revealed that the clinical features of COVID-19 may include asymptomatic/mild symptoms, neurological, cardiovascular complications, severe pneumonia and mortality. The most common features noticed are fever, dry cough, sore throat, shortness of breath, sputum production, fatigue, and myalgia. Recently, US health protection agency has also reported repeated shaking along with chills, loss of taste and smell in new case studies as additional symptoms. In addition to this, COVID-19 patients may show clinical signs like persistent pressure and pain in the chest, blue lips or face, confusion and GIT disturbances (diarrhea, nausea, vomiting and abdominal discomfort). The current ongoing pandemic has remarkably affected almost every age group of humans, starting from infants less than 3 months, adults, elder and older patients. Furthermore, the clinical presentations in these groups of COVID-19 infected patients were found to show considerable inter-individual variations. The findings also suggested that the comorbid conditions (heart injury, hyperglycemia, hypertension, neurodegenerative diseases) in elder/older patients further complicate the health of COVID-19 patients.

In the present book chapter, the clinical presentation of COVID-19 in pediatric, adults and geriatric group of population will be emphasized along with the higher susceptibility of COVID-19 in comorbid patients.

Keywords: ACE-2, Adolescents, Anosmia, Asymptomatic, Atypical symptoms, Comorbid, Comorbidity, Consolidations, Cutaneous, Dyspnea, Fatigue, Fever, Gastrointestinal, Ground glass opacities, Immunity, Incubation period, Neonates, Neurological, Pneumonia, Respiratory distress, Respiratory symptoms, SARS-CoV-2, Septic shock, Spikes, Vaccination.

---

* **Corresponding author Gurpreet Kaur:** Department of Pharmaceutical Sciences and Drug Research, Punjabi University, Patiala, Punjab, India, E-mail:kaurgpt@gmail.com

Neeraj Mittal, Sanjay Kumar Bhadada, O. P. Katare and Varun Garg (Eds.)
All rights reserved-© 2021 Bentham Science Publishers

INTRODUCTION

At the beginning of the COVID-19 outbreak, the clinicians have encountered a substantial diversity in the clinical presentations, such as different incubation periods among different age groups, noticeable variations in the onset of symptoms and degree of severity (moderate, serious and critical). Besides the most common respiratory symptoms, an array of complications has been found to be associated with Severe Acute Respiratory Syndrome Coronavirus-2 (SARS-CoV-2) infection. Moreover, asymptomatic (transmit virus but never have symptoms) and presymptomatic (transmit virus and symptoms appear later) transmissions have also raised concerns. The present chapter elaborates the typical and atypical clinical features discerned in original clinical cases of COVID-19 patients. Besides, the factors (age, Angiotensin-Converting Enzyme 2 (ACE2), gender, blood group, previous immunization, comorbidity) responsible for the high inter-individual variations of clinical outcomes have also been discussed in detail.

CLINICAL PRESENTATIONS OF COVID-19 INFECTION

In COVID-19 patients, it is found that after exposure, the virus takes an incubation period of 2-14 days. According to the findings of clinical cases, the COVID-19 infection starts showing its mild symptoms after a median incubation time period of approximately 5.1 days (McIntosh, 2020). However, Lauer and his coworker estimated that 97.5% of COVID-19 infected patients presented severe symptoms by 11.5 days (Lauer *et al.*, 2020). The diverse respiratory and non-respiratory symptoms observed to date are compiled in Table **1**.

Table 1. Respiratory and non-respiratory symptoms of COVID-19.

Respiratory Symptoms (Hassan *et al.*, 2020; Cascella *et al.*, 2020; Wang *et al.*, 2020)			
Mild Cases • Infection resides only in upper respiratory tract. • Fever, nasal congestion, dry cough, headache, sore throat and malaise.	**Moderate Cases** • Respiratory manifestations include cough, shortness of breath, and tachypnea.	**Severe Cases** • Patients are reported to have severe pneumonia. • Acute Respiratory Distress Syndrome (ARDS), $PaO_2/FiO_2 < 300$, $SpO_2 \leq 93\%$, tachypnea, severe dyspnea. • Fever can be absent or moderate.	**Acute Respiratory Distress Syndrome** • It indicates worsening/failure of the respiratory system. • ARDS can be of different types on the basis of values of PaO_2/FiO_2. Severe (≤ 100 mmHg). Moderate (100-200 mmHg). Mild (200-300 mmHg).

• Dyspnea is absent. • Radiographic manifestations are not present. • Most of the cases have been found to be mild. • Mild cases may deteriorate into severe cases if precautions will not be acquired.	• Severe symptoms are absent.	• In critical cases, cardiac injury, RNAaemia, respiratory failure or multiple organ dysfunction have also been found. • Comorbidities such as hypertension, diabetes, cancer, cardiovascular problems further increase the fatality rate in severe cases of COVID infection.	Its different values indicate different degrees of hypoxia. • Deterioration of ARDS can also be correlated with altered AST (aspartate transaminase) and ALT (alanine transaminase) levels. • Ground Glass Opacity (GGO) (86%), bilateral (76%), peripheral (33%) distribution, consolidation (29%), crazy paving (19%) are the prominent features found in computed tomography (CT) scan.
Non-Respiratory Symptoms (unusual Manifestations)			
Neurological	Altered mental state, musculoskeletal disturbance, acute necrotising encephalopathy ischaemic stroke, headache, dizziness, Guillain-Barre syndrome.		
Ocular	• In China, 32% of infected patients showed ocular manifestations, for example, chemosis and conjunctival hyperaemia. • Tears and conjunctival seepage have shown the presence of COVID-19. • In severe COVID-19 cases, pseudomembranous and hemorrhagic conjunctivitis was also found. • Development of ptechiae, tarsal pseudomembranous, mucous filaments in 63-year-old COVID-19 positive male. • External ocular infections could occur lately due to the spread of infection and physicians should take care if ocular complications exist for >2 weeks in COVID-19 patients (Navel, Chiambaretta and Dutheil, 2020).		
Taste and Smell	• Olfactory dysfunction (Anosmia) is typically found to be present only in the most severe cases. • Bilateral obstruction in olfactory clefts due to inflammation; however no abnormalities were found in olfactory bulbs and tracts (Giacomelli et al., 2020; Temmel et al., 2004; Eliezer et al., 2020). • Anosmia may persist with or without dysgeusia and manifest itself either in the early stage of progression or in patients with mild symptoms (Xydakis et al., 2020; Carrillo-Larco et al., 2020).		
Cardiovascular	Heart failure, cardiac arrhythmias, pacemaker conduction defects, infections such as myocarditis and myopericarditis, chest pain (Yang et al., 2020; Bonow et al., 2020; Inciardi et al., 2020; Driggin et al., 2020; Wang et al., 2020; Zhou et al., 2020).		
Hematological Symptoms	Hypercoagulable state in COVID-19 patients increased the threat of thrombotic occlusion		
	Mediastinal lymphadenopathy was also found in patients with a severe form of COVID-19 (Valette et al., 2020)		

(Table 1) cont.....

Cutaneous Manifestations	• Conjunctival hyperaemia and chemosis were disclosed in SARS-CoV-2 patients (Wu *et al.,* 2020). • Development of an erythematous, confluent, non-pruritic macula papular rash which started initially in the neck and trunk and spread to cheeks, palms, upper and lower extremities (Morey-Olive, 2020) • Low-grade fever accompanied by acute urticaria, rashes on face, upper extremities, trunk and lower extremities • COVID-19 infection induced chilblains (Kolivras *et al.,* 2020; Romani *et al.,* 2020).
Otolaryngological	Otitis media, tinnitus (Fidan *et al.,* 2020)

INTER-INDIVIDUAL VARIATIONS IN CLINICAL PRESENTATIONS DUE TO DIFFERENTIAL SUSCEPTIBILITY TOWARDS COVID-19

Patients with COVID-19 present a range of clinical presentations. Some are silent carriers (asymptomatic), few have only fever or regular cold, some experience reduced sense of taste and smell, while others need to get hospitalized and need the assistance of a ventilator to breathe. Such a mysterious wide range of clinical manifestations has forced the clinical researchers to find out the reasons behind the differential susceptibility in humans. Various risk factors can be discussed which may be responsible for the occurrence of a range of mild to severe symptoms. Some of these factors are described below:

Age: According to CDC reports, 14-21% and 31-59% of patients were in the age range of 20-44 and 75-84 years, respectively. It is important to discuss the clinical outcomes in individual groups such as neonates/infants, children, adults, elderly and older patients (Chen *et al.,* 2020, Liu *et al.,* 2020). Studies have revealed that children and young generation have mild symptoms with good prognosis as compared to middle-aged and elderly COVID-19 patients. The major outcomes from clinical cases in different age groups are discussed in the below sections:

Neonates or Newborns (Upto 1 Month); Infants (1 Month-2 Years), Children (2-10 Years)

Several reports have been put forth which showed that COVID-19 has not even spared the population of neonate group. During the initial stages of infection, the neonates were found to be asymptomatic, having low fever and normal chest imaging and may show only mild gastrointestinal symptoms. However, later on, these may progress to severe conditions (if having one or multiple comorbid conditions) (Yu and Chen, 2020). The innate immune system of children may be responsible for the lower susceptibility to COVID-19. The infant acquires the maternal antibodies through feeding, which the mother develops after exposure to infection (Carsetti *et al.*, 2020). However, a significant number of findings revealed that infants under the age of one year might have a higher risk of severe illness with COVID-19. This can be mainly due to their immature immune systems and smaller airways, which make them more likely to develop breathing issues with respiratory virus infections. Newborns can become infected with COVID-19 during childbirth or by exposure to sick caregivers after delivery (Sun *et al.*, 2020; Hagmann, 2020). Thus, it is advised by the American Academy of Pediatrics to temporarily separate the newborn from the mother with special care and monitoring of both for symptoms of infection (Amatya *et al.*, 2020).

Various pathogens have already been reported to transmit contagious diseases in the fetus from the mother *via* direct contact during delivery, across the placenta or during breastfeeding. The RT-PCR test conducted on ten neonates delivered to mothers with COVID-19 suggested a tendency of coronaviruses (CoVs) to undergo vertical transmission. The pharyngeal swab samples showed negative results from 1-9 days after birth. Likewise, similar negative results were reported in the samples of neonatal throat swab, breast milk, amniotic fluid and cord blood samples from six COVID-19 infected pregnant women. However, a positive case report of a newborn (30 h after birth) born to a confirmed COVID-19 mother on Feb 5, 2020 raised the concerns of vertical transmission among obstetricians and health agencies. There are mixed reports of transmission. Hence extensive studies are required to investigate the chances of horizontal or vertical transmission *via* contact through the birth canal and breastfeeding (Peng *et al.*, 2020).

Table **2** contains major clinical cases of newborns, infants and children across the world affected by COVID-19. A collective study of these clinical cases from all over the world explains the asymptomatic picture of COVID-19 in newborns, infants and children. A deep molecular level understanding is required to strengthen these facts. The role of the immune system, acquired immunity through vaccination and level of expression of ACE2 in this group of population is warranted to develop hope for future.

Table 2. Clinical case reports of COVID-19 in new borns, infants and children.

S.no.	Patients	Clinical Symptoms/Manifestations	Salient Point of Recovery Period	References
1.	Female neonate born after 35+3weeks of the gestation period	• Baby's mother was feeling fatigued, fever and shortness of breath.	• After seven days of persisting symptoms in the mother, the baby was delivered by cesarean section.	Peng *et al.*, 2020

(Table 2) cont.....

S.no.	Patients	Clinical Symptoms/Manifestations	Salient Point of Recovery Period	References
		• Multiple patchy nodular opacities and GGO in sub-pleural spaces was revealed through the chest CT scan. • RT-PCR testing of throat swab showed the presence of SARS-CoV-2.	• After birth, the baby presented moaning and periodic breathing and tachypnea. • Baby's chest X-ray demonstrated bilateral lung volume reduction, thus she was given pulmonary surfactant. Test for COVID-19 was performed on different swabs samples such as of throat, anal, serum, and urine. • Each time the test came out to be negative upto 14 days. • As a result, the baby was discharged after 14 days of observation in the hospital. • The virus was also not spotted in amniotic fluid, breast milk, serum, anal swab, placenta, cord blood. • This case report confirmed the unlikeliness of transmission of coronavirus to fetus from mother during pregnancy.	Peng *et al.*, 2020

(Table 2) cont.....

S.no.	Patients	Clinical Symptoms/Manifestations	Salient Point of Recovery Period	References
2	Female neonate born after a gestation period of 38 + 4 weeks	• Baby's mother was reported to have high fever with severe bilateral pneumonia. • Baby's father was found to exhibit fever and gastroenteritis since the birth of his baby girl. • RT-PCR test for COVID-19 was found to be positive in both mother and father. • Initially, the baby girl was negative but later on became positive (8 days after birth).	• The baby girl was monitored carefully and was detected with intermittent hyperpnoea, oxygen desaturation during deep sleep and feeding. • GGO in the right peripheral region was visualized by a chest radiograph. • The symptoms resolved after 24 hours, and remained asymptomatic even 13 days after birth. • RT-PCR test continued to be positive • The clinicians attributed the appearance of COVID-19 in newborn to the transmission of virus by direct contact with mother.	Diaz *et al.*, 2020
3.	26 days old male infant	• The infant experienced 2 paroxysmal episodes- upward rolling of the eyes, hypertonia and facial cyanosis during sleep. • In the hospital, he did not present any abnormal movements. • However, fever, nasal discharge and vomiting was noted. • He was breastfed continuously, normal bowel activity, no history of gastroesophageal reflux.	• In the hospital, the infant was found to have fever and watery stools. • All other viral antigens tests were found to be negative, however, tested positive for COVID-19. • The male infant was isolated under strict rules in a negative pressure room and visits of outsiders were restricted. • He showed favourable outcomes and was discharged with advice to maintain isolation and a strict follow-up.	Chacon-Aguilar, 2020

(Table 2) cont.....

S.no.	Patients	Clinical Symptoms/Manifestations	Salient Point of Recovery Period	References
4.	1 month old male having Cystic fibrosis (CF)	• Male infant was detected positive for COVID-19, however, he remained asymptomatic. • Later on, it was revealed that he was in close contact with his grandfather, who was also detected with SARS-CoV-2 infection. • He was isolated from his family members and remained asymptomatic, no fever or any other signs.	First case reporting the occurrence of COVID-19 infection in a child with CF; baby did not present any respiratory illness and was asymptomatic.	Poli and Timpano, 2020
5.	7-week-old baby	• The patient was showing symptoms of upper respiratory tract infection. • Diagnosis of nasal and pharyngeal swabs was made using different assays.	• Immunofluorescence assay and nucleic acid amplification assays did not detect any virus in the nasopharyngeal aspirate. • Only cell cultures of nasal or pharyngeal samples detected SARS-CoV-2 virus. • The baby did not demonstrate any worsening of respiratory symptoms and thus discharged after 3 days from the hospital.	Calderaro et al., 2020

(Table 2) cont.....

S.no.	Patients	Clinical Symptoms/Manifestations	Salient Point of Recovery Period	References
6.	3-month-old female patient	• The infant was presented to emergency with rhinorrhea and nasal congestion. • No cough, fever, diarrhea, vomiting, wheezing, or dyspnea was detected • On hospital day (HD) 3, she was reported with fever. • Nasopharyngeal swab samples revealed the presence of SARS-CoV-2.	• Chest radiographs were normal. • No dyspnea, normal breath sounds without rhonchi and crepitation • Heart rate, cardiac ultrasound was normal • Hematology reports for total white blood cell, neutrophil and lymphocyte count were also normal • The infant was put on azithromycin for 5 days • Her condition remained stable and the RT-PCR test was found to be negative after 8 and 11 days • This case represents mild upper respiratory symptoms upon COVID-19 infection and was attributed to its secondary transmission from a close family member • The infection even did not transmit to her mother despite close contacts	Le et al., 2020

(Table 2) cont.....

S.no.	Patients	Clinical Symptoms/Manifestations	Salient Point of Recovery Period	References
7.	5-month-old boy (history of cardiac arrest and type I-Hurler syndrome)	• Patient was experiencing irritability, cough, low-grade fever, vomiting, runny nose for the last 24 hours • Also presented with bibasal pulmonary subcrackles, pallor and respiratory distress • Biventricular hypertrophy and cardiomegaly without consolidations were observed in chest X-ray • CT scan and echocardiography showed dilatation of left ventricle and dysfunctioning of the left ventricle • RT-PCR test was positive	• After 3 days in the hospital, the infant was presented with high fever, respiratory distress, and extensive symmetric parahilar consolidations in pericardiac region and the left side of the pulmonary base was observed • A hyperinflammation state was found 3 to 4 days after the first onset of symptoms • No lymphopenia • He was on hydroxychloroquine, ceftriaxone and and remdesivir; however, the patient had a sudden cardiac arrest • In the intensive care unit, the infant encountered a second cardiac arrest, which proved fatal. • Heart failure or cardiac myopathies in SARS-Co--2 infection may worsen the conditions	Assaad *et al.,* 2020
8.	27 week old male infant	• At 35 weeks of age, the infant was presented with sneezing, dyspnea and poor feeding for the last two days • He was assessed to have septic shock, respiratory failure, severe lactic acidosis • Bilateral air space opacification was visible in chest X-ray	• Antimicrobial treatment including cefotaxime, amoxicillin, clarithromycin, gentamicin was prescribed • Antiviral remdesivir was prescribed intravenously • This is the first report of COVID-19 infection in the premature infant which developed multiple organ injury and altered status of inflammatory markers	Cook *et al.,* 2020

(Table 2) cont.....

S.no.	Patients	Clinical Symptoms/Manifestations	Salient Point of Recovery Period	References
9.	8-month-old male patient having complex hydrocephalus (shunt malfunctioning)	• The infant was having mild temperature, dry cough, and occipital cerebrospinal fluid collection (shunt malfunctioning). • Repeated vomiting. • Shunt disconnection was also evident in the head CT scan • Interstitial pneumonia was not present in chest X-ray • However, the test of SARS-CoV-2 was positive • Later on the infant started showing upper respiratory symptoms	• After four days of surgery, vomiting worsened and it was followed by second neurosurgical surgery of the shunt • During the second surgery, no respiratory complications were reported and the baby was extubated • In this case report, it was observed that major surgeries could be performed in babies and children who are paucisymptomatic with COVID-19	Carraba *et al.*, 2020
10.	4-year-old girl; was facing unilateral nasal obstruction for one week (patient was reported to place a green sponge into the right nasal cavity during bath time)	• Swelling and mild oozing observed in the anterior nasal cavity and right nare, respectively • In the following week, an increase in sneezing, mucous drainage, foul smell and nasal obstruction was noticed • Fragments of the green sponge were removed with forceps • SARS-CoV-2 was detected through the RT-PCR test	• After one week, the infant and her mother remained asymptomatic. • First report of an asymptomatic child who had undergone surgery in the upper airway	Diercks *et al.*, 2020
11.	55-month-old girl (undergone liver transplantation and coinfection with Epstein-Barr virus (EBV)	• COVID-19 infection was confirmed 5 months after the child had undergone liver transplantation • Was having rhinitis, fever, cough, and polypnea • Liver function tests were deteriorated; Signs of anicteric cholestasis and cytolysis were also found	• The patient recovered from COVID infection despite intake of tacrolimus (immunosuppressant; 8.8 ng/mL) • Nasopharyngeal swab samples became negative after 11 days • Authors suggested that worsening of COVID-19 was not associated with liver transplantation • EBV and COVID-19 co-infections have not been found to aggravate the clinical outcome.	Morand *et al.*, 2020

(Table 2) cont.....

S.no.	Patients	Clinical Symptoms/Manifestations	Salient Point of Recovery Period	References
12.	9-year-old male patient	• He was presented to emergency with continuous fever (38.9°C) for 3 days • There were no signs of coughing, shivering, sore throat, chest distress, abdominal pain, headaches, muscle aches and cyanosis • Chest CT scan was found to be normal, however, his SARS-CoV-2 nucleic acids test was found to be positive	• Clinical manifestations were not severe. • However, proper measures were taken for isolation to prevent further transmission of infection	Yin *et al.*, 2020

Adolescent (11-19 Years), Young (20-35 Years) and Middle Aged (36-59 Years) Patients

Liao *et al.* studied the demographic, epidemiological data from 46 COVID-19 patients in the age range of 10-35 years admitted in Chongqing Three Gorges Central Hospital. Out of 46 patients, young adults constituted a major fraction (69.56%) while adolescents comprised only 30.43% (Liao *et al.*, 2020). The data from this study suggested that no severe cases have been reported in adolescent group of patients except a few with comorbid conditions. Only 6.3% adolescent patients have been shown to be asymptomatic in comparison to 14.3% of young adults. In another study, only 7 adolescent patients showed GGO on chest CT as compared to 22 young adults. Besides, significant differences have been found in various biochemical indicators such as C-reactive protein, D-dimer, lactate dehydrogenase, alanine aminotransferase and total bilirubin with higher values in young adult patients as compared to adolescents (Liao *et al.*, 2020). The incubation period of COVID-19 has also noticed to vary in adolescents, young adults and older patients. A longer incubation period is reported to be associated with adolescents, young adults as compared to older patients. Unlike newborns and infants, adolescent and young adults tend to transmit the disease to their family relations very frequently. Huang and coworkers have recorded seven family-clustered cases of COVID-19 originating from asymptomatic patients. It was observed that transmission mainly occurred through close contact among patients without any travel history (Fig. 1). Furthermore, the onset of symptoms varied among all the patients excluding patient 4 and 5 who remained asymptomatic during the study. On the other hand, CT findings were discovered within one week of onset of symptoms in 4 patients. However, commonly found CT findings consistent with COVID-19 pneumonia were also visible in asymptomatic patients (Fig. 1). CT imaging manifestations include GGO with consolidation, multilobar involvement and crazy paving signs. The study also emphasized the importance of personalized CT screening at initial stages, which may manage the further spread of infection (Huang *et al.,* 2020).

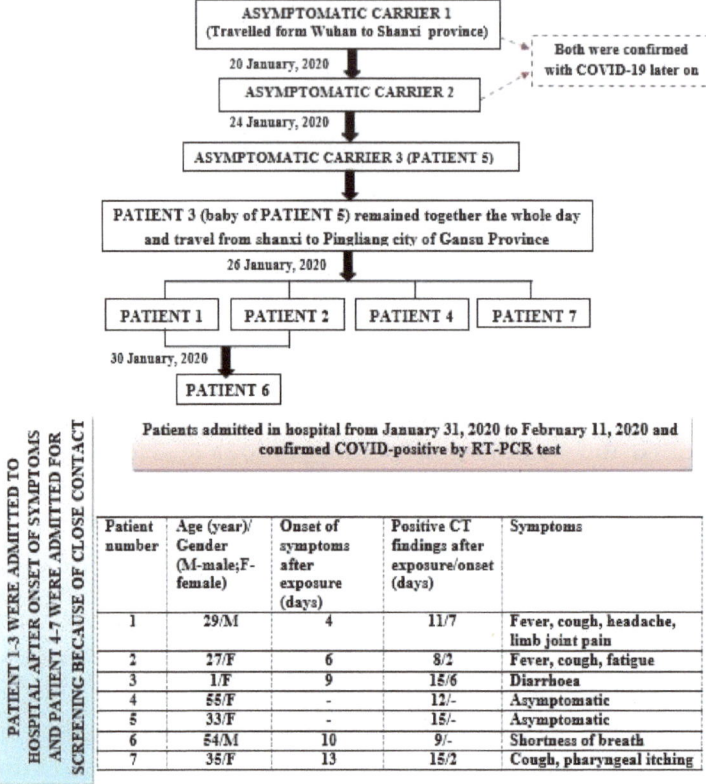

Fig. (1). Family-cluster cases of 7 COVID-19 positive patients. Figure elaborates the travel history, close contact among 7 patients, clinical characteristics and correlation between onset of symptoms and initial CT imaging features.

During the initial period of pandemic, most of the clinical reports indicated that higher number of patients were from the middle aged population with a mean incubation period and a serial interval incubation of 5.2 (range 0–14 days) and 7.5 days (2–17 days), respectively. In China, the proportion of confirmed cases involving younger patients was higher. According to the reports of Chinese CDC, approximately 4,168 confirmed COVID-19 patients with an age less than 30 years were reported till February 11, 2020. Similarly, younger individuals also constitute a major proportion of COVID-19 carriers in Italy, Japan and South Korea. The overseas travelling for study, business and work has been considered as the reason behind this hike in younger generation COVID cases (Liao *et al.,* 2020). The examples of clinical cases with atypical manifestation or presentation encountered till date have been discussed in Table 3. The clinical cases described the development of unknown pathologies along with COVID-19 or exacerbation of patient's conditions due to concomitant co-morbid states. The studies revealed that COVID-19 may also manifest neurological, cardiovascular, cutaneous, ocular, hematological and otolaryngological symptoms in addition to common pulmonary manifestations.

Table 3. Salient clinical manifestations documented in clinical cases of COVID-19 patients (Young and middle aged patients).

S. No.	Patients	Comorbid Condition	Clinical Symptoms/ Manifestations	Outcome From Study	References
1.	21-year-old male	Severe aplastic anaemia	• Pancytopenia was observed • Multiple intravenous transfusions of stem cells were done to establish haematopoietic function • He was presented with petechiae (red or purple dots on the skin) and epistaxis (Nose bleeding) • Apheresis platelets were transfused from a healthy donor to patient • It was later on intimated that the platelet donor was detected with COVID-19 infection • However, platelet donor and recipient both remained negative for SARS-CoV-2	COVID-19 patients should avoid donating blood in their recovery period; wait for about 28 days after resolution of symptoms or completion of therapy	Cho et al., 2020
2.	21-year-old male	Dependent on cocaine and methamphetamine with a smoking habit	• Fever, dyspnea, dry cough, fatigue, myalgia and diarrhea • No chills, nausea, vomiting, abdominal and chest pain • Positive test for parainfluenza virus • GGO was observed • Dyspnea worsened • SARS-CoV-2 was tested positive	Simultaneous infection of parainfluenza and COVID-19 virus can cause severe pneumonia which can further deteriorate to ARDS	Rodriguez et al., 2020

(Table 3) cont.....

S. No.	Patients	Comorbid Condition	Clinical Symptoms/ Manifestations	Outcome From Study	References
3.	29-year-old male	Tricuspid atresia	• Fevers, fatigue, cough and shortness of breath • Was in close contact with family member having COVID-19 • No reports of gastrointestinal or neurological symptoms, anosmia and taste disturbances • RT-PCR test was positive for COVID-19 • Chest X-ray revealed bilateral patch opacities	Hypoxic conditions developed after COVID-19 infection can complicate the case in adults with a congenital heart defect	Ahluwalia et al., 2020
4.	29-year-old	Obesity (BMI: 42 kg/m^2)	• Patient was suffering from fever, myalgia, non-productive cough, sore throat, malaise, respiratory distress, mild peripheral cyanosis from the past 8 days • Bilateral fine crackles was evidenced in lungs while consolidation was not present • SARS CoV-2 was tested positive again after 5 days • Bilateral, multifocal airspace opacities were observed in chest CT • EKG showed sinus tachycardia • Cardiac marker-creatine kinase-myocardial band initially increased and normalized after 3 days, however, cardiac troponin I, and myoglobin remained normal	COVID-19 infection increased the chances of occurrence of cardiac arrhythmias and failure	Loghin et al, 2020

(Table 3) cont.....

S. No.	Patients	Comorbid Condition	Clinical Symptoms/ Manifestations	Outcome From Study	References
5.	29-year-old woman	-	• Patient was experiencing fever, headaches, cough, shortness of breath and developed seizures in past few days • Neurologic exam notified decreased blink, global aphasia, facial palsy and spontaneous movement against gravity • Temporoparietal hemorrhagic venous infarct and thrombosis was observed in sinus by non-contrast head CT • Microcytic anemia was also detected (hemoglobin-5.5 g/dL) • The signals of MRI brain showed the presence of hemorrhagic infarct in different regions • Diplopia was complained • Bilateral 6th nerve palsies and papilledema was also detected	The study emphasized that young individuals are more prone to develop Venous Thrombo Embolism (VTE) along with neurologic complications	Klein *et al.*, 2020

(Table 3) cont.....

S. No.	Patients	Comorbid Condition	Clinical Symptoms/ Manifestations	Outcome From Study	References
6.	35-year-old female	--	• Patient was diagnosed with otalgia media accompanied by tinnitus • COVID-19 symptoms were absent • No comorbid diseases • Hyperemia and bulging tympanic membrane was noticed • Mild rhonchi was found in the lower region of the thorax • Hearing loss in right ear was measured by audiometry and tympanometry tests • Chest X-ray showed bilateral lung involvement • RT-PCR tests was positive for COVID-19	No classical symptoms of COVID-19 and instead presented an adult otitis media as an atypical manifestation	Fidan et al., 2020
7.	49-year-old male	--	• High fever was accompanied by dry cough, shortness of breath • However, symptoms such as nausea, vomiting, skin rash, sore throat were absent • EKG reports were found to be normal • Chest X ray showed middle lobe opacity • Noticed to have bradycardia, AV block and dissociation	Case report demonstrate an unusual outcome (transient high-degree AV block) in young COVID-19 patient without any previous cardiac comorbidities or conduction disease	Kir et al., 2020

(Table 3) cont.....

S. No.	Patients	Comorbid Condition	Clinical Symptoms/ Manifestations	Outcome From Study	References
			• Cardiac biomarkers including troponin I, NT-proBNP were normal. • Mild elevation in inflammatory markers, ferritin and C-reactive protein • RT-PCR test of nasopharyngeal swab indicated the presence of SARS-COV-2		
8.	33-year-old pregnant woman	Sickle cell disease, acute chest syndrome, necrosis in joints	• Presented with anemia • First nasal swab test was disclosed to be negative for COVID-19 • Patient was convinced to undergo surgical abortion at gestation period of 15 weeks (HD-11) • Placenta was evaluated for COVID-19 and the test resulted negative • On following days, patient was detected with hypotension and pneumonia • RT-PCR test was detected positive after 13 days of onset of symptoms	• RT-PCR test for COVID may show false negative results • COVID infection may transfer from healthcare workers to patients	Fang *et al.*, 2020
9.	33-year-old female; Gestational age- 34 weeks	--	• Patient was diagnosed with pancytopenia • Hemoperfusion improved anemia and thrombocytopenia • RT-PCR test was positive for COVID-19 • GGO with consolidation was revealed in upper part of right lobe • Higher creatinine levels were observed (up to 6.8 mg/dl)	COVID-19 possess the tendency to develop Acute Tubular Necrosis (ATN)	Taghizadieh *et al.*, 2020

(Table 3) cont.....

S. No.	Patients	Comorbid Condition	Clinical Symptoms/ Manifestations	Outcome From Study	References
10.	34-year-old man	HIV patient	• 14 days before admission hospital, he was presented with fever, cough, and dyspnea and was attributed to influenza A infection • He was treated for influenza and again had a acute onset of fever, chills, cough and shortness of breath (HD 1) • From HD 2-HD8, symptomatic worsening was observed by chest CT • On HD 9, bronchoscopy was done • Pathology reports indicated patchy chronic inflammation in alveolar tissue, intra-alveolar fibrin, pneumocyte hyperplasia leading to acute lung injury	• Patient experienced very uncommon symptoms during hospitalization • COVID-19 rapidly progressed the pulmonary disease and was diagnosed after 9 days of illness by bronchoscopic biopsy and BAL	Harkin *et al.*, 2020
11.	35-year-old woman	--	• Drug refractory seizures were observed along with headache, nausea, dizziness • There were no motor or sensory deficits • According to MRI reports, left anterior temporal lobectomy was achieved and postoperatively, she was tested positive for COVID-19 • Encephalitis was diagnosed 5 days post surgery indicating possibility of neuroinvasion of SARS-CoV-2	• The findings confirmed the occurrence of encephalitis in COVID-19 positive patient • COVID-19 (viral RNA) can invade in brain tissues	Efe *et al.*, 2020

(Table 3) cont.....

S. No.	Patients	Comorbid Condition	Clinical Symptoms/ Manifestations	Outcome From Study	References
12.	36-year-old woman (Gestation period-33 weeks)	Diabetes mellitus, asthma, maternal obesity and preeclampsia in her previous two pregnancies	• Presented with fever, muscle pain and dry cough for last four days • Sudden onset of vomiting, nausea and epigastric pain was observed with blood sugars > 200 mg/dl • Acute pancreatitis was diagnosed on HD 2 • Chest radiograph showed diffuse bilateral infiltrates • Persistent dry cough followed by development of dyspnea • COVID-19 test remained positive even after four weeks	Human pancreatitis can develop upon COVID-19 infection	Rabice et al., 2020
13.	39-year-old male	Diabetes Mellitus and hyperlipidemia	• Presented with high temperature and cough post visiting Italy and London and 8 days prior to hospital visit • Primary issues were restlessness, shivering and body aches • There were no signs of dyspnea, abdominal or chest pain, vomiting and diarrhea • Mild respiratory distress and Diaphoresis was also diagnosed • Heart was tachycardic without murmurs; Chest CT revealed GGO with consolidation • SARS-CoV-2 was found to be present in nasopharyngeal swab samples	Young COVID-19 patients with accompanying comorbid conditions presented worsening of respiratory and cardiovascular symptoms	Shah et al., 2020

(Table 3) cont.....

S. No.	Patients	Comorbid Condition	Clinical Symptoms/ Manifestations	Outcome From Study	References
14.	41-year-old male	Well controlled Human Immunodeficiency Syndrome (HIV) and recurrent Herpes Simplex Virus (HSV)	• Experienced illness six days prior to start of dry cough and intermittent fever • EKG showed tachycardia • Chest CT revealed diffused and patchy nodular ground glass infiltrates • Patient presented with acute encephalopathy, lumbar puncture revealed no white blood cells • On HD 2, detection of encephalopathy, agitation, left sided ptosis and occurrence of tonic-clonic seizure, tongue laceration subsequently led to respiratory arrest • COVID-19 testing was positive	COVID-19 may increase the chances of renal injury, tachycardia, tonic-clonic seizure	Haddad *et al.,* 2020

(Table 3) cont.....

S. No.	Patients	Comorbid Condition	Clinical Symptoms/ Manifestations	Outcome From Study	References
15.	42-year-old male	--	• Diagnosed 12 days earlier with mild symptoms of COVID-19 infection • Later on dyspnea worsened; chest pain, and hemoptysis was also manifested • Mild respiratory distress along with development of bibasilar rhonchi • EKG displayed slow flattening of T waves • Computerized Tomography Angiography (CTA) reports revealed that bilateral pulmonary emboli and consolidation was present in right lower lobe • Peripheral GGO was also noted	Hemoptysis has also been detected as an uncommon symptom of COVID-19 infection	Casey et al., 2020

(Table 3) cont.....

S. No.	Patients	Comorbid Condition	Clinical Symptoms/ Manifestations	Outcome From Study	References
16.	42-year-old-male	--	• Patient reported pain in abdominal, testicular, and back region for past 8 days • Was having fever two days before presentation • No signs of nausea, vomiting, rhinorrhea, sore throat, cough, and shortness of breath was observed • Chest radiographs revealed no abnormal findings, however, abdominal and pelvic region CT scan spotted pulmonary GGO and consolidation in lung bases • In addition, colitis was identified in descending and sigmoidal region of colon • Two days later, the patient was detected with COVID-19 infection	Both GGO and consolidations constitute the most common radiological findings in chest CT scan reports. It is estimated to be reported in approximately 88% of COVID-19 cases	Kim et al., 2020

(Table 3) cont.....

S. No.	Patients	Comorbid Condition	Clinical Symptoms/ Manifestations	Outcome From Study	References
17.	43-year-old man	--	• Headache, fever (100.0°F) • Chest X-ray showed absence of cardiopulmonary abnormality • Patient was presenting strange actions such as talking to himself, improper eating or drinking, frequent shakings and staring at wall, sweating without having fever • RT-PCR test came positive • CT scan of head showed no acute intracranial abnormality; upon lumbar puncture, no polymorphonuclear abnormalities were disclosed in cerebrospinal fluid • The patient was described to have diaphoresis, disturbed mental status, muscle rigidity, slowed verbal responses and inability to resist gravity in all limbs	Catatonia (three or more signs- staring, stupor, rigidity, mutism, posturing, and autonomic abnormalities) has also been associated with acute COVID-19	Caan *et al.*, 2020

(Table 3) cont.....

S. No.	Patients	Comorbid Condition	Clinical Symptoms/ Manifestations	Outcome From Study	References
18.	44-year-old woman	Diabetes Mellitus, hypertension, dyslipidemia, and chronic kidney disease	• Patient was noticed with fever, cough, vomiting and pain in flank region • High creatinine levels (4.0 mg/dL), presence of blood an d protein indicated acute kidney injury • Chest X-ray indicated sub-segmental atelectasis, pleural effusion on right side, and bilateral diffuse patchy opacities • COVID-19 PCR test was found to be positive • Renal functions deteriorate simultaneously • Sjogren-syndrome was evidenced *via* an autoimmune test • Kidney biopsy-bowman space showed epithelial hypertrophy and hyperplasia, collapsing glomerulopathy • APOL1 genotyping of biopsy material revealed the presence of homozygous allele (rs73885319) for the G1 risk	COVID-19 infection aggravates the kidney injury *via* direct infection or through cytokine storm occurring in sepsis	Larson *et al.*, 2020

(Table 3) cont.....

S. No.	Patients	Comorbid Condition	Clinical Symptoms/ Manifestations	Outcome From Study	References
19.	48-year-old man	Sleep-Disordered Breathing (SDB) and Obesity	• Severe COVID-19 infection presented by fever, cough, and progressive dyspnea • Bilateral patchy pulmonary infiltrates in middle and lower regions were detected through chest X-ray • SARS-CoV-2 RNA was positive • Septic shock was observed	Thrombotic complications tend to progress in COVID-19 patients accompanied with multiple comorbidities	Dumitrascu et al., 2020
20.	48-year-old man	Hepatitis B infection	• Worsening of constipation, lower abdominal pain, hypoactive bowel sounds, dyspnea, periumbilical tenderness were recorded • Elevated levels of procalcitonin • GGO in right upper lung was also identified on examination • Surgery was performed to ameliorate acute sigmoid colonic obstruction • Pathological reports revealed adenocarcinoma T4aN0M0	COVID-19 RNA has been detected in fecal matter	Huang et al., 2020
21.	Man in his 50s	Hypertension, kidney failure, chronic hepatitis B virus infection	• Symptoms such as non-productive cough persisted for about 7 days • Patient was admitted 2 weeks later upon progression to hypoxemia without fever and myalgia • Elevation in C-reactive protein and pro-calcitonin • Throat swab samples revealed the presence of SARS-CoV-2 infection	COVID-19 infection presented very mild symptoms despite multiple comorbid conditions	Tang et al., 2020

Elderly (>60 Years) and Older (>80 Years) Patients

Geriatric population constitutes a major group of individuals. Geriatric patients have a lower immunity and the presence of comorbid conditions makes them more susceptible to bacterial/viral infections (Feng *et al.*, 2012; Low *et al.*, 2019). The prevalent medical demonstrations of COVID-19 infection in older patients are high temperature, dry cough, dyspnea and tiredness. Furthermore, some patients may develop septic shock and ARDS (Chen *et al.*, 2020; Xu *et al.*, 2020; Deng *et al*, 2020; Yang *et al.*, 2020a; Guan *et al.*, 2020). The other severe acute complications include pneumonia and acute cardiac injury. The elderly population is also highly vulnerable to COVID-19 infection and high mortality rate is reported in them (Sun *et al.*, 2020).

COVID-19 pandemic exhibited a global fatality rate of 2-5% (Ji *et al.*, 2020; Mahase Elisabeth, 2020; Wu *et al.*, 2020; Wu and McGoogan, 2020; Sun *et al.*, 2020). Nonetheless, the fatality rate in the geriatric population has been found to be 8.0% (70–79 years) and 14.8% (80 years) (Wu and McGoogan, 2020). The higher proportion of comorbidities, a weaker immune system in patients older than 80 years renders them highly susceptible to COVID-19 infection. The commonly occurring comorbidities include hypertension, diabetes mellitus, cardiac diseases, COPD, and cerebrovascular disease (6.5%) (Yang *et al.*, 2020b, Chen *et al.*, 2020). The distinct range of typical and atypical clinical manifestations found in clinical cases of COVID-19 positive elder and older patients are summarized in Table 4.

Table 4. Respiratory and non-respiratory (typical/atypical) clinical presentations in COVID-19 positive elder and older patients.

S. No.	Covid-19 Patient	Comorbid Condition (If Any)	Major Clinical Presentation Including Typical Symptoms	References
1.	51 year old male	---	Hypertensive nephropathy, diarrhea, fever, fatigue, dyspnea, abdominal pain, lymphopenia, GGO followed by consolidation.	Wang *et al.*, 2020
2.	51 year old male	Mounier-Kuhn Syndrome (MKS)	Fever, dyspnea, deterioration of chronic coughs, GGO and bronchiectasis.	Jafari *et al.*, 2020
3.	53 year old male	High blood pressure, diabetes and chronic renal failure	Dyspnea, palpitation, diarrhea, black stool along with gastrointestinal bleeding, epigastric pain, No fever and cough.	Gulen *et al.*, 2020

(Table 4) cont.....

S. No.	Covid-19 Patient	Comorbid Condition (If Any)	Major Clinical Presentation Including Typical Symptoms	References
4.	55 year old male	---	Abdominal pain and nausea for 8 days without vomiting, diarrhea, fever and any respiratory symptoms, bilateral, multifocal areas of GGO having rounded and crazy paving morphology	Sendi *et al.*, 2020
5.	56 year old male	Active smoker	Cough, rise in temperature and respiratory distress; Chest radiograph showed pneumothorax on the left side; antracotic pigmentation on the lung surface	Aiolfi *et al.*, 2020
6.	57 year old	---	Headache and malaise, no fever, respiratory or gastrointestinal symptoms, thrombocytopenia	Sadr *et al.*, 2020
7.	61 year old male	---	Cutaneous rashes which persisted for the last 4 days; cough, dyspnea along with anxiety, headache, pain in the throat, restlessness, nasal congestion, urticarial rash and erythematous papules on thighs and forearms	Quintana-Castanedo *et al.*, 2020
8.	61 year old female	Type II diabetes mellitus	Dry cough and non-radiating, sharp periumbilical pain	Mahan *et al.*, 2020
9.	61 year old male	---	Cough, fever, acute respiratory distress, GGO, bilateral pulmonary consolidations	Zubovic *et al.*, 2020
10.	62 year old male	High blood pressure, ischemic heart disease and diabetes	Persistent hiccups for four days, GGO	Prince *et al.*, 2020
11.	62 year old female	Hypertensive, prediabetic, dyslipidemic, transient ischemic attack	2-week history of cough and cold including shortness of breath, severe dysarthia, weakness in right upper and lower extremity	Oliver *et al.*, 2020
12.	62 year old male	Gallstone	Fever (persisting for last 8 days); cough and distress in the chest (persisting for last 6 days); GGO appeared in bilateral lungs later on	Wang and Hu, 2020
13.	62 year old male	---	Fevers, malaise, and dyspnea; chest radiograph revealed airspace opacities in the lung; worsening of bilateral opacities led to refractory hypoxemic conditions	Horowitz *et al.*, 2020

(Table 4) cont.....

S. No.	Covid-19 Patient	Comorbid Condition (If Any)	Major Clinical Presentation Including Typical Symptoms	References
14.	63 year old female	Smoker, recurrent adenocarcinoma, undergoing Stereotactic ablative radiotherapy for thoracic malignancy	She remained asymptomatic upto 18 days and still she was COVID positive	Samson *et al.*, 2020
15.	64 year old female	Smoker; COPD; cT1bN0M0 Non-small cell lung cancer (NSCLC) and was undergoing radiotherapy	Cough, shortness of breath, increased fatigue, post-tussive emesis and GGO in the right lower lobe	Samson *et al.*, 2020
16.	65 year old male	Abdominal aortic aneurysm, crohn's disease, hypertension, coronary artery disease, myocardial infarction, hypothyroidism, gout, lower back and hip pain	Type III Crawford thoracoabdominal aneurysm (TAAA) was detected, diarrohea with pain, fever and respiratory distress	Resch *et al.*, 2020
17.	66 year old female	Small-cell lung cancer (T1bN2M0, Stage IIIA) and was undergoing radiation therapy, obstructive sleep apnea, emphysema	Non-productive cough, dyspnea, however, fever and fatigue were absent	Samson *et al.*, 2020
18.	67 year old female	Left ventricular ejection fraction (LVEF), Cardiomyopathy	Cough, shortness of breath, left shoulder pain and serious cardiac complications	Dabbagh *et al.*, 2020
19.	65 year old male	----	Cough, fever, dyspnea, acute progressive symmetric ascending quadriparesis indicating Guillain Barne Syndrome (GBS), neurological manifestations-acute weakness of distal lower extremities, facial paresis bilaterally	Sedaghat *et al.*, 2020
20.	68 year old female	Chronic kidney disease	High temperature, elevated inflammatory markers and Chest X-ray revealed consolidation in both lungs	Abdelnour *et al.*, 2020
21.	70 year old male	COPD, coronary heart disease, arterial hypertension, diabetes mellitus, obstructive sleep apnea syndrome and obesity (body mass index: 38 kg/m^2)	Intermittent fever (> 38.5 °C), productive cough, dyspnea which persists for one week, bilateral basal coarse reticular opacities and GGO	Prattes *et al.*, 2020

(Table 4) cont.....

S. No.	Covid-19 Patient	Comorbid Condition (If Any)	Major Clinical Presentation Including Typical Symptoms	References
22.	70 year old male	Diabetes Mellitus	Fatigue, fever, and respiratory distress, bilateral, subpleural GGO, left-side pneumothorax	Aiolfi *et al.*, 2020
23.	71 year old male	----	Fever, nonproductive cough, dyspnea and myalgia for last 10 days, coarse crackles in the basal part of lungs, multifocal infiltrates developed later on. Hypoxemia and respiratory alkalosis was also observed	Kaur *et al.*, 2020
24.	71 year old male	Hypertension, chronic kidney disease, overactive bladder and seizure	Tingling and numbness in lower extremities, no respiratory problems or fever. Later on pneumonia was diagnosed in chest X-ray	Chan *et al.*, 2020
25.	71 year old female	---	Productive cough, shortness of breath, fever, maculo-papular rashes were found on the trunk similar to Grover disease	Sachdeva *et al.*, 2020
26.	72 year old male	Diabetes, hypertension, andobesity	Cough with blood-tinged sputum. Fever, sharp pain in the head, diarrhea, myalgia, ageusia, anosmia were absent. Chest X-ray revealed peripheral pulmonary opacities, kidney injury and silent hypoxia	Wilkerson *et al.*, 72
27.	72 year old male	Diabetes Mellitus and Glucose-6-phosphate dehydrogenase deficiency	Experiencing fever, nasal congestion, dry cough and dyspnea for the last 10 days, right lung GGO, severe hypoxia and metabolic acidosis, which led to cardiopulmonary arrest and death	Chhetri *et al.*, 2020
28.	73 year old male	Had undergone surgery for the treatment of T2aN0 NSCLC in 2016	Malignancy was detected in nodules, asymptomatic for typical COVID symptoms, presence of GGO was also verified in lower lobes	Polverari *et al.*, 2020
29.	73 year old female	Breast cancer, obesity, hypertension and thrombosis	Fever, severe lung damage (50-75%); GGO having a crazy paving pattern. However, pulmonary embolism was absent	Grellier *et al.*, 2020

(Table 4) cont.....

S. No.	Covid-19 Patient	Comorbid Condition (If Any)	Major Clinical Presentation Including Typical Symptoms	References
30.	73 year old male	Hyperlipidemia	Abdominal and epigastric pain accompanied by nausea, later on, the patient developed cough, chest pain, dyspnea, became tachypneic and hypoxic, consolidations were also revealed	Alkhafaji et al, 2020
31.	75 year old female	Ischemic heart disease, hypertension and acid reflux disease	Loss of appetite, weakness, however, the patient denied having any respiratory symptoms, fever, myalgia, chills and rigors, the appearance of GGO, crackles and rhonchi in lungs was also observed	Chan et al., 2020
32.	76 year old male	---	Altered mental status- decrease interaction, confusions and lethargy, dry cough	Jansen et al., 2020
33.	77 year old female	---	Fever, cough, enlargement in lymph nodal region of the neck, maculopapular exanthem and the macular hemorrhagic rash was diagnosed on the trunk and legs, No signs of pneumonia	Sachdeva et al., 2020
34.	78 year old female	Hypertension, postencephalitic, epilepsy, Herpes Simplex Virus-1 (HSV-1)	Involuntary muscular jerks on face and limbs, right central facial nerve palsy, aphasia, focal status epilepticus, pronation and drifting in arm and leg, respectively, left temporoparietal lobe was found to exhibit gliosis and atrophy, No fever and interstitial pneumonia	Vollono et al., 2020
35.	78 year old male	Hypertension	Chest pain, atrial fibrillation (150 beat/min), shortness of breath, GGO with consolidation in the right lower lobe, pericardial effusion and subsegmental atelectasis	Cizgici et al., 2020
36.	79 year old female	---	Fever, acute dyspnea, epigastric pain, GGO but no pulmonary embolism, arterial and venous abdominal thrombosis	Barry et al., 2020
37.	79 year old female	Diabetes, hyperlipidemia and hypertension	Slurred speech, left-sided weakness, aphasia, acute thromboembolic disease, no fever, bilateral peripheral, upper lobe GGO	Gill et al., 2020

(Table 4) cont.....

S. No.	Covid-19 Patient	Comorbid Condition (If Any)	Major Clinical Presentation Including Typical Symptoms	References
38.	81 year old female	---	Morning and evening fever, bilateral progression, consolidation in the left lobe, ARDS, GGO in both lobes	Zubovic et al., 2020
39.	82 year old female	---	Fever, shortness of breath, persistent cough, bilateral GGO in lower lobes	Ucpinar et al., 2020
40.	86 year old male	13 Chronic cases: Hypertension level III, senile heart valve disorders, lacunar infarction, unstable angina, cardiomegaly, hypoproteinemia, cerebral arteriosclerosis, cardiac function level II, hypertensive cardiopathy, chronic pancreatitis, calcification of aortic valve, diabetes mellitus, chronic kidney disease stage II, and typical GGO	Fever, cough, typical GGO in both lungs	Tu et al., 2020

ACE2

The gene (21 kb) located on chromosome 17 encodes a 170 kDa protein known as ACE (Angiotensin Converting Enzyme). It is a transmembrane enzyme, abundantly present on the outer membrane of enterocytes, epithelial cells of alveoli, endothelial and smooth muscle cells of arteries and veins. These transmembrane proteins are consisted of 805-amino acid long carboxypeptidase along with an outer N-terminus (17-amino acids) and intracellular C-terminus (Donoghue *et al.*, 2000, Tipnis *et al.*, 2000). The polymorphic form ACE17 helps in conversion of inactive angiotensin I (decapeptide) into active angiotensin II (octapeptide). The angiotensin I and II play an important part in maintaining homeostasis of blood pressure *via* inactivating the bradykinin vasodilator to counterbalance the vasoconstrictive action of angiotensin II. Aldosterone release is stimulated by angiotensin II, which further prompts the kidney in absorbing sodium and water (Devaux *et al.*, 2020).

The existence of polymorphic form of ACE2 gene was initially confirmed in the population of China during a cohort study on Nicotine Dependence in teens. The wide range of genetic polymorphism in ACE2 gene has been strongly associated with occurrence of arterial hypertension, diabetes mellitus, cerebral stroke, coronary artery disease, heart septal wall thickness and ventricular hypertrophy

(Lu et al., 2012, Chen et al., 2016, Zhang et al., 2018, Pinheiro et al., 2019, Luo et al., 2019). The three ACE2 variants- rs4240157, rs4646155, rs4830542 and other rs2074192, rs233575, and rs2158083 have been noticed to be correlated with hypertension (HT) and variations of blood pressure, respectively. An association of the latter mutations has also been found with HT in a study of 246 HT patients in India. In addition, Brazilian and African-American patients also revealed existence of polymorphism in ACE2 (Devaux et al., 2020).

SARS-CoV and SARS-CoV-2 share phylogenetic similarities and exploit same ACE2 human cell receptor. The existence of different polymorphic forms of ACE2 worldwide may be the rationale behind the different geographical distribution of SARS-CoV infection across the globe. The polymorphism affects the perceptivity of people towards SARS-CoV-2 infection and the resulting symptomatic outcomes. During early stage infection of SARS-CoV-2, virus spread inside body tissues and impairs the ACE2 function. The binding of virus with peptide domain of ACE2 produces steric hindrance and down regulates the ACE2 mRNA expression. However, in severe cases of COVID-19, virus attacks on ACE2 other than lung resulting in multi-organ failure. Thus, it is suggested that quantification of AngII and ACE2 can be adapted as biological markers for monitoring susceptibility of COVID-19. The interaction between ACE2 and spike protein is expected to enhance or reduce depending upon the binding compatibility of spike (S)-protein of SARS-CoV-2 with ACE2 and ultimately affecting the ability of virus to infect host cell.

Gender

COVID-19 exhibits a strong gender susceptibility difference. Such difference in gender susceptibility can be correlated to the different polymorphic forms of ACE2. The gene located on X chromosome of male generally encode ACE2 protein which can be attributed to the higher ACE2 expression in lungs of male compared with women (Smith et al., 2020). Similarly, in males the angiotensin II converts to angiotensin I at higher levels. About 66-75% severe clinical cases reported till date indicated higher proportion of men in comparison to women. In China, approximately 58% of the admitted patients were revealed to be male. Similar patterns were observed in Italy and USA. According to meta-analysis directed by Fu and coworkers, 29-77% of infected patients were male. The higher proportion of COVID-19 males was also spotted in Asia, South America, and New York. However, more women tested positive in Canada and European countries (Fu et al., 2020).

The hospitalization rates were also higher for males than female ranging from 55 to 62% in all countries. It is recorded in Europe that approximately 73% of patients admitted in ICU were men. The proportion of death ranged from 59-69% among men in comparison to women. In China, the death rates for men and women were found to be 2.8 and 1.7%, respectively. Similar higher death rates in men were estimated in Australia, Denmark, Austria, France, Seattle, Germany, Belgium, Italy, Europe, and New York. In Italy, the mortality rate of COVID-19 was also higher at all ages for men than women. Furthermore, men estimated for 60.3% deaths while women for 39.7% in New York (Rozenberg et al., 2020).

Brener has explained the association of male predominance and androgen regulation in COVID-19 cases. The proteolytic activation of S-protein of SARS-COV-2 by Transmembrane Serine Protease 2 (TMPRSS2) assists the latter's entry inside cells. TMPRSS2 enzyme is abundantly present in high grade prostate cancers and prostate epithelium. Similar male predominance was observed in pandemic influenza A and was attributed to the presence of TMPRSS2 in host cells. This concept can be considered as a strong reason behind the scarcity of COVID-19 cases in preadolescents, as they lack androgens and cellular proteases TMPRSS2. However, factor such as smoking has been found to affect men by COVID significantly as smoking tends to raise the ratio of androgens to estrogen (Brenner, 2020).

Blood Group

Biological markers may portray a crucial part in predicting susceptibility to COVID-19. The susceptibility of various viral infections has also been associated with different ABO blood groups in past such as in hepatitis B and Norwalk. It was also noticeable during SARS-CoV attack in 2003 that individuals with blood group O were less sensitive towards infection (Lindesmith et al., 2003 and Cheng et al., 2005, Batool et al., 2017). The blood groups of patients thus can act as biological marker for COVID-19 infection. Different blood groups have been studied as one of the responsible aspect for different medical outcomes in COVID patients. Zhao and his coworkers originally studied the correlation between COVID-19 and ABO blood group. An investigation was performed to determine the blood group of 1,775 COVID-19 infected patients admitted in Wuhan Jinyintan Hospital. The ABO distribution study revealed that 37.75% patients were spotted with blood group A as compared to 25.80% patients having blood group O. The results revealed that blood group A patients are more vulnerable to COVID-19 infection as compared to lower risk for blood group O. In addition, the proportion of blood group A (41.26%) was higher than blood group O (25.24%) in 206 dead patients. Another study performed on 113 patients in Renmin Hospital, Wuhan also revealed similar results. The blood group O was conjoined with lessened chance of infection as related to blood group A (Zhao et al., 2020). In consonance with above investigations, higher proportions of blood group A was also detected among 265 patients admitted in Central hospital of Wuhan (Li et al., 2020). The research carried out by Patrice and coworkers attributed the reduced susceptibility of blood group O to the decreased adhesion of S-protein of coronavirus to ACE-2 receptor by anti-A antibodies (Guillon et al., 2008). However, these speculations need further elucidation to reveal the interrelation between COVID-19 susceptibility and patient blood groups.

In addition, the lower susceptibility in blood group O patients, can also be correlated to decreased risk of cardiac complications and thrombotic disorders in comparison to other blood groups (O'Sullivan et al., 2020). Otherwise, micro thrombi may disseminate through lung vasculature and contribute to emergence of ARDS. In ABO(H) blood groups, the red blood cells (RBCs) show carbohydrate structures which are usually coincided as antigens present on RBCs. The later have not only detected on RBCs but on platelets, plasma glycoproteins such as von Willebrand factor and factor VIII and endothelial cells (O'Sullivan et al., 2020). These factors interact among themselves in complex pattern and play a conspicuous part in activating the pathogenesis of SARS-CoV-2 infection.

Lansiaux and his coworkers analyzed β-thalassemic heterozygote population for their susceptibility to COVID infection in three different regions (Puglia, Sardinia, Sicilia) of Italy employing multiple linear regression. They hypothesized that persons suffering from thalassemia have shown immunity against COVID-19 (Lansiaux et al., 2020). However, these studies are required to be performed on large population of thalassemia patients for longer period of time. Similarly, it is requisite to establish correlation between COVID-19 and other blood pathologies.

Previous Immunization

Albert Calmette and Camille Guerin were the first to introduce Bacillus Calmette-Guerin (BCG) vaccine employing attenuated strain of *Mycobacterium bovis*. Clinically, it was administered in humans in 1921 for the treatment of tuberculosis. It is mainly indicated in neonates and infants to protect against tuberculosis, meningitis and disseminated tuberculosis (Colditz et al., 1995; Redelman-Sidi et al., 2014). Further, it has been reported that its immunomodulatory properties have non-specific (off-target) effects on immune system which is helpful for fighting against infections other than respiratory infections. BCG vaccine is also used as an adjuvant immunotherapeutic agent and for curing bladder cancer (Goodridge et al., 2016; Pollard et al., 2017).

In clinical studies, BCG-Danish has been found to reduce the mortality by 38% in neonates (Guinea-Bissau) and 73% in adolescents (South Africa) suffering from pneumonia, sepsis or infection in respiratory tract (Nemes et al., 2018; Curtis et al., 2020). It has also showed a reduction in cases of yellow fever, viraemia (volunteers in the Netherlands), mengovirus (encephalomyocarditis virus) infection (Old *et al.,* 1961; Floch *et al.,* 1976). In addition, such vaccines have the tendency to induce epigenetic and metabolic alterations which can help in attaining trained immunity by upgrade the existing immune system (Netea *et al.,* 2020). On the basis of above speculations, different vaccinations have been considered to demonstrate beneficial effects against COVID-19 infection. The concept has nevertheless various limitations and is required to research at larger levels and in high risk populations.

The frequency of COVID-19 infection in neonates and children is very low. The frequent vaccinations and infections in neonates, infants and children have been considered as the major key factor in development of innate immunity system (Lyu *et al.,* 2020). The clinical cases discussed in this chapter (Table 2) also elaborate that mild symptomatic cases have very low chances of transmission to other children or adults. Lyu and coworkers also focused that administration of vaccines for pneumonia, influenza, and tuberculosis, may act as protection shield against COVID-19 (Lyu *et al.,* 2020).

COMORBIDITY

It is a well known that COVID-19 infection have proven fatal in patient with Comorbid conditions. The investigations performed by Niu *et al.* also revealed that COVID-19 has exaggerated the severity of comorbid conditions in elder and older patients (Niu *et al.,* 2020). The common and uncommon clinical manifestations in different age groups have been documented in different clinical studies as described in Tables **2**, **3** and **4** .

CONCLUSION

COVID-19 pandemic has not only manifested itself in the form of respiratory symptoms but a myriad of other uncommon presentations also. Different age groups may present different manifestations such as asymptomatic or mild symptoms in infants, children or adult, severe and atypical presentations in elder and older group. The atypical symptoms observed in COVID-19 patients include cardiovascular, hematological, renal, cutaneous, ocular, otolaryngological alterations. Although the young population has encountered the infection in higher number, however, the severity and fatality rate is higher in older patients. Silent (asymptomatic/presymptomatic) carriers of COVID-19 also pose an additional concern regarding the silent transmission/spread of COVID-19 infection. The scientific community has continuously updated the occurrence of typical/atypical presentation of COVID-19 infection. Their knowledge may help in future clinical cases in preventing any delay in early diagnosis and unknown transmission to non-infected individuals.

LIST OF ABBREVIATIONS

ACE2	Angiotensin Converting Enzyme 2
ALT	Alanine Transaminase
ARDS	Acute Respiratory Distress Syndrome
AST	Aspartate Transaminase
ATN	Acute Tubular Necrosis
BCG	Bacillus Calmette–Guerin
CT	Computed Tomography
CF	Cystic Fibrosis
COPD	Chronic Obstructive Pulmonary Disease
CoV	Coronavirus
CTA	Computerized Tomography Angiography
EBV	Epstein–Barr virus
ECG/EKG	Electrocardiography
FLAIR	Fluid-Attenuated Inversion Recovery
GBS	Guillain Barne syndrome
GERD	Gateroesophageal Reflux Disease
GGO	Ground Glass Opacities
HIV	Human Immunodeficiency Syndrome
HSV	Herpes Simplex Virus
HBsAg	Hepatitis B Antigen
HD	Hospital Day
HT	Hypertension
LVEF	Left Ventricular Ejection Fraction
MKS	Mounier-Kuhn Syndrome
NBS	New Born Screening
NSCLC	Non-Small Cell Lung Cancer
RT-PCR	Reverse Transcriptase-Polymerase Chain Reaction
SARS-CoV-2	Severe Acute Respiratory Syndrome Coronavirus-2
TAAA	Thoraco-Abdominal Aneurysm
TMPRSS2	Transmembrane Protease Serine 2
VTE	Venus Thromoboembolism

CONSENT FOR PUBLICATION

Not applicable.

CONFLICT OF INTEREST

The author declares no conflict of interest, financial or otherwise.

ACKNOWLEDGEMENTS

Declared none.

REFERENCES

Abdelnour, LH & Abdalla, ME (2020) Progression of CXR features on a COVID-19 survivor. *IDCases,* 21, e00834.
[http://dx.doi.org/10.1016/j.idcr.2020.e00834] [PMID: 32461911]

Ahluwalia, N, Love, B, Chan, A & Zaidi, AN (2020) COVID-19 in an adult with tricuspid atresia S/P fontan palliation. *JACC Case Rep.*
[http://dx.doi.org/10.1016/j.jaccas.2020.05.013]

Aiolfi, A, Biraghi, T, Montisci, A, Bonitta, G, Micheletto, G, Donatelli, F, Cirri, S & Bona, D (2020) Management of persistent pneumothorax with thoracoscopy and blebs resection in COVID-19 patients. *Ann Thorac Surg,* 110, e413-5.
[http://dx.doi.org/10.1016/j.athoracsur.2020.04.011]

Amatya, S, Corr, TE, Gandhi, CK, Glass, KM, Kresch, MJ, Mujsce, DJ, Oji-Mmuo, CN, Mola, SJ, Murray, YL, Palmer, TW, Singh, M, Fricchione, A, Arnold, J, Prentice, D, Bridgeman, CR, Smith, BM, Gavigan, PJ, Ericson, JE, Miller, JR, Pauli, JM, Williams, DC, McSherry, GD, Legro, RS, Iriana, SM & Kaiser, JR (2020) Management of newborns exposed to mothers with confirmed or suspected COVID-19. *J Perinatol,* 40, 987-96.
[http://dx.doi.org/10.1038/s41372-020-0695-0] [PMID: 32439956]

Batool, Z, Durrani, SH & Tariq, S (2017) Association of ABO and Rh blood group types to hepatitis B, hepatitis C, HIV and Syphillis infection, a five years experience in healthy blood donors in a tertiary care hospital. *J Ayub Med Coll Abbottabad,* 29, 90-2.
[PMID: 28712183]

Bonow, RO, Fonarow, GC, O'Gara, PT & Yancy, CW (2020) Association of coronavirus disease 2019 (COVID-19) with myocardial injury and mortality. *JAMA Cardiol,* 5, 751-3.
[http://dx.doi.org/10.1001/jamacardio.2020.1105]

Bosch, BJ, Bartelink, W & Rottier, PJ (2008) Cathepsin L functionally cleaves the severe acute respiratory syndrome coronavirus class I fusion protein upstream of rather than adjacent to the fusion peptide. *J Virol,* 82, 8887-90.
[http://dx.doi.org/10.1128/JVI.00415-08] [PMID: 18562523]

Brenner, SR (2020) Covid-19, TMPRSS2, and whether android regulation affects pandemic virus gender incidence and age distribution of disease. *Med Hypotheses,* 140, 109773.
[http://dx.doi.org/10.1016/j.mehy.2020.109773] [PMID: 32339776]

Caan, MP, Lim, CT & Howard, M (2020) A case of catatonia in a man with COVID-19. *Psychosomatics,* 61, 556-60.
[http://dx.doi.org/10.1016/j.psym.2020.05.021]

Calderaro, A, Arcangeletti, MC, De Conto, F, Buttrini, M, Montagna, P, Montecchini, S, Ferraglia, F, Pinardi, F & Chezzi, C (2020) SARS-CoV-2 infection diagnosed only by cell culture isolation before the

local outbreak in an Italian seven-week-old suckling baby. *Int J Infect Dis,* 96, 387-9.
[http://dx.doi.org/10.1016/j.ijid.2020.05.035] [PMID: 32417248]

Carrabba, G, Tariciotti, L, Guez, S, Calderini, E & Locatelli, M (2020) Neurosurgery in an infant with COVID-19. *Lancet,* 395, e76.
[http://dx.doi.org/10.1016/S0140-6736(20)30927-2] [PMID: 32333840]

Carrillo-Larco, RM & Altez-Fernandez, C (2020) Anosmia and dysgeusia in COVID-19: A systematic review. *Wellcome Open Res,* 5, 94.
[http://dx.doi.org/10.12688/wellcomeopenres.15917.1] [PMID: 32587902]

Carsetti, R, Quintarelli, C, Quinti, I, Piano Mortari, E, Zumla, A, Ippolito, G & Locatelli, F (2020) The immune system of children: the key to understanding SARS-CoV-2 susceptibility? *Lancet Child Adolesc Health,* 4, 414-6.
[http://dx.doi.org/10.1016/S2352-4642(20)30135-8] [PMID: 32458804]

Cascella, M, Rajnik, M, Cuomo, A, Dulebohn, SC & Di Napoli, R (2020) *Features, Evaluation and Treatment Coronavirus (COVID-19).* StatPearls Publishing Treasure Island, FL.

Casey, K, Iteen, A, Nicolini, R & Auten, J (2020) COVID-19 pneumonia with hemoptysis: Acute segmental pulmonary emboli associated with novel coronavirus infection. *Am J Emerg Med,* 38, 1544.e1-3.
[http://dx.doi.org/10.1016/j.ajem.2020.04.011] [PMID: 32312574]

Chan, KH, Farouji, I, Harnoud, AA & Slim, J (2020) Weakness and elevated creatinine kinase as the initial presentation of coronavirus disease 2019 (COVID-19). *Am J Emerg Med,* 38, 1548.e1-3.

Chen, N, Zhou, M, Dong, X, Qu, J, Gong, F, Han, Y, Qiu, Y, Wang, J, Liu, Y, Wei, Y, Xia, J, Yu, T, Zhang, X & Zhang, L (2020) Epidemiological and clinical characteristics of 99 cases of 2019 novel coronavirus pneumonia in Wuhan, China: a descriptive study. *Lancet,* 395, 507-13.
[http://dx.doi.org/10.1016/S0140-6736(20)30211-7] [PMID: 32007143]

Chen, YY, Liu, D, Zhang, P, Zhong, JC, Zhang, CJ, Wu, SL, Zhang, YQ, Liu, GZ, He, M, Jin, LJ & Yu, HM (2016) Impact of ACE2 gene polymorphism on antihypertensive efficacy of ACE inhibitors. *J Hum Hypertens,* 30, 766-71.
[http://dx.doi.org/10.1038/jhh.2016.24] [PMID: 27121444]

Chen, Z, Fan, H, Cai, J, Li, Y, Wu, B, Hou, Y, Xu, S, Zhou, F, Liu, Y, Xuan, W, Hu, H & Sun, J (2020) High-resolution computed tomography manifestations of COVID-19 infections in patients of different ages. *Eur J Radiol,* 126, 108972.
[http://dx.doi.org/10.1016/j.ejrad.2020.108972] [PMID: 32240913]

Cheng, Y, Cheng, G, Chui, CH, Lau, FY, Chan, PK, Ng, MH, Sung, JJ & Wong, RS (2005) ABO blood group and susceptibility to severe acute respiratory syndrome. *JAMA,* 293, 1450-1.
[PMID: 15784866]

Chhetri, S, Khamis, F, Pandak, N, Al Khalili, H, Said, E & Petersen, E (2020) A fatal case of COVID-19 due to metabolic acidosis following dysregulate inflammatory response (cytokine storm). *IDCases,* 21, e00829.
[http://dx.doi.org/10.1016/j.idcr.2020.e00829] [PMID: 32483525]

Cho, HJ, Koo, JW, Roh, SK, Kim, YK, Suh, JS, Moon, JH, Sohn, SK & Baek, DW (2020) COVID-19 transmission and blood transfusion: A case report. *J Infect Public Health,* 13, 1678-9.
[http://dx.doi.org/10.1016/j.jiph.2020.05.001] [PMID: 32405329]

Cizgici, AY, Zencirkiran Agus, H & Yildiz, M (2020) COVID-19 myopericarditis: It should be kept in mind in today's conditions. *Am J Emerg Med,* 38, 1547.e5-6.
[http://dx.doi.org/10.1016/j.ajem.2020.04.080] [PMID: 32360119]

Co, COC, Yu, JRT, Laxamana, LC & David-Ona, DIA (2020) Intravenous thrombolysis for stroke in a COVID-19 positive filipino patient a case report. *J Clin Neurosci,* 77, 234-6.
[http://dx.doi.org/10.1016/j.jocn.2020.05.006]

Colditz, GA, Berkey, CS, Mosteller, F, Brewer, TF, Wilson, ME, Burdick, E & Fineberg, HV (1995) The efficacy of bacillus Calmette-Guérin vaccination of newborns and infants in the prevention of tuberculosis:

meta-analyses of the published literature. *Pediatrics,* 96, 29-35.
[PMID: 7596718]

Cook, J, Harman, K, Zoica, B, Verma, A, D'Silva, P & Gupta, A (2020) Horizontal transmission of severe acute respiratory syndrome coronavirus 2 to a premature infant: multiple organ injury and association with markers of inflammation. *Lancet Child Adolesc Health,* 4, 548-51.
[http://dx.doi.org/10.1016/S2352-4642(20)30166-8] [PMID: 32442422]

Curtis, N, Sparrow, A, Ghebreyesus, TA & Netea, MG (2020) Considering BCG vaccination to reduce the impact of COVID-19. *Lancet,* 395, 1545-6.
[http://dx.doi.org/10.1016/S0140-6736(20)31025-4] [PMID: 32359402]

Dabbagh, MF, Aurora, L, D'Souza, P, Weinmann, AJ, Bhargava, P & Basir, MB (2020) Cardiac tamponade secondary to COVID-19. *JACC Case Rep,* 2, 1326-30.

de Barry, O, Mekki, A, Diffre, C, Seror, M, El Hajjam, M & Carlier, RY (2020) Arterial and venous abdominal thrombosis in a 79-year-old woman with COVID-19 pneumonia. *Radiol Case Rep,* 15, 1054-7.
[http://dx.doi.org/10.1016/j.radcr.2020.04.055] [PMID: 32351657]

Deng, SQ & Peng, HJ (2020) Characteristics of and public health responses to the coronavirus disease 2019 outbreak in China. *J Clin Med,* 9, 575.
[http://dx.doi.org/10.3390/jcm9020575] [PMID: 32093211]

Diaz, CA, Maestro, ML, Pumarega, MTM, Anton, BF & Alonso, CP (2020) First case of neonatal infection due to COVID 19 in Spain. *An Pediatr (Engl Ed)* 237-8.

Donoghue, M, Hsieh, F, Baronas, E, Godbout, K, Gosselin, M, Stagliano, N, Donovan, M, Woolf, B, Robison, K, Jeyaseelan, R, Breitbart, RE & Acton, S (2000) A novel angiotensin-converting enzyme-related carboxypeptidase (ACE2) converts angiotensin I to angiotensin 1-9. *Circ Res,* 87, E1-9.
[http://dx.doi.org/10.1161/01.RES.87.5.e1] [PMID: 10969042]

Driggin, E, Madhavan, MV, Bikdeli, B, Chuich, T, Laracy, J, Biondi-Zoccai, G, Brown, TS, Der Nigoghossian, C, Zidar, DA, Haythe, J, Brodie, D, Beckman, JA, Kirtane, AJ, Stone, GW, Krumholz, HM & Parikh, SA (2020) Cardiovascular considerations for patients, health care workers, and health systems during the COVID-19 pandemic. *J Am Coll Cardiol,* 75, 2352-71.
[http://dx.doi.org/10.1016/j.jacc.2020.03.031] [PMID: 32201335]

Dumitrascu, OM, Volod, O, Bose, S, Wang, Y, Biousse, V & Lyden, PD (2020) Acute ophthalmic artery occlusion in a COVID-19 patient on apixaban. *J Stroke Cerebrovasc Dis,* 29, 104982.
[http://dx.doi.org/10.1016/j.jstrokecerebrovasdis.2020.104982]

Efe, IE, Aydin, OU, Alabulut, A, Celik, O & Aydin, K (2020) COVID-19-associated encephalitis mimicking glial tumor: A case report. *World Neurosurg,* 140, 46-8.

El Assaad, I, Hood-Pishchany, MI, Kheir, J, Mistry, K, Dixit, A, Halyabar, O, Mah, DY, Meyer-Macaulay, C & Cheng, H (2020) Complete heart block, severe ventricular dysfunction and myocardial inflammation in a child with COVID-19 infection. *JACC Case Rep,* 2, 1351-5.

Eliezer, M, Hautefort, C, Hamel, AL, Verillaud, B, Herman, P, Houdart, E & Eloit, C (2020) Sudden and complete olfactory loss function as a possible symptom of COVID-19. *JAMA Otolaryngol Head Neck Surg,* 146, 674-5.
[http://dx.doi.org/10.1001/jamaoto.2020.0832]

Fang, NZ, Castaño, PM & Davis, A (2020) A hospital-based COVID-19 abortion case in the early phase of the pandemic. *Contraception,* 102, 137-8.
[http://dx.doi.org/10.1016/j.contraception.2020.05.005] [PMID: 32416144]

Feng, Z, Liu, C, Guan, X & Mor, V (2012) China's rapidly aging population creates policy challenges in shaping a viable long-term care system. *Health Aff (Millwood),* 31, 2764-73.
[http://dx.doi.org/10.1377/hlthaff.2012.0535] [PMID: 23213161]

Fidan, V (2020) New type of corona virus induced acute otitis media in adult. *Am J Otolaryngol,* 41, 102487.

[http://dx.doi.org/10.1016/j.amjoto.2020.102487] [PMID: 32336572]

Floc'h, F & Werner, GH (1976) Increased resistance to virus infections of mice inoculated with BCG (Bacillus calmette-guérin). *Ann Immunol (Paris),* 127, 173-86.
[PMID: 180868]

Fu, L, Wang, B, Yuan, T, Chen, X, Ao, Y, Fitzpatrick, T, Li, P, Zhou, Y, Lin, Y, Duan, Q & Luo, G (2020) Clinical characteristics of coronavirus disease 2019 (COVID-19) in China: a systematic review and meta-analysis. *J Infect,* 80, 656-65.

Giacomelli, A, Pezzati, L, Conti, F, Bernacchia, D, Siano, M, Oreni, L, Rusconi, S, Gervasoni, C, Ridolfo, AL, Rizzardini, G, Antinori, S & Galli, M (2020) Self-reported olfactory and taste disorders in patients with severe acute respiratory coronavirus 2 infection: A cross-sectional study. *Clin Infect Dis,* 71, 889-90.
[http://dx.doi.org/10.1093/cid/ciaa330] [PMID: 32215618]

Goodridge, HS, Ahmed, SS, Curtis, N, Kollmann, TR, Levy, O, Netea, MG, Pollard, AJ, van Crevel, R & Wilson, CB (2016) Harnessing the beneficial heterologous effects of vaccination. *Nat Rev Immunol,* 16, 392-400.
[http://dx.doi.org/10.1038/nri.2016.43] [PMID: 27157064]

Grellier, N, Hadhri, A, Bendavid, J, Adou, M, Demory, A, Bouchereau, S, Hassani, W, Hervé, ML, Mahé, M, Colson-Durand, L & Belkacemi, Y (2020) Regional lymph node irradiation in breast cancer may worsen lung damage in COVID-19 positive patients. *Adv Radiat Oncol,* 5, 722-6.

Guan, WJ, Ni, ZY, Hu, Y, Liang, WH, Ou, CQ, He, JX, Liu, L, Shan, H, Lei, CL, Hui, DSC, Du, B, Li, LJ, Zeng, G, Yuen, KY, Chen, RC, Tang, CL, Wang, T, Chen, PY, Xiang, J, Li, SY, Wang, JL, Liang, ZJ, Peng, YX, Wei, L, Liu, Y, Hu, YH, Peng, P, Wang, JM, Liu, JY, Chen, Z, Li, G, Zheng, ZJ, Qiu, SQ, Luo, J, Ye, CJ, Zhu, SY & Zhong, NS China Medical Treatment Expert Group for Covid-19 (2020) Clinical characteristics of coronavirus disease 2019 in China. *N Engl J Med,* 382, 1708-20.
[http://dx.doi.org/10.1056/NEJMoa2002032] [PMID: 32109013]

Guillon, P, Clément, M, Sébille, V, Rivain, JG, Chou, CF, Ruvoën-Clouet, N & Le Pendu, J (2008) Inhibition of the interaction between the SARS-CoV spike protein and its cellular receptor by anti-histo-blood group antibodies. *Glycobiology,* 18, 1085-93.
[http://dx.doi.org/10.1093/glycob/cwn093] [PMID: 18818423]

Gulen, M (2020) Uncommon presentation of Covid-19: gastrointestinal bleeding. *Clin Res Hepatol Gastroenterol,* 44, e72-6.
[http://dx.doi.org/10.1016/j.clinre.2020.05.001]

Haddad, S, Tayyar, R, Risch, L, Churchill, G, Fares, E, Choe, M & Montemuro, P (2020) Encephalopathy and seizure activity in a COVID-19 well controlled HIV patient. *IDCases,* 21, e00814.
[http://dx.doi.org/10.1016/j.idcr.2020.e00814] [PMID: 32426230]

Hagmann, SHF (2020) COVID-19 in children: More than meets the eye. *Travel Med Infect Dis,* 34, 101649.
[http://dx.doi.org/10.1016/j.tmaid.2020.101649] [PMID: 32234457]

Harkin, TJ, Rurak, KM, Martins, J, Eber, C, Szporn, AH & Beasley, MB (2020) Delayed diagnosis of COVID-19 in a 34-year-old man with atypical presentation. *Lancet Respir Med,* 8, 644-6.
[http://dx.doi.org/10.1016/S2213-2600(20)30232-0]

Hassan, SA, Sheikh, FN, Jamal, S, Ezeh, JK & Akhtar, A (2020) Coronavirus (COVID-19): A review of clinical features, diagnosis, and treatment. *Cureus,* 12, e7355.
[http://dx.doi.org/10.7759/cureus.7355] [PMID: 32328367]

Horowitz, JM, Yuriditsky, E, Henderson, IJ, Stachel, MW, Kwok, B & Saric, M (2020) Clot in transit on transesophageal echocardiography in a prone patient with COVID-19 acute respiratory distress syndrome. *CASE (Phila),* 4, 200-3.

Huang, L, Jiang, J, Li, X, Zhou, Y, Xu, M & Zhou, J (2020) Initial CT imaging characters of an imported family cluster of COVID-19. *Clin Imaging,* 65, 78-81.
[http://dx.doi.org/10.1016/j.clinimag.2020.04.010]

Huang, Z, Yan, J, Jin, T, Huang, X, Zeng, G, Adashek, ML, Wang, X, Li, J, Zhou, D & Wu, Z (2020) The challenges of urgent radical sigmoid colorectal cancer resection in a COVID-19 patient-a case report. *Int J Surg Case Rep,* 71, 147-50.
[http://dx.doi.org/10.1016/j.ijscr.2020.04.088]

Inciardi, RM, Lupi, L, Zaccone, G, Italia, L, Raffo, M, Tomasoni, D, Cani, DS, Cerini, M, Farina, D, Gavazzi, E & Maroldi, R (2020) Cardiac involvement in a patient with coronavirus disease 2019 (COVID-19). *JAMA Cardiol,* 5, 819-24.
[http://dx.doi.org/10.1001/jamacardio.2020.1096]

Jafari, R, Cegolon, L, Dehghanpoor, F, Javanbakht, M, Izadi, M, Saadat, SH, Otoukesh, B & Einollahi, B (2020) Early manifestation of ARDS in COVID-19 infection in a 51-year-old man affected by Mounier-Kuhn syndrome. *Heart Lung,* 49, 855-7.

Jansen, JH & Day, RL (2020) A novel presentation of COVID-19 *via* community acquired infection. *Vis J Emerg Med,* 20, 100760.
[http://dx.doi.org/10.1016/j.visj.2020.100760]

Ji, Y, Ma, Z, Peppelenbosch, MP & Pan, Q (2020) Potential association between COVID-19 mortality and health-care resource availability. *Lancet Glob Health,* 8, e480.
[http://dx.doi.org/10.1016/S2214-109X(20)30068-1] [PMID: 32109372]

Kaur, P, Qaqa, F, Ramahi, A, Shamoon, Y, Singhal, M, Shamoon, F, Maroules, M & Singh, B (2020) Acute upper limb ischemia in a patient with COVID-19. *Hematology/Oncology and Stem Cell Therapy.*
[http://dx.doi.org/10.1016/j.hemonc.2020.05.001]

Kim, J, Thomsen, T, Sell, N & Goldsmith, AJ (2020) Abdominal and testicular pain: An atypical presentation of COVID-19. *Am J Emerg Med.*
[http://dx.doi.org/10.1016/j.ajem.2020.03.052]

Kir, D, Mohan, C & Sancassani, R (2020) Heart brake-an unusual cardiac manifestation of coronavirus disease 2019 (COVID-19). *JACC Case Rep.*

Klein, DE, Libman, R, Kirsch, C & Arora, R (2020) Cerebral venous thrombosis: atypical presentation of COVID-19 in the young. *Journal of Stroke and Cerebrovascular Diseases.*

Kolivras, A, Dehavay, F, Delplace, D, Feoli, F, Meiers, I, Milone, L, Olemans, C, Sass, U, Theunis, A, Thompson, CT & Van De Borne, L (2020) Coronavirus (COVID-19) infection–induced chilblains: A case report with histopathologic findings. *JAAD Case Reports.*
[http://dx.doi.org/10.1016/j.jdcr.2020.04.011]

Lansiaux, E, Pébaÿ, PP, Picard, JL & Son-Forget, J (2020) COVID-19: beta-thalassemia subjects immunised? *Med Hypotheses,* 142, 109827.
[http://dx.doi.org/10.1016/j.mehy.2020.109827] [PMID: 32447232]

Larsen, CP, Bourne, TD, Wilson, JD, Saqqa, O & Moh'd, A, S (2020) Collapsing glomerulopathy in a patient with coronavirus disease 2019 (COVID-19). *Kidney International Reports.*

Lauer, SA, Grantz, KH, Bi, Q, Jones, FK, Zheng, Q, Meredith, HR, Azman, AS, Reich, NG & Lessler, J (2020) The incubation period of coronavirus disease 2019 (COVID-19) from publicly reported confirmed cases: estimation and application. *Ann Intern Med,* 172, 577-82.
[http://dx.doi.org/10.7326/M20-0504] [PMID: 32150748]

Le, HT, Nguyen, LV, Tran, DM, Do, HT, Tran, HT, Le, YT & Phan, PH (2020) The first infant case of COVID-19 acquired from a secondary transmission in Vietnam. *Lancet Child Adolesc Health,* 4, 405-6.
[http://dx.doi.org/10.1016/S2352-4642(20)30091-2] [PMID: 32213326]

Li, J, Wang, X, Chen, J, Cai, Y, Deng, A & Yang, M (2020) Association betweenABOblood groups and risk of SARS-CoV-2 pneumonia. *Br J Haematol,* 190, 24-7.
[http://dx.doi.org/10.1111/bjh.16797] [PMID: 32379894]

Liao, J, Fan, S, Chen, J, Wu, J, Xu, S, Guo, Y, Li, C, Zhang, X, Wu, C, Mou, H, Song, C, Li, F, Wu, G,

Zhang, J, Guo, L, Liu, H, Lv, J, Xu, L & Lang, C (2020) Epidemiological and clinical characteristics of COVID-19 in adolescents and young adults. *Innovation (N Y)*, 1, 100001.
[http://dx.doi.org/10.1016/j.xinn.2020.04.001] [PMID: 33554183]

Lindesmith, L, Moe, C, Marionneau, S, Ruvoen, N, Jiang, X, Lindblad, L, Stewart, P, LePendu, J & Baric, R (2003) Human susceptibility and resistance to Norwalk virus infection. *Nat Med*, 9, 548-53.
[http://dx.doi.org/10.1038/nm860] [PMID: 12692541]

Liu, Y, Gu, Z, Xia, S, Shi, B, Zhou, XN, Shi, Y & Liu, J (2020) What are the underlying transmission patterns of COVID-19 outbreak?–an age-specific social contact characterization. *EClinical Medicine*, 100354.
[http://dx.doi.org/10.1016/j.eclinm.2020.100354]

Low, LL, Kwan, YH, Ko, MSM, Yeam, CT, Lee, VSY, Tan, WB & Thumboo, J (2019) Epidemiologic characteristics of multimorbidity and sociodemographic factors associated with multimorbidity in a rapidly aging asian country. *JAMA Netw Open*, 2, e1915245.
[http://dx.doi.org/10.1001/jamanetworkopen.2019.15245] [PMID: 31722030]

Lu, N, Yang, Y, Wang, Y, Liu, Y, Fu, G, Chen, D, Dai, H, Fan, X, Hui, R & Zheng, Y (2012) ACE2 gene polymorphism and essential hypertension: an updated meta-analysis involving 11,051 subjects. *Mol Biol Rep*, 39, 6581-9.
[http://dx.doi.org/10.1007/s11033-012-1487-1] [PMID: 22297693]

Luo, Y, Liu, C, Guan, T, Li, Y, Lai, Y, Li, F, Zhao, H, Maimaiti, T & Zeyaweiding, A (2019) Correction: Association of ACE2 genetic polymorphisms with hypertension-related target organ damages in south Xinjiang. *Hypertens Res*, 42, 744-4.
[http://dx.doi.org/10.1038/s41440-019-0205-y] [PMID: 30675038]

Lyu, J, Miao, T, Dong, J, Cao, R, Li, Y & Chen, Q (2020) Reflection on lower rates of COVID-19 in children: Does childhood immunizations offer unexpected protection? *Med Hypotheses*, 143, 109842.
[http://dx.doi.org/10.1016/j.mehy.2020.109842] [PMID: 32425304]

Mahan, K, Kabrhel, C & Goldsmith, AJ (2020) Abdominal pain in a patient with COVID-19 infection: A case of multiple thromboemboli. *Am J Emerg Med*, 38, 2245.e3-5.
[http://dx.doi.org/10.1016/j.ajem.2020.05.054] [PMID: 32513452]

Mahase, E (2020) Coronavirus: COVID-19 has killed more people than SARS and MERS combined, despite lower case fatality rate. *BMJ*, 368, m641.
[http://dx.doi.org/10.1136/bmj.m641]

McIntosh, K, Hirsch, MS & Bloom, A (2020) Coronavirus disease 2019 (COVID-19). *Situation Report-72 by World Health Organisation.*

Mjaess, G, Karam, A, Aoun, F, Albisinni, S & Roumeguère, T (2020) COVID-19 and the male susceptibility: the role of ACE2, TMPRSS2 and the androgen receptor. *Prog Urol*, 30, 484-7.
[http://dx.doi.org/10.1016/j.purol.2020.05.007] [PMID: 32620366]

Morand, A, Roquelaure, B, Colson, P, Amrane, S, Bosdure, E, Raoult, D, Lagier, JC & Fabre, A (2020) Child with liver transplant recovers from COVID-19 infection. A case report. *Arch Pediatr*, 27, 275-6.
[http://dx.doi.org/10.1016/j.arcped.2020.05.004] [PMID: 32402433]

Morey-Olive, M, Espiau, M, Mercadal-Hally, M, Lera-Carballo, E & García-Patos, V (2020) Cutaneous manifestations in the current pandemic of coronavirus infection disease (COVID 2019). *Anales De Pediatria.*

Navel, V, Chiambaretta, F & Dutheil, F (2020) Haemorrhagic conjunctivitis with pseudomembranous related to SARS-CoV-2. *Am J Ophthalmol Case Rep*, 19, 100735.
[http://dx.doi.org/10.1016/j.ajoc.2020.100735] [PMID: 32377594]

Nemes, E, Geldenhuys, H, Rozot, V, Rutkowski, KT, Ratangee, F, Bilek, N, Mabwe, S, Makhethe, L, Erasmus, M, Toefy, A, Mulenga, H, Hanekom, WA, Self, SG, Bekker, LG, Ryall, R, Gurunathan, S, DiazGranados, CA, Andersen, P, Kromann, I, Evans, T, Ellis, RD, Landry, B, Hokey, DA, Hopkins, R, Ginsberg, AM, Scriba, TJ & Hatherill, M C-040-404 Study Team (2018) Prevention of *M. tuberculosis*

infection with H4: IC31 vaccine or BCG revaccination. *N Engl J Med,* 379, 138-49.
[http://dx.doi.org/10.1056/NEJMoa1714021] [PMID: 29996082]

Netea, MG, Domínguez-Andrés, J, Barreiro, LB, Chavakis, T, Divangahi, M, Fuchs, E, Joosten, LAB, van der Meer, JWM, Mhlanga, MM, Mulder, WJM, Riksen, NP, Schlitzer, A, Schultze, JL, Stabell Benn, C, Sun, JC, Xavier, RJ & Latz, E (2020) Defining trained immunity and its role in health and disease. *Nat Rev Immunol,* 20, 375-88.
[http://dx.doi.org/10.1038/s41577-020-0285-6] [PMID: 32132681]

Niu, S, Tian, S, Lou, J, Kang, X, Zhang, L, Lian, H & Zhang, J (2020) Clinical characteristics of older patients infected with COVID-19: A descriptive study. *Arch Gerontol Geriatr,* 89, 104058.
[http://dx.doi.org/10.1016/j.archger.2020.104058] [PMID: 32339960]

O'Sullivan, JM, Ward, S, Fogarty, H & O'Donnell, JS (2020) More on "association between ABO blood groups and risk of SARS-CoV-2 pneumonia. *Br J Haematol,* 190, 24-7.
[http://dx.doi.org/10.1111/bjh.16845]

Old, LJ, Benacerraf, B, Clarke, DA, Carswell, EA & Stockert, E (1961) The role of the reticuloendothelial system in the host reaction to neoplasia. *Cancer Res,* 21, 1281-300.
[PMID: 14481701]

Peng, Z, Wang, J, Mo, Y, Duan, W, Xiang, G, Yi, M, Bao, L & Shi, Y (2020) Unlikely SARS-CoV-2 vertical transmission from mother to child: A case report. *J Infect Public Health,* 13, 818-20.
[http://dx.doi.org/10.1016/j.jiph.2020.04.004] [PMID: 32305459]

Pinheiro, DS, Santos, RS, Jardim, PCBV, Silva, EG, Reis, AAS, Pedrino, GR & Ulhoa, CJ (2019) The combination of ACE I/D and ACE2 G8790A polymorphisms revels susceptibility to hypertension: A genetic association study in Brazilian patients. *PLoS One,* 14, e0221248.
[http://dx.doi.org/10.1371/journal.pone.0221248] [PMID: 31430320]

Poli, P, Timpano, S, Goffredo, M, Padoan, R & Badolato, R (2020) Asymptomatic case of Covid-19 in an infant with cystic fibrosis. *J Cyst Fibros,* 19, e18.
[http://dx.doi.org/10.1016/j.jcf.2020.03.017] [PMID: 32303430]

Pollard, AJ, Finn, A & Curtis, N (2017) Non-specific effects of vaccines: plausible and potentially important, but implications uncertain. *Arch Dis Child,* 102, 1077-81.
[http://dx.doi.org/10.1136/archdischild-2015-310282] [PMID: 28501809]

Polverari, G, Arena, V, Ceci, F, Pelosi, E, Ianniello, A, Poli, E, Sandri, A & Penna, D (2020) ^{18}F-Fluorodeoxyglucose uptake in patient with asymptomatic severe acute respiratory syndrome Coronavirus 2 (Coronavirus Disease 2019) referred to positron emission tomography/computed tomography for NSCLC restaging. *J Thorac Oncol,* 15, 1078-80.
[http://dx.doi.org/10.1016/j.jtho.2020.03.022] [PMID: 32243920]

Prattes, J, Valentin, T, Hoenigl, M, Talakic, E, Reisinger, AC & Eller, P (2020) Invasive pulmonary aspergillosis complicating COVID-19 in the ICU-A case report. *Med Mycol Case Rep,* 31, 2-5.
[PMID: 32395423]

Prince, G & Sergel, M (2020) Persistent hiccups as an atypical presenting complaint of COVID-19. *Am J Emerg Med,* 38, 1546.e5-6.

Quintana-Castanedo, L, Feito-Rodríguez, M, Valero-López, I, Chiloeches-Fernández, C, Sendagorta-Cudós, E & Herranz-Pinto, P (2020) Urticarial exanthem as early diagnostic clue for COVID-19 infection. *JAAD Case Rep,* 6, 498-9.
[http://dx.doi.org/10.1016/j.jdcr.2020.04.026] [PMID: 32352022]

Rabice, SR, Altshuler, PC, Bovet, C, Sullivan, C & Gagnon, AJ (2020) COVID-19 infection presenting as pancreatitis in a pregnant woman: A case report. *Case Rep Womens Health,* 27, e00228.
[http://dx.doi.org/10.1016/j.crwh.2020.e00228] [PMID: 32537425]

Redelman-Sidi, G, Glickman, MS & Bochner, BH (2014) The mechanism of action of BCG therapy for bladder cancer--a current perspective. *Nat Rev Urol,* 11, 153-62.

[http://dx.doi.org/10.1038/nrurol.2014.15] [PMID: 24492433]

Resch, T, Vogt, K & Md, NE (2020) A typical COVID-19 presentation in patient undergoing staged TAAA repair. *J Vasc Surg Cases Innov,* 6, 337-9.

Rodriguez, JA, Rubio-Gomez, H, Roa, AA, Miller, N & Eckardt, PA (2020) Co-Infection with SARS-COV-2 and Parainfluenza in a young adult patient with pneumonia: Case Report. *IDCases,* 20, e00762.
[http://dx.doi.org/10.1016/j.idcr.2020.e00762] [PMID: 32368493]

Romani, J, Baselga, E, Mitja, O, Riera-Marti, N, Garbayo, P, Vicente, A, Casals, M, Fumado, V, Fortuny, C & Calzado, S (2020) Chilblain and acral purpuric lesions in Spain during COVID confinement: Retrospective analysis of 12 cases. *Actas Dermo-sifiliograficas.*

Sachdeva, M, Gianotti, R, Shah, M, Lucia, B, Tosi, D, Veraldi, S, Ziv, M, Leshem, E & Dodiuk-Gad, RP (2020) Cutaneous manifestations of COVID-19: Report of three cases and a review of literature. *J Dermatol Sci,* 98, 75-81.
[http://dx.doi.org/10.1016/j.jdermsci.2020.04.011]

Sadr, S, SeyedAlinaghi, S, Ghiasvand, F, Hassan Nezhad, M, Javadian, N, Hossienzade, R & Jafari, F (2020) Isolated severe thrombocytopenia in a patient with COVID-19: A case report. *IDCases,* 21, e00820.
[http://dx.doi.org/10.1016/j.idcr.2020.e00820] [PMID: 32483524]

Sendi, AA, Saggat, DF & Alzahrani, SJ (2020) Incidental typical COVID-19 appearance on the lung bases, visualized at abdominal CT for a patient that presented with abdominal pain and nausea. *Radiol Case Rep,* 15, 1238-41.
[http://dx.doi.org/10.1016/j.radcr.2020.05.039] [PMID: 32542102]

Samson, P, Ning, MS, Shaverdian, N, Shepherd, AF, Gomez, DR, McGinnis, GJ, Nitsch, PL, Chmura, S, O'Reilly, MS, Lee, P, Chang, JY, Robinson, C & Lin, SH (2020) Clinical and Radiographic Presentations of COVID-19 Among Patients Receiving Radiation Therapy for Thoracic Malignancies. *Adv Radiat Oncol,* 5, 700-4.
[http://dx.doi.org/10.1016/j.adro.2020.04.020] [PMID: 32395673]

Sedaghat, Z & Karimi, N (2020) Guillain Barre syndrome associated with COVID-19 infection: A case report. *J Clin Neurosci,* 76, 233-5.
[http://dx.doi.org/10.1016/j.jocn.2020.04.062] [PMID: 32312628]

Rozenberg, S, Vandromme, J & Martin, C (2020) Are we equal in adversity? Does Covid-19 affect women and men differently? *Maturitas,* 138, 62-8.
[http://dx.doi.org/10.1016/j.maturitas.2020.05.009] [PMID: 32425315]

Shah, K, Kamler, J, Phan, A & Toy, D (2020) Imaging & other potential predictors of deterioration in COVID-19. *Am J Emerg Med,* 38, 1547.e1-4.
[http://dx.doi.org/10.1016/j.ajem.2020.04.075]

Smith, JC & Sheltzer, JM (2020) Cigarette smoke triggers the expansion of a subpopulation of respiratory epithelial cells that express the SARS-CoV-2 receptor ACE2. *BioRxiv.*
[http://dx.doi.org/10.1101/2020.03.28.013672]

Sun, M, Xu, G, Yang, Y, Tao, Y, Pian-Smith, M, Madhavan, V, Xie, Z & Zhang, J (2020) Evidence of mother-to-newborn infection with COVID-19. *Br J Anaesth,* 125, e245-7.

Sun, P, Qie, S, Liu, Z, Ren, J & Xi, JJ (2020) Clinical characteristics of 50466 patients with 2019-nCoV infection. *MedRxiv.*

Taghizadieh, A, Mikaeili, H, Ahmadi, M & Valizadeh, H (2020) Acute kidney injury in pregnant women following SARS-CoV-2 infection: A case report from Iran. *Respir Med Case Rep,* 30, 101090.
[http://dx.doi.org/10.1016/j.rmcr.2020.101090] [PMID: 32405454]

Tang, B, Li, S, Xiong, Y, Tian, M, Yu, J, Xu, L, Zhang, L, Li, Z, Ma, J, Wen, F & Feng, Z (2020) Coronavirus disease 2019 (COVID-19) pneumonia in a hemodialysis patient. *Kidney Med,* 2, 354-8.
[http://dx.doi.org/10.1016/j.xkme.2020.03.001]

Temmel, AF, Quint, C, Schickinger-Fischer, B, Klimek, L, Stoller, E & Hummel, T (2002) Characteristics of olfactory disorders in relation to major causes of olfactory loss. *Arch Otolaryngol Head Neck Surg,* 128, 635-41.
[http://dx.doi.org/10.1001/archotol.128.6.635] [PMID: 12049556]

Tipnis, SR, Hooper, NM, Hyde, R, Karran, E, Christie, G & Turner, AJ (2000) A human homolog of angiotensin-converting enzyme. Cloning and functional expression as a captopril-insensitive carboxypeptidase. *J Biol Chem,* 275, 33238-43.
[http://dx.doi.org/10.1074/jbc.M002615200] [PMID: 10924499]

Tu, Y, Fang, J, Yin, M, Yu, W & Li, Y (2020) A Cured COVID-19 case of 86-year-old with 13 chronic diseases: A Case Report. *JTO Clin Res Rep,* 1, 100038.

Ucpinar, BA, Sahin, C & Yanc, U (2020) Spontaneous pneumothorax and subcutaneous emphysema in COVID-19 patient: Case report. *J Infect Public Health,* 13, 887-9.

Valette, X, du Cheyron, D & Goursaud, S (2020) Mediastinal lymphadenopathy in patients with severe COVID-19. *Lancet Infect Dis,* 20, 1230.
[http://dx.doi.org/10.1016/S1473-3099(20)30310-8]

Vegar-Zubovic, S, Izetbegovic, S, Zukic, F, Jusufbegovic, M, Kristic, S & Prevljak, S (2020) A case series of chest imaging manifestation of COVID-19. *Radiography (Lond),* 26, e319-21.

Vetter, P, Vu, DL, L'Huillier, AG, Schibler, M, Kaiser, L & Jacquerioz, F (2020) Clinical features of COVID-19. *BMJ,* 369, m1470.
[http://dx.doi.org/10.1136/bmj.m1470]

Vollono, C, Rollo, E, Romozzi, M, Frisullo, G, Servidei, S, Borghetti, A & Calabresi, P (2020) Focal status epilepticus as unique clinical feature of COVID-19: A case report. *Seizure.*

Wang, D, Hu, B, Hu, C, Zhu, F, Liu, X, Zhang, J, Wang, B, Xiang, H, Cheng, Z, Xiong, Y, Zhao, Y, Li, Y, Wang, X & Peng, Z (2020) Clinical characteristics of 138 hospitalized patients with 2019 novel coronavirus–infected pneumonia in Wuhan, China. *JAMA,* 323, 1061-9.
[http://dx.doi.org/10.1001/jama.2020.1585] [PMID: 32031570]

Wang, Q & Hu, Z (2020) Successful recovery of severe COVID-19 with cytokine storm treating with extracorporeal blood purification. *Int J Infect Dis,* 96, 618-20.
[http://dx.doi.org/10.1016/j.ijid.2020.05.065] [PMID: 32470601]

Wang, R, Liao, C, He, H, Hu, C, Wei, Z, Hong, Z, Zhang, C, Liao, M & Shui, H (2020) COVID-19 in hemodialysis patients: a report of 5 cases. *Am J Kidney Dis,* 76, 141-3.
[http://dx.doi.org/10.1053/j.ajkd.2020.03.009] [PMID: 32240718]

Wang, Y, Wang, Y, Chen, Y & Qin, Q (2020) Unique epidemiological and clinical features of the emerging 2019 novel coronavirus pneumonia (COVID-19) implicate special control measures. *J Med Virol,* 92, 568-76.
[http://dx.doi.org/10.1002/jmv.25748] [PMID: 32134116]

Wilkerson, RG, Adler, JD, Shah, NG & Brown, R (2020) Silent hypoxia: A harbinger of clinical deterioration in patients with COVID-19. *Am J Emerg Med.*
[http://dx.doi.org/10.1016/j.ajem.2020.05.044]

Wu, J, Liu, J, Zhao, X, Liu, C, Wang, W, Wang, D, Xu, W, Zhang, C, Yu, J, Jiang, B & Cao, H (2020) Clinical characteristics of imported cases of COVID-19 in Jiangsu province: a multicenter descriptive study. *Clin Infect Dis,* 10.
[http://dx.doi.org/10.1093/cid/ciaa199] [PMID: 32109279]

Wu, P, Duan, F, Luo, C, Liu, Q, Qu, X & Liang, L (2020) Characteristics of ocular findings of patients with coronavirus disease 2019 (COVID-19) in hubei province, China. *JAMA Ophthalmol,* 138, 575-8.
[http://dx.doi.org/10.1001/jamaophthalmol.2020.1291]

Wu, Z & McGoogan, JM (2020) Characteristics of and important lessons from the coronavirus disease 2019 (COVID-19) outbreak in China: summary of a report of 72 314 cases from the Chinese Center for Disease

Control and Prevention. *JAMA,* 323, 1239-42.
[http://dx.doi.org/10.1001/jama.2020.2648] [PMID: 32091533]

Xu, X, Yu, C, Qu, J, Zhang, L, Jiang, S, Huang, D, Chen, B, Zhang, Z, Guan, W, Ling, Z, Jiang, R, Hu, T, Ding, Y, Lin, L, Gan, Q, Luo, L, Tang, X & Liu, J (2020) Imaging and clinical features of patients with 2019 novel coronavirus SARS-CoV-2. *Eur J Nucl Med Mol Imaging,* 47, 1275-80.
[http://dx.doi.org/10.1007/s00259-020-04735-9] [PMID: 32107577]

Xydakis, MS, Dehgani-Mobaraki, P, Holbrook, EH, Geisthoff, UW, Bauer, C, Hautefort, C, Herman, P, Manley, GT, Lyon, DM & Hopkins, C (2020) Smell and taste dysfunction in patients with COVID-19. *Lancet Infect Dis,* 20, 1015-6.
[http://dx.doi.org/10.1016/S1473-3099(20)30293-0]

Yang, W, Cao, Q, Qin, L, Wang, X, Cheng, Z, Pan, A, Dai, J, Sun, Q, Zhao, F, Qu, J & Yan, F (2020) Clinical characteristics and imaging manifestations of the 2019 novel coronavirus disease (COVID-19): A multi-center study in Wenzhou city, Zhejiang, China. *J Infect,* 80, 388-93.
[http://dx.doi.org/10.1016/j.jinf.2020.02.016]

Yang, X, Yu, Y, Xu, J, Shu, H, Xia, J, Liu, H, Wu, Y, Zhang, L, Yu, Z, Fang, M, Yu, T, Wang, Y, Pan, S, Zou, X, Yuan, S & Shang, Y (2020) Clinical course and outcomes of critically ill patients with SARS-CoV-2 pneumonia in Wuhan, China: a single-centered, retrospective, observational study. *Lancet Respir Med,* 8, 475-81.
[http://dx.doi.org/10.1016/S2213-2600(20)30079-5] [PMID: 32105632]

Yin, X, Dong, L, Zhang, Y, Bian, W & Li, H (2020) A mild type of childhood Covid-19-A case report. *Radiol Infect Dis,* 7, 78-80.
[http://dx.doi.org/10.1016/j.jrid.2020.03.004]

Yu, Y & Chen, P (2020) Coronavirus disease 2019 (COVID-19) in neonates and children from China: a review. *Front Pediatr,* 8, 287-99.
[http://dx.doi.org/10.3389/fped.2020.00287] [PMID: 32574286]

Zhang, Q, Cong, M, Wang, N, Li, X, Zhang, H, Zhang, K, Jin, M, Wu, N, Qiu, C & Li, J (2018) Association of angiotensin-converting enzyme 2 gene polymorphism and enzymatic activity with essential hypertension in different gender: A case-control study. *Medicine (Baltimore),* 97, e12917.
[http://dx.doi.org/10.1097/MD.0000000000012917] [PMID: 30335025]

Zhao, J, Yang, Y, Huang, HP, Li, D, Gu, DF, Lu, XF, Zhang, Z, Liu, L, Liu, T, Liu, YK & He, YJ (2020) Relationship between the ABO blood group and the COVID-19 susceptibility. *MedRxiv.*

Zhou, F, Yu, T, Du, R, Fan, G, Liu, Y, Liu, Z, Xiang, J, Wang, Y, Song, B, Gu, X, Guan, L, Wei, Y, Li, H, Wu, X, Xu, J, Tu, S, Zhang, Y, Chen, H & Cao, B (2020) Clinical course and risk factors for mortality of adult inpatients with COVID-19 in Wuhan, China: a retrospective cohort study. *Lancet,* 395, 1054-62.
[http://dx.doi.org/10.1016/S0140-6736(20)30566-3] [PMID: 32171076]

CHAPTER 6

Diagnosis

Richa Deshpande[1,#], Aishwarya Joshi[1,#], Nikunj Tandel[1] and Rajeev K. Tyagi[2,*]

[1] Institute of Science, Nirma University, Ahmedabad, Gujarat, India

[2] Biomedical Parasitology and Nano-immunology Lab, CSIR Institute of Microbal Technology (imtech), Chandigarh, India

Abstract: Diagnosis of COVID-19 is supremely valuable in unraveling the complex dynamics involved in SARS-CoV-2 infection and in vaccine development. With an extremely high transmission rate, and initial symptoms similar to other human respiratory viruses, there has been a tremendous urge to develop and supply accurate and rapid procedures for testing the presence of SARS-CoV-2 in a plethora of patient specimens. Scientific and healthcare communities globally have been racing to develop critically needed test kits and ensure ample supply worldwide. Containing the spread of COVID-19 poses multiple challenges, including being able to correctly identify asymptomatic viral carriers that result in the silent spread of the virus, and diagnosing the infection at early stages. Current strategies employ molecular and serological testing techniques in lower and upper respiratory tract samples. The first type detects the presence of viral genetic material and can diagnose an active COVID-19 infection, whereas serological immunoassays detect viral antibodies, which can help identify individuals who have developed an adaptive immune response to the virus, as part of an active or prior infection. The newly authorized antigen tests are designed for the rapid detection of viral antigenic proteins. More elaborative diagnostic testing based on viral genomic sequencing can determine the rate and degree of mutational variability associated with SARS-CoV-2 and identifying newly emerging viral strains for more effective vaccine development. The chapter also highlights the role of rapid, easy-to use point-of-care diagnostic tests in alleviating the challenge posed by the strain on the healthcare system and mitigating the cost of care for both individuals and the government.

Keywords: Antibody, Antigen, Biomarker, Biosensor, Chest CT, COVID-19, CRISPR, Cytokine, Detection, Diagnosis, ELISA, Hematological analysis, Immunoassay, Isothermal amplification, Microarray, POC tests, RT-PCR, SARS-CoV-2, Serology, Viral RNA.

---

[*] **Corresponding author Rajeev K. Tygai:** Biomedical Parasitology and Nano-immunology Lab, Council of Scientific and Industrial ResearchInstitute of Microbial Technology, Sector-39A, Chandigarh-160036, India; Tel: 91-172 6665278 (Off), 91-172-6665279 (Lab), 91-9899554047 (Cell); E-mail:rajeevtyagi@imtech.res.in and rajeev.gru@gmail.com

[#] These authors contributed equally

Neeraj Mittal, Sanjay Kumar Bhadada, O. P. Katare and Varun Garg (Eds.)
All rights reserved-© 2021 Bentham Science Publishers

COVID-19: A PANDEMIC DISEASE

With the current stage of the pandemic and the associated challenges presenting major hurdles, it is evident that highly sensitized and precise diagnostic measures for COVID-19 are paramount for rationalizing infection control initiatives, as well as for case identification and contact tracing (Chan *et al.*, 2020). There is an urgent necessity for rapid yet accurate SARS-CoV-2 diagnostic methods, with emphasis on what type of tests are available in the region, under what in circumstances these tests can be used, and who should be tested (Patel *et al.*, 2020).

Similar to other infectious diseases, effective COVID-19 diagnosis relies on various parameters such as patient history, respective epidemiological conditions, clinical symptoms, and, radiological and hematological analysis. However, standard guidelines state two categories of COVID-19 tests; viral RNA tests (molecular tests) to detect the presence of SARS-CoV-2 in an active infection state, and serological tests to identify whether the subject (patient) has been exposed earlier/previously to the virus and the presence of virus-specific antibodies in the serum (Li *et al.*, 2020b). Some techniques are onerous and technically taxing, hence, there is an urgent need for rapid, cost-effective, and selectively diagnostic point-of-care (POC) tests for COVID-19 capable of providing quick yet accurate, results within a duration of possibly a few minutes (Moitra *et al.*, 2020). These POC tests allow medical diagnostic testing at the time and place of patient care while offering extra benefits of speed of diagnosis and ease of use. The current POC tests available in the market utilize the aforementioned diagnosis strategies of nucleic acid detection and analysis of antigen and/or antibodies in various sample specimens (mostly nasopharyngeal swabs). POC tests are pictured to supplement laboratory testing and enable testing to be available for remote communities and populations that lack readily accessible laboratory settings. In such secluded, crisis-struck locations, small and portable mobile POC platforms are optimal for deployment, although they are lower throughput and run one sample at a time in a specified time-frame of 5-30 minutes. They can be of great value to test moderately symptomatic patients outside clinical settings (Yang *et al.*, 2020). Higher throughput, facility-based POC platforms are also available for use in hospitals and medical centers for diagnosing top-priority specimens, such as that of frontline healthcare workers and critically-ill patients. Although POC tests are a handy component of the rapid diagnostic strategy to battle the ongoing outbreak, they are strictly recommended to be used only in conjunction with PCR-based detection. Laboratory testing undoubtedly remains the foremost testing mechanism because of the presence of complex technology specifically designed to perform a sizeable number of tests at a time. Thus, parallel use of these serology-based detection techniques alongside molecular techniques is the way forward for mitigating the global, as well as regional load of the disease (CDC-Fact-Sheet, 2019).

COVID-19: EARLY DETECTION BASED ON SYMPTOMS

Clinical Analysis

Clinical presentation of COVID-19 is vague as symptoms coincide with other seasonal respiratory infections simultaneously circulating in the respective territorial population. It is observed that infected patients present with symptoms ranging in severity. Fever (37.5° C and above) must be carefully interpreted as even in severe cases; it can be present in moderation or even absent. Upper respiratory tract viral infection, noted as the leading symptom, was reported in more than 80% infected patients which also include mild fever, dry cough, soreness of the throat with probable nasal congestion, headache, fatigue, or malaise. Patients with moderate infection present symptoms like shortness of breath or tachypnea in children in addition to mild symptoms. On the other hand, highly infected patients are diagnosed with severe pneumonia, having fever associated with severe dyspnea, respiratory distress, cyanosis in children, tachypnea, and hypoxia (Cascella *et al.*, 2020). Particularly, a chest computed tomography (CT) is the expert's recommendation for the severely infected individuals and works as an auxiliary tool alongside other standard diagnostic methods. The current pandemic status depicts that it has no age-limits as it affects the newly-born and the aged people; however, those who have crossed the age of 50 are at a relatively higher risk. Additionally, patients with a history of other comorbidities such as cardiovascular disease, diabetes, lung disease, and other types of immune suppression are also at the risk of getting an infection due to their compromised immune system. Despite measurements of the severity and other symptomatic conditions, the identification marks for the COVID-19 cases, epidemiological circumstances of the respective locations and other parameters may vary from place to place, other factors which affect the diagnosis and identification of the patients (Harapan *et al.*, 2020).

According to WHO, screening for the routine causes of respiratory illness, which delineates the season of the respective location, is the rudimentary step as and when the patient first appears with the symptoms. If a sample yields a negative result, it should be sent to a referral laboratory for SARS-CoV-2 detection. Real-time RT-PCR assay is the preferred molecular test for detecting SARS-CoV-2 infection in a clinical specimen, while serology-based techniques are used as adjunct tools. Specimen for testing must be collected from both the upper respiratory tract (*i.e.*, nasopharyngeal (NP) and oropharyngeal (OP) swabs) as well as the lower respiratory tract (*i.e.*, expectorated sputum, endotracheal aspirate, or bronchoalveolar lavage (BAL)), depending on the symptom shown by the patient. NP and OP swabs are preferred since they are better for the patient to tolerate, safe to collect and yield higher diagnostic results. To evaluate patients suspected of having pneumonia, self-collected saliva and nasal washes may be alternative upper respiratory tract specimen (Tang et al., 2020).

Hematological Analysis

To better identify the status of infection, other laboratory examinations of blood and plasma specimen are taken into consideration. These include liver and renal function tests, urine routine test, erythrocyte sedimentation rate (ESR), coagulation image, myocardial enzyme, myoglobin, C-reactive protein (CRP), procalcitonin (PCT), lactate dehydrogenase (LDH), D-dimer. Additionally, inflammatory factors such as interleukins (IL-6, IL-10, tumor necrosis factor- α (TNF-α), interferon γ (IFN-γ)), 11 items of tuberculosis subgroup, complement, anti-acid staining are also analyzed (Jin et al., 2020). Blood gas analysis, in combination with analysis of lactic acid, is performed to determine the oxygenation of moderately and severely ill patients. The increased level of liver enzymes (alanine aminotransferase (ALT) and aspartate aminotransferase (AST)), muscle enzyme, ESR and myoglobin has also been reported in certain patients (Zhongnan Hospital of Wuhan University) (Jin et al., 2020). The detection of CRP and PCT is important to check for the history of bacterial infection in the lung. D-dimer was found to be significantly high, in accordance with microthrombotic formation and frequent clotting disorders in peripheral blood vessels of severely infected patients. In the early stage of the infection, a steady or decreased total white blood cell (WBC) and lymphocyte count are also observed in peripheral blood samples (Cascella et al., 2020). A study of 41 infected patients admitted to the Jin Yin-tan Hospital in Wuhan, China, showed that the detection of other cytokines and chemokines, specifically IL-1β, IL-1 receptor antagonist (IL-1RA), IL-2, IL-4, IL-5, IL-7, IL-8 (or CXCL8), IL-9, IL-12 heterodimer p70 (IL-12p70), IL-13, IL-15, IL-17A, Eotaxin (or CCL11), basic fibroblastic growth factor (FGF2), granulocyte colony-stimulating factor (GCSF or CSF3), granulocyte-macrophage colony-stimulating factor (GMCSF or CSF2), IFN-γ induced protein (IP-10 or CXCL10), monocyte chemo-attractant protein (MCP1 or CCL2), macrophage inflammatory protein MIP-1α (or CCL3) and MIP-1β (or CCL4), platelet-derived growth factor subunit-B (PDGFB), regulated upon activation, normal T-Cell expressed and presumably secreted chemokine (RANTES or CCL5) and vascular endothelial growth factor-A (VEGFA) in plasma samples may help in preliminary evaluation of the patient's immune status. It was also noted that COVID-19 patients had increased amounts of IL-1β, IFN-γ, IP10, and MCP1, thus activating T-helper-1 (Th1) cell responses. Moreover, higher concentrations of GCSF, IP-10, MCP1, MIP-1α, and TNF-α were observed in patients requiring ICU admission when compared to those that do not, indicating that the cytokine storm is related to disease severity. SARS-CoV-2 infection also initiated a surge in secretion of T-helper-2 (Th2) cytokines (IL-4 and IL-10) responsible for suppressing inflammation (Huang *et al.*, 2020).

Chest CT

The National Health Commission of the People's Republic of China published the diagnosis and treatment program (6th version), stating that the diagnosis of SARS-CoV-2 pneumonia on the basis of radiologic observations is one of the diagnostic criteria for COVID-19, with CT scan being the preferred modality. Accurate diagnosis based on chest CT examinations could indicate isolation of the virus and plays a vital role in the management of patients with suspected SARS-CoV-2 pneumonia. Singular or multiple areas of ground-glass opacities (GGO) and consolidation are two predominant signs of lesions on CT images of COVID-19 patients (Li *et al.*, 2020a).

Studies show CT imaging demonstrates five stages of COVID-19 in accordance with the time of onset and the body's response to the virus (Jin *et al.*, 2020).

1. ***Ultra-early Stage***: The stage where patients have no significant clinical manifestations but positive reports of throat swab for SARS-CoV-2 within 1–2 weeks post-exposure. Major imaging manifestations include single, double or scattered focal GGO and patchy GGO surrounding nodules in the central lobule. Middle and lower lobes of lung show patchy consolidation and signs of intra-bronchial air bronchogram.
2. ***Early Stage***: The period of 1–3 days post clinical manifestations (fever, cough, fatigue, dry cough, *etc.*). The alveolar septal capillary shows dilatation and congestion, along with interlobular interstitial edema and exudation of fluid in alveolar cavity. Images showed scattered (single or multiple) patchy or agglomerated GGO, separated by grid-like or honeycomb-like thickening of interlobular septa.
3. ***Rapid Progression Stage***: The period of about 3–7 days after onset of clinical manifestations, where numerous cell-rich exudates collect in the alveolar cavity, with aggravated alveolar and interstitial edema due to vascular expansion and exudation in the interstitium. CT scan shows a large-scale, fused light consolidation containing air-bronchogram.
4. ***Consolidation Stage***: Around 7–14 days after appearance of clinical manifestations, in which the alveolar cavity shows fibrous exudation and the alveolar wall shows no capillary congestion. CT images show lesser density and smaller range of multiple patchy consolidations in comparison to the previous stage.

5. ***Dissipation Stage***: A period of approximately 2 and 3 weeks post onset, during which there was further reduction in lesion range and CT scans showed strip-like opacity or patchy consolidation. As time progressed, interlobular septum showed grid-like thickening, bronchial wall showed thickening and strip-like twist and some scattered patchy consolidations (Jin *et al.*, 2020).

Usage of chest CT to diagnose COVID-19 is a controversial matter although detailed features of CT images of the disease have been reported. Very few are available in public forum which creates the scarcity in the appropriate understanding of the disease. With CT examination of SARS-CoV-2 pneumonia, suspected individuals can be further isolated and given the right treatment timely so that the patient management can be optimized, especially in communities or hospitals of developing and underdeveloped countries where they have the limited resources for nucleic acid testing kits. Also, it is a relevant tool for radiologists to identify that the CT findings of COVID-19 can be correlated with and compared to images of diseases caused by other viruses, such as Adenovirus, and those within the same family such as SARS-CoV and MERS-CoV. However, CT is still a limited option for the identification of newly discovered viruses like the SARS-CoV-2 (Li *et al.*, 2020a).

COVID-19: MOLECULAR DETECTION OF VIRUS

Since the outbreak in December 2019, early diagnosis of COVID-19 has not only been a significant challenge, but also a critical factor in disease prevention and progression control. However, clinical characteristics alone are not sufficient to base the diagnosis of COVID-19, especially if patients present early and ultra-early stage symptoms (Tahamtan and Ardebili, 2020). In conjunction with medical diagnostic advancements, reliable laboratory detection techniques are of utmost importance to expedite public health interventions. In general cases of acute respiratory infections, nucleic acid detection-based approaches are routinely utilized to detect pathogenic agents collected from respiratory secretion specimen. The feasibility of introducing rapid and reliable nucleic acid tests at the time of global health emergencies *via* the collaboration between public and academic laboratories was previously demonstrated in cases of other human viruses like SARS, Chikungunya (Panning *et al.*, 2009) and Zika virus (Corman *et al.*, 2016). In these situations, for establishing assays and assessing their performance, virus isolates were accessible as a reference. However, in the current scenario of COVID-19, such virus isolates from diseased patients have not yet been pre-established as per the international public health community guidelines (Corman *et al.*, 2020).

Numerous SARS-CoV-2 nucleic acid detection kits have been designed and have obtained rapid approval as multiple suspected cases having typical clinical COVID-19 characteristics with related CT images went undiagnosed. Due to the overcrowded situation in many healthcare centers, more number of suspected and confirmed cases could not be efficiently identified, isolated or treated (Zeng et al., 2020). Amidst such nucleic acid tests, the polymerase chain reaction (PCR) method is referred to as the 'gold standard' for the detection of specific human viruses. At present, it has been discovered that real-time reverse transcriptase-PCR (RT-PCR) is immensely valuable for detection of SARS-CoV-2 due to the advantage of being a highly specific yet simple qualitative assay with adequate sensitivity for rapidly diagnosing infections in early stages. Thereby, 'criterion-referenced' real-time RT-PCR tests can potentially be regarded as a prime technique to diagnose COVID-19 causative agent, *i.e.*, SARS-CoV-2. Besides basic PCR, several novel molecular tests that employ non-PCR-related techniques and assays also reportedly have enhanced specificity and sensitivity. Such tests include nucleic acid amplification under isothermal conditions (such as loop mediated isothermal amplification-LAMP) and nucleic acid sequence-based amplification which are intricately developed to rapidly detect coronavirus RNA (Shen *et al.*, 2020). Moreover, POC tests employing nucleic acid detection strategies have been developed to enhance the accuracy and effectiveness of current testing strategies.

RT-PCR Based Assays

The most preferred and dependable test for diagnosis of COVID-19 is RT-PCR test, carried out using upper (NP and OP swabs) and lower (expectorated sputum, endotracheal aspirate or BAL) respiratory tract specimen, blood, urine and feces. Different manufacturers use a variety of molecular targets within the SARS-Co--2 positive-sense, single-stranded RNA genome, includes structural proteins and several spike protein (S), envelope protein (E), transmembrane protein (M), helicase (Hel), and nucleocapsid protein (N) (Kang *et al.*, 2020). Additionally, some tests target species-specific accessory genes essential for viral replication, such as hemagglutinin-esterase (HE), RNA-dependent RNA polymerase (RdRp) and open reading frames *ORF1a* and *ORF1b* (open reading frame 1a/b) (Tang *et al.*, 2020).

Recently developed RT-PCR assays targeting three genes, *i.e.*, RNA-dependent RNA polymerase/helicase (*RdRp/Hel*), *S*, and nucleocapsid (*N1* and *N2*), of SARS-CoV-2. Amongst these, the COVID-19 *RdRp/Hel* assay yielded the lowest *in vitro* detection limit, but was advised to confirm positive results. However, in comparison to the *RdRp* assay, the *E* gene assay shows higher sensitivity in combination with the single-step RT-PCR system and is sufficient to detect

SARS-CoV-2 RNA (Zhai et al., 2020). To identify patients in early stages, two single-step quantitative RT-PCR (qRT-PCR) assays were designed to detect two other targets of the SARS-CoV-2 genome that are highly conserved amongst *Sarbecoviruses*; the *ORF1b* and the *N* gene of expected amplicon sizes of 132bp and 110bp respectively (Chu et al., 2020). Although there has been no attestation that either sequence regions are advantageous for clinical diagnostic testing, it is preferred that a minimum of two molecular targets should be included in the RT-PCR assays to prevent possible cross-reaction and probable genetic drift of SARS-CoV-2 (Tang et al., 2020). Researchers in various countries have devised real-time RT-PCR assays based on different combinations of these targets. In the United States, the CDC (Center for Disease Control) recommended two loci in the *N* gene, which has reportedly been performing well (Holshue et al., 2020). Hong Kong used two targets for RT-PCR assays; initial screening using the *N* gene, followed by *ORF1b* for confirmation (Chan et al., 2020). The combination of *E* and *RdRp* genes were selected in the territory of Germany (Corman et al., 2020).

The viral load kinetics suggests the variations in different location of individual patients. Optimum type of samples and timing for maximumviral load during the course of SARS-CoV-2infection are yet to be revealed (Tahamtan and Ardebili, 2020). In a study conducted by Wang et al., different clinical specimen of 205 patients with confirmed COVID-19 were tested by RT-PCR, targeting the *ORF1ab* gene. Maximum positivity was obtained in BAL specimens (93%), accompanied by sputum specimen (72%), NP swab (63%), and OP swab (32%) (Wang et al., 2020). In NP swabs of most cases of symptomatic SARS-CoV-2 infection, viral RNA can be detected and measured (by cycle threshold (Ct)) on day-1 of symptoms and reaches to the peak within a week. Ct is defined as the number of replication cycles needed to yield a fluorescent signal; lower the Ct values, greater the viral RNA load in a sample. If the Ct value is lesser than 40, the patient is clinically declared as "PCR positive". By the third week, this positivity gradually starts to decline and subsequently becomes undetectable. For critically ill and hospitalized patients, Ct values are lower than that of mild to moderate cases, and positive PCR results may be persistantfor more than 21 days after infection onset, whereas majority mild cases produce negative results. However, PCR positivity indicates only the presence of viral RNA, but may not compulsorily imply viability of the virus in the sample (Sethuraman et al., 2020).

Despite the higher sensitivity and specificity of RT-PCR, the usage of these assays heavily relay on the method of sample collection and their transport to the respective COVID-19 testing laboratories. Missing the time window of viral replication, incorrect sample collection timing in comparison to illness onset and lack of efficient sampling technique can confer to false-negative results. Occasionally, this could also occur due to technical errors and contamination of reagents or samples. At this stage of the pandemic, FNRs can have serious consequences by allowing infected patients to spread the infection and hampering the measures to contain rapid spread of the virus (Guo *et al.*, 2020). All the commonly used diagnostic methods are illustrated in below given (Fig. **1**).

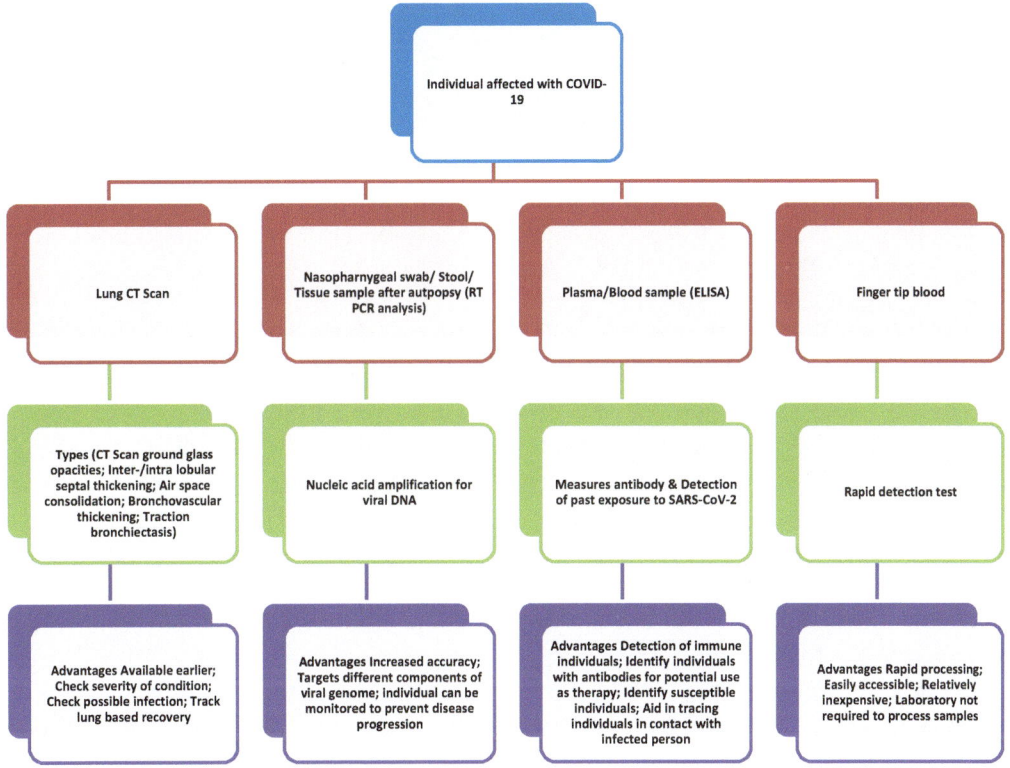

Fig. (1). Diagnostic methods and their advantages for COVID-19 (Iyer *et al.*, 2020).

Loop Mediated Isothermal Amplification (LAMP)

In PCR, double-stranded DNA is denatured using heat, and the products are used to promote the next few rounds of DNA synthesis. LAMP is a novel nucleic acid amplification technique that does not require initial heat denaturation and thus, proceeds rapidly to amplify fewer copies of nucleic acid to multiple-fold in under an hour under isothermal conditions and with increased specificity (Shen *et al.*, 2020). Isothermal conditions can be provided by a simple water bath or heating block, thus making LAMP much approachable to use, especially in the area where prompt action is required for the immediate diagnosis due to the episodes of severe illness of COVID-19 (Notomi *et al.*, 2000). Similar to the principle of RT-PCR, it uses reverse transcriptase enzyme to obtain complementary DNA (cDNA) from a RNA template, which is further amplified by DNA polymerase with a set of two specially designed inner and two outer primers (Wong *et al.*, 2018). The initial steps require all four kinds of primers, followed by usage of only inner primers for strand displacement of DNA. Each inner primer (forward inner primer (FIP) and the backward inner primer (BIP)) comprises of a pair of distinct sequences that correspond to the sense and antisense sequences of the target DNA; one is used for priming in the initial phaseand the other for self-priming in later phases (Notomi *et al.*, 2000). The amplified product can then be identified *via* photometry or by quantifying the turbidity caused by magnesium pyrophosphate precipitate as a byproduct of DNA amplification (Carter *et al.*, 2020).

LAMP-based detection methods have previously been developed and applied in diagnosis of the SARS-CoV and MERS-CoV. In 2004, Poon *et al.* reported and demonstrated how a simple LAMP assay is a feasible technology for the immediate diagnosis of SARS-CoV. Comparative study showed that SARS-CoV detection rates and LAMP assay sensitivity is equivalent to that of conventional PCR-based methods (Poon *et al.*, 2004). Later on, Shirato *et al.* developed LAMP-based assay for the detection and epidemiologic surveillance of MERS-CoV. Here the detection of amplicons was carried out by precipitation of magnesium pyrophosphate or by naked-eye observation of fluorescence signals, eliminating the requirement for any specialized instruments. As few as 3.4 copies of MERS-CoV RNA could be detected without any cross-reaction with other respiratory viruses (Shirato *et al.*, 2014). Recently, Zhang *et al.* described a simple colorimetric LAMP-based assay for rapid detection of SARS-CoV-2 from direct tissue or cell lysate without an RNA purification step as the sample input (Zhang *et al.*, 2020b).

In addition to enhancing the accuracy in diagnosis, the RT-LAMP can also be used as an epidemiologic surveillance tool for viral infections. It is a pioneering nucleic acid amplification technique and works as a simple yet rapid diagnostic tool for detection and identification of infectious pathogens (Fig. **2**). LAMP is also an advantageous real-time assay for use in developing countries due to its easy-to-use approach in any field, under any circumstances and environment (Wong *et al.*, 2018).

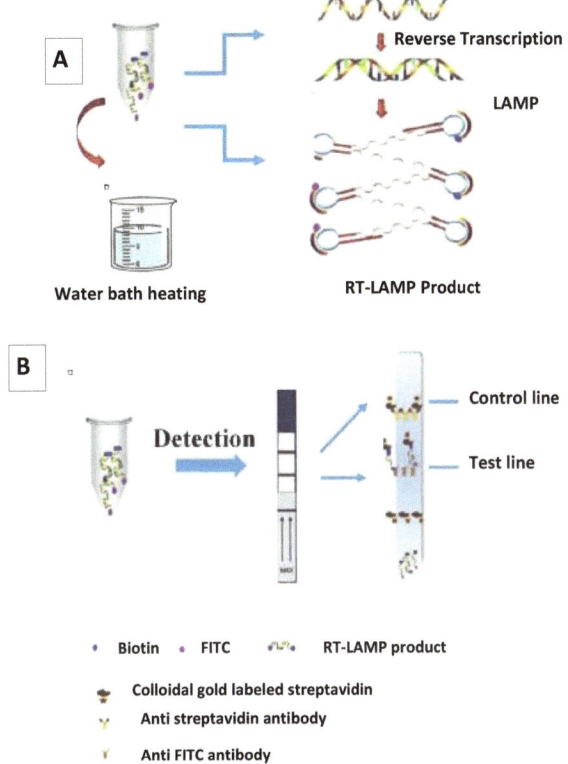

Fig. (2). Schematic illustration of the RT-LAMP-VF assay. **(A)** amplification reaction for RT-LAMP and **(B)** detection on visualization strip [Adapted with permission from (Shen *et al.*, 2020)].

CRISPR-Isothermal Amplification Based Assays

Microbial clustered regularly interspaced short palindromic repeats (CRISPR) based diagnosis (CRISPR-Dx) can rapidly diagnose nucleic acids with increased sensitivity and single-base specificity(Gootenberg *et al.*, 2017). Having CRISPR array processing activity, the RNA-targeting CRISPR associated (*Cas*) enzyme '*Cas13*' targets and cleaves RNA and release individual CRISPR RNA (crRNAs). Additionally, *Cas13* has concomitant cleavage activity that has been utilized for specialized diagnostic applications, such as specific high-sensitivity enzymatic reporter unlocking (SHERLOCK) (Gootenberg *et al.*, 2018, Freije *et al.*, 2019). SHERLOCK uses the combination of recombinase-mediated isothermal pre-amplification orrecombinase polymerase amplification (RPA), and *Cas13* for multiplexed, ultra-sensitive detection of single molecules of nucleic acids. Two guide RNAs were designed based on the SARS-CoV-2 RNA sequence, each recognizing the *S* gene and the *ORF1ab* gene respectively. To maximize the accuracy, sequences most specific for SARS-CoV-2 are selected to minimize the interference from other respiratory virus genomes (Kang *et al.*, 2020). Broughton *et al.* reported the development of a quick (less than 40 minute), simple yet accurate CRISPR-Cas12-based lateral flow assay, termed as DETECTR (DNA Endonuclease-Targeted CRISPR Trans Reporter), for diagnosis of SARS-CoV-2 RNA from respiratory swab specimen (Broughton *et al.*, 2020).

Microarrays

The microarray is a high-throughput detection method where the target RNA produces cDNA by reverse transcription, followed by loading of these specific probe-labeled cDNA into wells of microarray plates. The surfaces of these microarray chips contain fixed solid-phase oligonucleotides. If the cDNAs hybridize, they remain bound to the surface and the unbound DNAs get washed away. In this way, presence of virus-specific nucleic acids can be detected by target-specific probes (Carter *et al.*, 2020). The microarray assays have previously been able to identify SARS-CoV genomic mutations and up to 24 associated single nucleotide polymorphisms (SNP) in the SARS-CoVgene with an accuracy of 100% (Guo *et al.*, 2014). Due to its superior design for rapid diagnosis, microarray assays are capable of detecting a broad range of human viruses and can be accessed at or near patient POC in the future (Shen *et al.*, 2020). In a study conducted by Luna *et al.*, an inexpensive, non-fluorescent, low-density oligonucleotide array was designed for detecting the complete Coronavirus genus with a sensitivity equivalent to that of real-time RT-PCR (de Souza Luna *et al.*, 2007). Another study evaluated the mobile analysis platform (MAP), which is a compact, portable, near-POC diagnostic platform utilizing disposable assay-specific microfluidic cards. It is a promising technology for rapid, accurate automated detection and differentiation of several pathogens in clinical specimen (Hardick *et al.*, 2018).

Metagenomic Sequencing Based Methods

Metagenomic sequencing is used evaluate the background microbiome of infected patients. To identify SARS-CoV-2, this technique combines the use of amplicon-based sequencing with metagenomics sequencing(Moore *et al.*, 2020). This approach enables the rapid identification of SARS-CoV-2 as well as secondary infection causing pathogens, and study of potential contact tracing, molecular epidemiology, and viral evolution. Metagenomic approaches like sequence-independent single primer amplification (SISPA) check for sequence divergence. With relevance to the current SARS-CoV-2 outbreak, this technology is particularly useful in assessing rate of mutation and detecting probable recombination with other human Coronaviruses; both have direct impact on development and efficacy of vaccines and antivirals (Carter *et al.*, 2020). Moore *et al.* used amplicon and metagenomics 'MinION' sequencing technique to rapidly obtain the genomic sequencing of SARS-CoV-2 and other pathogens in NP swabs of COVID-19 patients by the ISARIC 4C consortium. For the amplicon-based system, 16 primer binding sites from specific conserved regions in the SARS-CoV-2 genome were chosen to amplify about 1000bp fragments having a roughly 200bp overlapping region. These primer sets generated 30 amplicons from the cDNA, which were then sequenced using MinION (Moore *et al.*, 2020).

Shotgun metagenomics is a comprehensive sequencing technique that collectively examines all organisms present in complex samples without concerns of highly mutagenic regions that can be challenging to detect *via* other assays (Ai *et al.*, 2020). It provides an in-depth, almost complete sequence of the viral genome, highlighting valuable details such as virus function and biology that further aid immensely in implementing effective surveillance strategies to prevent transmission and infection (Carter *et al.*, 2020). Illumina developed a next-generation shotgun metagenomics sequencing platform that can detect and collectively assess multiple strains of pathogenic organisms (including Coronaviruses) present in samples of varying complexities. The workflow involves the TruSeqRibo-Zero Gold rRNA depletion kit for sample preparation, TruSeq Stranded Total RNA Library Prep for library preparation, the Illumina-benchtop sequencing system, and the LRM resequencing module or IDbyDNAExplify platform for final data analysis (Carter *et al.*, 2020).

Gold Nanoparticles-Based Colorimetric Assay

In terms of reliability, reproducibility and selectivity, many assays fail when testing viral load at its early representation or viral gene mutations during its ongoing spread. Thus, there is a need for sophisticated diagnostics to test patient samples, preferably without any access to advanced instruments (Moitra *et al.*, 2020). Colorimetric bioassays incorporating nanotechnology can be conveniently used to design biosensors with an easy-to-use platform with visual output. Gold nanoparticles (AuNPs) have been a recent trend for use in such colorimetric-based biosensing applications because of their immanent photostability, high extinction coefficient and localized surface plasmon resonance (SPR), *i.e.*, the optical property which represents a color with maximal absorbance wavelength (Kim *et al.*, 2019). AuNPs have been utilized in colorimetric assays for the detection of a broad range of chemical and biological targets like small molecules, metal ions, proteins and nucleic acids, where the change in particle color is generated by sensitive reactivity of the nano-sized particles to the external conditions (Zeng *et al.*, 2020). However, this technique implements the production of single-stranded DNA probes and gradual denaturation and annealing after PCR. Shokri*et al.*, 2017 developed a simple colorimetric bioassay for the visual detection of DNA or RNA targets on the basis of unmodified AuNP aggregation using disulfide self-assembly of terminally-modified DNA. The study showed that the resulting products exhibited a great affinity for the surface of AuNPs and also conferred protection from salt-induced aggregation (Shokri et al., 2017). Based on a similar approach, Kim et al., proposed a colorimetric assay to detect the presence of MERS (Kim et al., 2019).

On a similar basis, Moitra*et al.*, reported a colorimetric assay using AuNPs capped with aptly designed thiol-modified antisense oligonucleotides (ASOs) exclusively for the SARS-CoV-2 *N* gene, which could be useful for detecting positive COVID-19 cases within 10 minutes from isolated RNA samples. These AuNPs selectively agglomerate in the presence of their target SARS-CoV-2 RNA sequence and demonstrate a change in the SRP. *RNaseH*-mediated cleavage of the RNA strand from the RNA−DNA hybrid forms a visually detectable precipitate. The assay can also be optimized to target other regions of the viral genome, such as the *S*, *E* and *M* genes, for pre-clinical or POC screening and to achieve utmost sensitivity with the least number of false positives (Moitra et al., 2020). The currently available different molecular-based methods with their target of the gene have been summarized in Table 1 (See in the later section-including the test serology-based test).

Table 1. The list of commercially available SARS-CoV-2 Diagnostic Kits.

Manufacturer	Test Name	Test Type	Principle of Detection	Target for Detection Gene
1 drop Inc.	1copy ™ COVID-19 qPCR Multi Kit	Molecular- based	RT-PCR	*RdRp* and *E*
Abbott Diagnostics Scarborough, Inc.	ID NOW COVID-19	Molecular-based, POC	ITAP	*RdRp*
ArcDia International Oy Ltd. (Ivaska et al., 2013)	mariPOC® COVID-19 tests	Antigendetection, POC	-	-
AtilaBioSystems, Inc.	iAMP® COVID-19 Detection Kit	Molecular-based	ITAP	*ORF1ab* and *N*
Becton, Dickinson and Company	BD SARS-CoV-2 Reagents for BD MAX™ System	Molecular-based	RT-PCR	*N1* and *N2*
BioCore Co. Ltd.	BioCore 2019-nCoV Real Time PCR Kit	Molecular-based	RT-PCR	*N* and *RdRp*
BioMedomics Inc. (BioMedomics, 2020)	COVID-19 IgM/IgGRapid Test	Serology-based, IgG/IgM, POC	LFIA	-
Cepheid	Xpert® Xpress SARS-CoV-2	Molecular-based, POC	RT-PCR	*N2* and *E*

(Table 1) cont.....

Manufacturer	Test Name	Test Type	Principle of Detection	Target for Detection Gene
ColorGenomics	SARS-CoV-2 LAMP Diagnostic Assay	Molecular-based	ITAP	*N, E* and *ORF1a*
CueHealth Inc.	Cue™ COVID-19 Test	Molecular-based, POC	ITAP	*N*
DiaSorin, Inc. (DiaSorin, 2020)	LIAISON® SARS-CoV-2 S1/S2 IgG	Serology-based, IgG	CLIA	*S1/S2* proteins
EmoryMedicalLaboratories(Suthar *et al.*, 2020)	SARS-CoV-2 RBD IgG	Serology-based, IgG	ELISA	*S1 RBD* proteins
GeteinBiotech, Inc. (Assaygenie, 2020)	COVID-19 Rapid POC CE-IVD Test	Serology-based, IgG/IgM, POC	Chromatographic LFIA	*S* and *N* proteins
Goldsite Diagnostics Inc. (Goldsite, 2020)	SARS-CoV-2 IgG/IgM Kit (TRFIA)	Serology-based, IgG/IgM, POC	TRFIA	*S* and *N* proteins
Hangzhou LaiheBiotech Co., Ltd.	LYHER Novel Coronavirus (2019-nCoV) IgM/IgGAntibody Combo Test Kit (Colloidal Gold)	Serology-based, IgG/IgM	LFIA	*S1* protein
Illumina Inc.	Illumina®COVIDSeq™ Test	Molecular-based	MetagenomicSequencing	-
Jiangsu Bioperfectus Technologies Co. Ltd.	COVID-19 Coronavirus Real Time PCR Kit	Molecular-based	RT-PCR	*ORF1ab* and *N*
KilpestIndia Ltd. DBA 3B BlackbioBiotech	TRUPCR® SARS-CoV-2 KIT	Molecular-based	RT-PCR	*E, N* and *RdRp*
Mammoth Biosciences, Inc.	SARS-CoV-2 DETECTR	Molecular-based	CRISPR-ITAP	*N2* and *E*
Mesa Biotech Inc.	Accula™ SARS-Cov-2 Test	Molecular-based, POC	RT-PCR	*N*
Ortho-Clinical Diagnostics, Inc. (OCD-Vitros, 2020)	VITROS ImmunodiagnosticProducts Anti-SARS-CoV-2 Total Reagent Pack	Serology-based, Total Antibody	Immunometric, CLIA	*S1* protein
PlexBio Co. Ltd.	IntelliPlex™ SARS-CoV-2 Detection Kit	Molecular-based	RT-PCR	*E, N* and *RdRp*
PreciGenome LLC.	FastPlex Triplex SARS-CoV-2 Detection Kit (RT-Digital PCR)	Molecular-based	RT-PCR	*ORF1ab* and *N*
QIAGEN	QIAstat-Dx® Respiratory SARS-CoV2 Panel	Molecular-based	RT-PCR	*RdRp* and *E*
Roche Diagnostics (Roche, 2020)	Elecsys Anti-SARS-CoV-2	Serology-based	ECLIA	*N* protein
SeasunBiomaterials	AQ-TOP™ COVID-19 RapidDetection Kit	Molecular-based	ITAP	*ORF1ab*
Shenzhen MindrayBio-MedicalElectronics Co., Ltd. (Nuccetelli *et al.*, 2020)	SARS-CoV-2 IgM	Serology-based, IgM	CLIA	-

(Table 1) cont.....

Manufacturer	Test Name	Test Type	Principle of Detection	Target for Detection Gene
Sherlock Biosciences, Inc.	Sherlock™ CRISPR SARS-CoV-2 kit	Molecular-based	CRISPR-ITAP	*ORF1ab* and *N*
Snibe Diagnostics (Isabel *et al.*, 2020)	MAGLUMI IgG/IgM de 2019-nCoV	Serology-based, IgG/IgM	CLIA	*S* and *N* protein
TBG Biotechnology Corp.	ExProbe™ SARS-CoV-2 Testing Kit	Molecular-based	RT-PCR	*E, N* and *RdRp*
Siemens Healthcare Diagnostics Inc.	SARS-CoV-2 Total Antibodyassay (CV2T)	Serology-based, Total Antibody	CLIA	*S1 RBD* protein
Quidel Corporation	Sofia 2 SARS Antigen FIA	Antigendetection, POC	LFIA	*N*protein

ITAP: Isothermal amplification, CRISPR-ITAP: CRISPR-Isothermal Amplification, ECLIA: Electro-chemiluminescence Immunoassay, CLIA: Chemiluminescent Immunoassay, ELISA: Enzyme-linked Immunosorbent Assay, LFIA: Lateral Flow Immunoassay, TRFIA: Time-resolved Fluorescence Immunoassay.

COVID-19: SERIOLOGICAL AND IMMUNOLOGICAL BASED DETECTION

In the current scenario for the diagnosis of COVID-19, PCR-based techniques and deep sequencing are prevalent methods for detecting the SARS-CoV-2 viral infection. Nevertheless, these methods are greatly dependent upon the presence of the viral genome in an adequate amount so as to be amplified; further, if the time window for viral replication is overlooked, false-positive results can arise. Likewise, erroneous sample collection can hinder the efficacy of qPCR-based assays, giving rise to false-negative results, which can augment the dire consequences of the current pandemic. Hence, auxiliary screening methods that enable us to detect infection in spite of low viral titers can prove to be extremely valuable (Guo *et al.*, 2020). Serological testing is generally regarded as the investigation of blood serum or plasma for the ubiety of IgM and IgG, but the term has been functionally broadened to encompass the analyses of other biological fluids such as saliva and sputum (Carter *et al.*, 2020). Immunoassays can provide information not only on the active viral infection (as in the case of qPCR-based detection), but also on past exposures to the virus. Several companies have ventured into this approach for developing SARS-CoV-2 detection kits. These assays are designed such that they mainly target those proteins in the virus that have extensively been established as suitably immunogenic – the S protein (being the most exposed protein in the virus), the N protein (for its abundant expression during an infection), and the receptor-binding domain (*RBD*) on the viral spike protein (Lee *et al.*, 2020).

Serological testing can prove to be a key strategy in guiding successful public health practices to contain the pandemic. Besides rapid identification of COVID-19 positive cases, it can help us largely in the aspect of contact-tracing and in defining case-clusters, particularly in highly dense populations (Xu *et al.*, 2020). Serological testing can also enable us to go beyond these immediate uses of case identification and containment. Serological testing on the population scale can enable researchers to evaluate the total number of individuals mounting an immune response, including those infections that had a sub-clinical manifestation or those that occurred in the past (Lee *et al.*, 2020). This information can point out four cardinals pertaining to the disease epidemiology; primarily, it can help estimate major epidemiological variables (for instance, the attack rate of the disease, or its case-fatality rate), which facilitates an assessment of the burden of community transmission; next, it can direct the strategic placement of frontline workers to mitigate the viral exposure to susceptible individuals in the population; further, the information can also be used to evaluate the consequences of non-pharmaceutical interventions at the population level; lastly, it can enable identification of those individuals who set off a robust immune response to SARS-CoV-2, such that their antibody isolates can be utilized in convalescent plasma therapy (Winter and Hegde, 2020) (Fig. **3**).

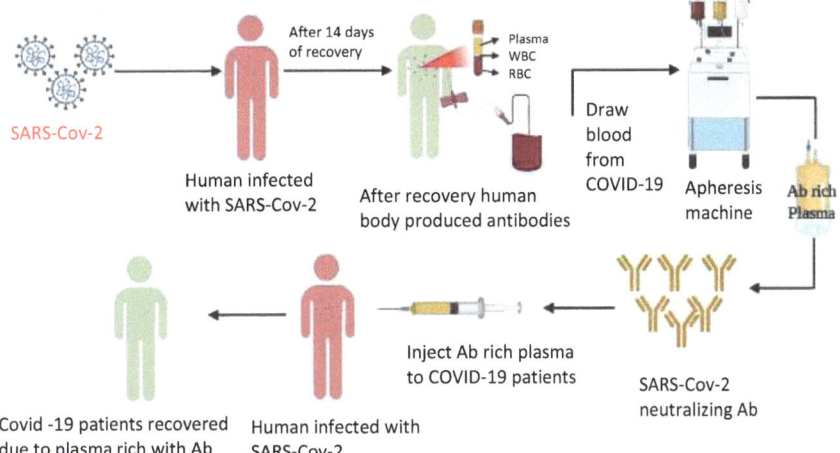

Fig. (3). Convalescent plasma (CP) therapy: The figure illustrates the process and importance of CP therapy to treat COVID-19 disease. CP therapy is immunotherapy where the humoral antibody (Ab) from the recovered patients to the severely affected diseased patients. In CP therapy, as the SARS-CoV-2 affected is infected the Ab spans out and marks the virus as an intruding agent into the human system. This, in future, will trigger the white blood cells to identify the SARS-CoV-2 virus, which deactivates the viral function in the human body. In this procedure, almost 1ltr of blood will be collected from the recovered patients and approximately 250 ml of plasma will be injected to the COVID-19 diseased patients. This might reduce the COVID-19 disease symptoms, give relief to the patients and would get recovered from this dreadful infection [Adapted with permission from (Iyer *et al.*, 2020)].

Despite being fast, robust and easy to carry out, immunological/serological assays have certain limitations. The incapacity of immunoassays to detect infection during the very early stage, because immunoglobulins are generated only after a few days of exposure to antigen, is a major drawback; in view of this, a recent infection might depict false-negative outcomes with serological testing. Another setback with the usage of serological assays might arise with the possibility of cross-reactivity, a factor that crucially influences the specificity and the sensitivity of an immunoassay (Lee *et al.*, 2020). Hence, serological testing is an indispensable measure that should be taken, at least in complementation with nucleic acid testing so as to account for a close window of detection between a positive PCR test and seroconversion to anti-SARS-CoV-2 IgG. This can also help address additional use cases such as to support return-to-work, immunity passport initiatives and studies aimed at the evaluation of therapeutic/vaccine candidates (F. hoffmann-la roche ltd, 2020).

BIOMARKER IDENTIFICATION: APPROACH OF SEROLOGICAL PLATFORM

Antibody Biomarkers

Numerous serological immunoassays have been developed so far for the recognition of SARS-CoV-2 proteins and for that of anti-SARS-CoV-2 antibodies in the serum or plasma. The most widely employed biomarkers in the currently available immunoassays are immunoglobulins, IgM and IgG (Vashist, 2020). IgM is the first antibody produced by the host immune system in response to the initial exposure to an antigen(Schroeder Jr and Cavacini, 2010). On the other hand, IgG, the most commonly found immunoglobulin isotype in the blood, is produced after the processes of class-switching and affinity maturation, and participates predominantly in the secondary immune responses (Vidarsson *et al.*, 2014). IgM is first detectable in serum a few days after infection, lasting for a few weeks after which class-switching to IgG takes place (Carter *et al.*, 2020). A few recent studies have pointed out that IgM can be detected as early as 3 days post-infection onset, but peaks between two to three weeks post infection onset; contrastingly, IgGis detectable 4 days post-infection onset and the levels peak no sooner than 17 days post-infection onset (Zhang *et al.*, 2020a, Long *et al.*, 2020). Thus, it follows that IgM can be an indicator of early stage of the infection whereas IgG, that of current or former infection. IgG might also be indicative of post-infection immunity (Carter *et al.*, 2020).

A study reporting acute antibody responses to SARS-CoV-2 in 285 COVID-19 patients also showed that 100 percent of patients tested positive for anti-SARS-

CoV-2 IgG within 19 days post-onset of symptoms. The study also reported plateauing of IgM and IgG titers within 6 days post seroconversion (Long et al., 2020). Other investigations have shown significant rates of seropositivity for antibodies against various SARS-CoV-2 viral proteins. To et al. carried out serological analyses for samples available not less than 14 days post onset of symptoms; they reported 94% and 88% seropositivity for anti-nucleoprotein IgG and IgM, respectively. In the case of anti-*RBD* immunoglobulins, 100% seropositivity for IgG and 94% seropositivity for IgM was reported (Kang et al., 2020). Another study assessing for the seropositivity of the spike-binding immunoglobulins reported the detection of SARS-CoV-2-specific neutralizing antibodies correlating to the *S1, S2* and *RBD* regions on the tenth to fifteenth-day post disease onset; the findings also suggested a highly variable correlation of immunoglobulin titres with parameters such as age, blood CRP levels, lymphocyte count (Wu et al., 2020).

In a nutshell, three major types of antibodies, on the basis of maturity, are taken into consideration. Immature antibodies appear in the initial stage of infection, serving the purpose of bringing about an initial host response to begin grasping the virus/antigen. It is not necessary that immature antibodies will effectively recognize the antigen. IgM, immature IgA and immature IgG fall under this category. Secondly, there are neutralizing antibodies that participate in the advanced stage of the infection, as well as during convalescence. These are a subset of mature immunoglobulins and can very effectively neutralize the virus, rendering it ineffective against the host. Lastly, mature antibodies that appear only in the convalescent phase are also late immunoglobulins and these can effectively recognize the virus. These mature antibodies hold significance in hosting the viral memory for future recognition and mounting a secondary immune response. Targeting mature antibodies for sero-immunological assays may account for an increase in their specificity.

Antigen Biomarkers

In supplementation with molecular assays, rapid antigen testing that allows detection of the viral antigens can also be used (Carter et al., 2020). Among the SARS-CoV-2 viral proteins, the spike proteins (S1 and S2), the receptor-binding domain (*RBD*) and the nucleocapsid are utilized as antigen biomarkers for several assays. Recombinant counterparts and biotinylated versions of these antigens have also been made commercially available. Besides these, recombinant SARS-CoV-2 methyltransferase, recombinant SARS-CoV-2 NSP9, and recombinant SARS-CoV-2 Plpro are also commercially available. The viral papain-like cysteine protease (Plpro) is involved in deubiquitinating and deISGylating activities and plays a key role in the innate immune response to the infection. The protease is associated with the inhibition of cytokine and chemokine production in the host system. These features make the protease a significant target and a reasonable biomarker for SARS-CoV-2 infection (Rut *et al.*, 2020).

Besides viral antigens, studies have reported that levels of several cancer biomarker antigens such as the carcinoembryonic antigen (CEA) and carbohydrate antigens (CA) are frequently observed to be elevated in lung inflammatory pathologies. This observation has entailed the conjecture that SARS-CoV-2-induced acute lung insult may be linked with elevated levels of these cancer biomarkers (Wei *et al.*, 2020).

Procalcitonin and Interleukin-6 as Prognostic COVID-19 Biomarkers

As suggested by the name, procalcitonin (PCT) is a pro-hormone whose metabolism produces calcitonin. The hormone calcitonin plays a role in calcium homeostasis. In a health individual, procalcitonin is virtually seronegative; notwithstanding this, in sepsis condition PCT has been known to be released from hepatocytes and peripheral blood mononuclear cells (Creamer *et al.*, 2019). PCT is considered to be a specific indicator of invasive bacterial infections, microbial products and pro-inflammatory mediators of host immunity. These conditions trigger a generalized induction of calcitonin mRNA and subsequent release of calcitonin precursors through a non-regulated constitutive pathway. This leads to PCT release from parenchymal tissue throughout the body resulting in a major elevation of PCT levels in circulation (Hesselink *et al.*, 2009). The production and release of this prohormone is actively sustained by enhanced concentrations of IL-1B, TNF-α and IL-6 but inhibited by IFN-γ which is a hallmark in patients afflicted with viral infections. Thus, it follows that in COVID-19 patients with non-complicated infection, the PCT level would remain within the reference range; an elevation of this biomarker can be indicative of a bacterial co-infection that might steer the disease towards a more severe manifestation (Lippi and Plebani, 2020).

Cytokines are of utmost significance in the regulation of inflammation and immune responses (Zhang and An, 2007). Among these, because of its pleiotropic nature, IL-6 serves a heavy implication in disease modulation (Tanaka *et al.*, 2014). Reports have suggested an increase in IL-6 levels in patients with respiratory dysfunction, which may entail the possibility of shared contraption in cytokine-mediated lung damage associated with COVID-19 infection (Herold *et al.*, 2020). Aggressive manifestation of SARS-CoV-2 infection can be linked to rapid viral replication that tends to invade the lower respiratory tract leading to elevated IL-6 mediated respiratory distress. It is known that ultimately it is the cytokine storm that deteriorates the prognosis of COVID-19 patients. Hence, it is reasonable that assessing IL-6 as a prognostic biomarker for COVID-19 patients seeking medical aid, might recommend valuable directions in the course of therapeutic interventions (Ulhaq and Soraya, 2020).

SEROLOGICAL AND IMMUNOLOGICAL ASSAYS

The determination of SARS-CoV-2 exposure depends heavily on the finding of IgM and IgG specific to the aforementioned viral antigens. Several approaches can be adopted for this purpose and each platform carries a unique set of advantages as well as inadequacies associated with it. Assays can be tailored and optimized according to the objective of a detection kit (Carter *et al.*, 2020); diagnostic companies all around the globe are focusing on the conception of high-throughput serology kits for detection of SARS-CoV-2 infection using the platforms described in this section.

Enzyme-linked Immunosorbent Assay (ELISA)

Enzyme-linked immunosorbent assay (ELISA) is an immunological assay and is vastly applied for the quantitative and/or qualitative estimation of antibodies, antigens, and other proteins in biological samples. The assay is based on the principle of antigen capture using a specific antibody, or vice versa, coupled to an enzyme-substrate reaction for detection/quantitation of target molecule (Yolken, 1980). ELISA assays are designed such that they can be utilized in different formats – direct, indirect, sandwich, and competitive ELISA. Direct ELISA is a format wherein an antigen is immobilized on the multi-well plate surface and detected using a primary antibody (specific to the antigen) that is directly conjugated to an enzyme. The benefit of a direct ELISA assay is that it relatively less-time consuming and lesser amount of reagents are invested. The disadvantage associated with this format is that there is a high chance of background noise, besides lower flexibility arising due to necessary conjugation of the primary antibody. Similarly, in the indirect assay the antigen is immobilized on the well-plate surface. The distinction comes with a two-step process in the indirect ELISA assay: (i) a primary antibody specific to the immobilized antigen adheres to the target molecule; (ii) a secondary antibody conjugated with an enzyme adheres to the primary antibody for detection. A major advantage that the indirect ELISA format offers is that of signal amplification owing to the ability of numerous secondary antibodies to bind to the primary antibody, providing high flexibility. However, this might also account for potential cross-reactivity arising from the use of secondary antibodies (Yolken, 1980, Carter *et al.*, 2020, Horlock, 2016).

Sandwich ELISA is widely utilized format, requiring two antibodies (regarded as matched antibody pairs) such that they are specific to the same antigen, but to two distinctive regions on the antigen. One of the matched antibody pair is coated on the well-plate surface, posing as the capture antibody to mediate antigen immobilization. The other antibody is conjugated to the enzyme for detection/quantitation of the antigen. This format is expedient in terms of the high specificity, sensitivity as well as high flexibility (Gonzalez et al., 2008). However, the design of such an assay often proves to be demanding as finding two antibodies specific to two distinct regions on the antigen can be a challenging task (Sakamoto et al., 2018). Another format, i.e., competitive ELISA measures the antigen titer by detecting signal interference. All of the previously described configurations can be modified to the competitive assay. By this set up, the test antigen contends with a reference antigen (pre-coated on the well plate) to bind to a limited volume of antibody conjugated with the enzyme. Prior to addition to the wells, the sample is incubated with the antibody-enzyme conjugate. Only the free unbound antibodies will be presented for binding to the reference antigen. Thus, the greater the antigen in the sample, the weaker is the signal detected (Yolken, 1980).

Lateral Flow Immunoassay

The lateral flow immunoassay (LFIA) is similar to ELISA in its layout as the base carries an immobilized target capturing entity, generally an antibody or an antigen. It is a qualitative assay based on the principle of chromatography. There are four major components in the assembly, viz. sample pad, conjugate pad, absorbent pad and nitrocellulose membrane. Generally a fluid sample is applied to the substrate which lets the fluid flow through a strip region of anchored antigen (Carter et al., 2020). Two formats of this assay are most frequently used depending on the target analyte to be tested. The competitive format is generally performed when the target to be tested has low molecular weight and/or exhibits a single antigenic determinant (Koczula and Gallotta, 2016). The analyte is complexed with a protein and coated on the test zone of a nitrocellulose membrane. The conjugate pad contains the detection antibody conjugated with a nanoparticle. If the analyte is present in the sample, it will adhere to the antibodies in the conjugate pad. Hence, as the flow advances towards the test line, the antibody-nanoparticle conjugate will not be free to bind to the previously immobilized analyte (in the test line). Another specific antibody-coated strip of area on the membrane forms the control zone, responsible for the capture of excess antibody complex; thus, the color band pertaining to this zone will always appear irrespective of the presence of analyte in the sample. This acts as a confirmation for correct development of assay. In the absence of the analyte in the sample, the antibody-nanoparticle conjugates will be free to bind to the analyte molecules on the test line, yielding a signal in the form of a second, colored band (O'Farrell, 2009).

The sandwich format of this immunoassay is employed for the detection of higher molecular weight proteins which have minimum two unique epitopes (Koczula and Gallotta, 2016). The antibody specific to one of these epitopes is conjugated with the nanoparticle, and the antibody specific to the second distinct epitope (on the analyte) is immobilized on the test line on the membrane. If the sample is positive for the analyte, binding will be observed with both, the antibody-nanoparticle conjugate, as well as with the antibody immobilized on the test line. In this format, the positive sample will yield two bands – one at the test line, another at the control line indicative of proper functioning of the assay (O'Farrell, 2009).

A group had also developed the IgM and IgG combined LFIA and tested against the blood samples of 397 PCR confirmed COVID-19 cases togetherwith 128 negative patients. It has shown the 88.66% sensitivity and around 90.63% specificity which confirm their suitabllity with compare to individual IgG and IgM test (Li *et al.*, 2020b) (Fig. 4).

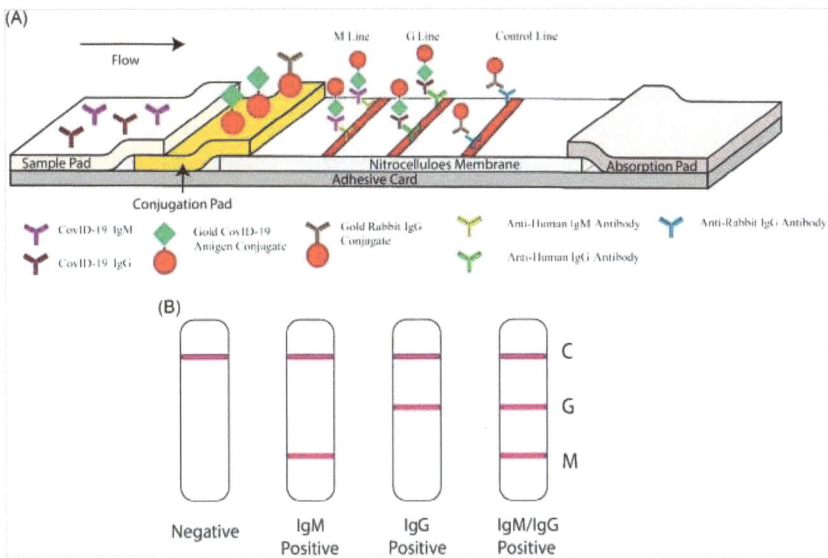

Fig. (4). Schematic illustration of rapid SARS-CoV-2 IgM-IgGcombinedantibody test. **A**, Schematicdiagram of the detectiondevice; **B**, an illustration of differenttestingresults; **C**, means control line; G, meansIgG line; M, meansIgM line. IgG, immunoglobulin G; IgM, immunoglobulin M; SARS-CoV-2, severe acute respiratory syndrome coronavirus 2 [Adapted from (Li *et al.*, 2020b)].

The result of the study confirms the functionality and suitability in different symptomatic and asymptomatic conditions which includes the various settings of laboratories. The lateral flow immunoassay provides a platform for the development of most POC tests because of ease of handling, and simple interpretation of results besides it being a rapid diagnostic test assay that provides results within 10 to 30 minutes (Carter *et al.*, 2020, St John and Price, 2014).

Nanoparticles (NPs) have widely been used as reporter molecules in the lateral flow immunoassay. It is natural that particles larger in size, will give a stronger signal visible to the eye. However, the bulkiness of larger particles hinders the flow, thus reducing the window of opportunity for the binding event to happen. Hence, nanoparticles are most suitably employed as reporter molecules in this assay. Gold nanoparticles are among the commonly employed NPs because of two reasons – they have exceptional light absorbing property, and they provide strong surface for binding antibodies and other proteins leading to formation of robust conjugates (Ngom *et al.*, 2010).

Neutralization Assays

Plaque reduction neutralization assays (PRNA) are based on the occurrence of virus-antibody interaction in a test tube or a microwellplate. Next, antibody response to viral infection is assessed by plating the mixture on cells susceptible to the virus of interest. A semi-solid medium is used to overlay the cells, restricting the spread of progeny virus. Plaques will be formed in the localized area on the plate where productive viral infection of the cells has taken place. The number of plaques is counted and compared with the initial viral concentration in order to infer the percentage reduction in total viral infectivity. In the original assay, the test serum is serially diluted and the viral load is kept constant and end-point titers are calculated for each dilution of serum at selected percentage reduction of viral activity. A modified neutralization assay based on the PRNA assay has been designed, *viz.* serum neutralization assay, wherein log serum neutralization index is used to evaluate the potency of the test serum to inhibit viral infection in susceptible cells. Contrarily to PRNA, in the serum neutralization assay, the serum concentration is held constant and it is the challenge dose of the virus that is serially increased. It is advantageous over the original assay in the fact that undiluted serum is tested which may be a better measure of the serum capacity (WHO, 2007).

The duration taken to obtain results with this test is generally 4-5 days; nevertheless, recent advances have enabled to reduce this duration to a few hours. A major drawback associated with this approach for diagnosis is that cell culture facilities and highly-skilled personnel are required. For detecting a pathogen as pernicious as SARS-CoV-2, laboratory infrastructure with biosafety level III is indeed. Nevertheless, these assays can prove to be tremendously helpful in determining the competence of neutralizing antibodies for convalescent plasma therapy and that for vaccine development (Carter *et al.*, 2020).

Luminescence-based Immunoassays

In a luminescent immunoassay a fixed quantity of labeled antigen is made to compete with varying quantities of sample antigen to bind to a limited number of specific antibodies. The conjugate on the labeled antigen acts as a light-generating entity. Following incubation, the labeled antigen-antibody complex is separated from the assay mixture by either of a variety of techniques- chromatography, ion-exchange, immunoprecipitation using a secondary antibody, *etc*. The next step is to determine the luminescence emitted by by the bound fraction or that of the free fraction *via* a monitoring reaction. The result obtained is mapped on a standard curve to infer the concentration of the unlabeled antigen (Schroeder, 1982). Luminogenic conjugates that are commonly coupled to the antigen of interest include luciferase, NAD, ATP and isoluminol that are covalently coupled *via* stable amide bonds(Yeh and Ai, 2019). Luminescence detection is carried out using luminometers. Three detection systems for this assay are very widely used – (i) NADH is used with long-chain fatty acid and a bacterial luciferase, (ii) isoluminol with microperoxidase and a peroxide, and (iii) ATP with luciferin and firefly luciferase (Schroeder, 1982).

A research group has reported developing a peptide-based luminescent immunoassay to detect SARS-CoV-2 specific IgG and IgM. The peptide they have used is derived from the viral S protein. They report significant specificity exhibited by the peptide inferred from no cross-reactivity observed in 167 sera samples obtained from non-COVID-19 patients afflicted with other pathogens; this may be attributed to the low homology of the region encoding for the particular peptide among other coronaviruses (Cai *et al.*, 2020).

Biosensor Tests

Biosensors are devices that perceive a target biological analyte in the sample or in the surrounding. These are composed of three components - one that recognizes the target analyte to produce a signal, a signal transducer, and a reader (Carter *et al.*, 2020). Several biosensor platforms for immunoassays have been developed over the past few decades. Electrochemical biosensors, localized surface plasmon resonance, surface enhanced Raman scattering, and piezoelectric microcantilever sensors are major types of biosensors (Mehrotra, 2016). Biosensors can potentially offer rapid, sensitive and accurate early detection of target molecules. Electrochemical biosensors are low cost, simple in design and miniaturization and one of the most widely used approaches (Cui and Zhou, 2020). Electrochemical biosensors based on electrochemical impedance spectroscopy (EIS) are commonly used in biomedical devices. Advances in technology have enabled modifications of the sensor surface using nanofabrication in order to increase the sensitivity of EIS. This approach has been utilized to detect interactions between CLEC5A and dengue virus (Cheng et al., 2012). Surface enhanced Raman scattering-based biosensors have a distinct advantage in that it is an ultra-sensitive molecular spectroscopy method, devoid from interference with water. Biosensors based on this phenomenon can detect even trace amounts of analyte (Cui and Zhou, 2020). Surface plasmonic resonance is an emerging technology that evaluates interference with light incident on a solid boundary, brought about by regional disturbances like the adsorption of an antigen or that of an antibody (Carter et al., 2020).

Several platforms employing biosensors have also been established for the immunoassay based detection of SARS-CoV-2. A group has reported proof-o--concept development of biosensor-mediated detection of the SARS-CoV-2 S1 protein. Their design is centered on the technique of molecular identification through membrane engineering. It is a cell-based assay which enables detection of analytes on the basis of specific, selective interaction of target analytes with cellular biorecognition elements. The surface of these cellular biorecognition elements is modified to facilitate detection, via electroinsertion of antibodies specific to the target analyte (Mavrikou et al., 2020). Another group has reported a field effect transistor-based biosensor device for the detection of SARS-CoV-2 in clinical samples. It was developed by layering FET graphene sheet with anti-SARS-CoV-2 spike antibody. The study demonstrated limit of detection of their construct to be 1fg/mL in phosphate buffer saline and 100 fg/mL in clinical transport medium. Further they reported that the biosensor could differentiate SARS-CoV-2 spike protein from MERS-CoV spike protein (Seo et al., 2020).

Rapid Antigen Tests

Rapid antigen tests depend on specific monoclonal antibodies to facilitate the capture of viral antigens from the serum sample. Rapid antigen detection tests are not limited to any individual type of format, but rather encompass a wide range of formats such as colorimetric enzyme immunoassays, chemiluminescence assays, as well as lateral flow assays, etc. (Carter et al., 2020). One such rapid antigen test for SARS-CoV has been developed using the colorimetric enzyme immunoassay (ELISA) format. The assay employs a cocktail of three different types of monoclonal antibodies for antigen capture and yet another type of rabbit polyclonal antibodies for the purpose of detection of the antigen (Che et al., 2004). A rapid antigen test based on the format of lateral flow assay for the detection of SARS-CoV-2 has been reported. However, the study reports the development of only a half-strip lateral flow assay, which is a successful first step towards the development of a lateral flow platform (Grant et al., 2020).

Currently available rapid antigen test assays for influenza virus and syncytial respiratory virus detection are attributed with suboptimal sensitivity. It is understood that this challenge might present for the detection of SARS-CoV-2. Prototypes of these rapid antigen tests for novel coronaviruses have not been convened with regulatory approval, but attempts towards the development and enhancement of the same are ongoing (Cheng *et al.*, 2020).

CONCLUDING REMARKS

The onset of COVID-19 has resulted in an ever-increasing demand for efficient and rapid SARS-CoV-2 diagnostic and screening strategies that are substantial for controlling transmission of the infection. To speed up the rate of diagnosis and simultaneously obtain accurate results, there is a strong focus on developing cost-efficient POC kits that can be produced on a large scale for mass distribution worldwide (Carter *et al.*, 2020). Current standards of COVID-19 diagnostics involve nucleic acid (viral DNA or RNA) detection strategies as well as immunological (or serological) detection of IgG and IgM antibodies. SARS-Co--2 screening also relies on the clinical symptoms observed in suspected patients, followed by confirmation of the status of the infection by molecular detection methods, specifically RT-PCR (Zhang *et al.*, 2020b). Although RT-PCR has been approved as a confirmatory test, other molecular techniques such as isothermal amplification assays, hybridization microarrays, metagenomics-based sequencing and CRISPR-associated assays are also being developed and approved for rapid and accurate SARS-CoV-2 testing. Complementary to these techniques, serological and immunological testing of not only symptomatic, but also asymptomatic patients is vital for assessing the body's immune response before, during and after the course of infection. The presence of specific antibodies against SARS-CoV-2 can be detected and studied for vaccine formulation for both, immunity against the virus and treatment of various stages of infection (Carter *et al.*, 2020).

Ever since the emergence of COVID-19, significant progress has been made in the diagnostics sector for the development of accurate, sensitive and rapid strategies to detect SARS-CoV-2 in a variety of clinical specimen (Zhang *et al.*, 2020b). The availability of test kits on a global scale, the requirement of technical expertise and access to high-throughput and elaborate laboratory facilities still remain a matter of concern. Despite the numerous challenges, constant efforts are being taken by various organizations to collaborate globally and facilitate the share of knowledge and resources for development of newer and more advanced SARS-CoV-2 diagnostic techniques.

LIST OF ABBREVIATIONS

ALT	Alanine aminotransferase
ARDS	Acute respitatorydistress syndrome
AST	Aspartateaminotransferase
AuNPs	Gold nanoparticle
BAL	Bronchoalveolar lavage
BIP	Backwardinnerprimer
CA	Carbohydrate antigen
CDC	Center for Disease Control
cDNA	complementary DNA
CEA	Carcinoembryogenicantigen
CoV	Coronaviruses
CP	Convalescent plasma
CRISPR	Clusteredregularlyinterspaced short palindromicrepeats
CRP	C-reactiveprotein
CRS	Cytokine release syndrome
CT	Computedtomography
EIS	Electrochemicalimpedancespectroscopy
ELISA	Enzyme-LinkedImmunosorbentAssay
ESR	Erythrocytesedimentation rate
FGF2	Fibroblasticgrowth factor
FIP	Forwardinnerprimer
GCSF	Granulocyte colony-stimulating factor
GMCSF	Granulocyte-macrophage colony-stimulating factor
HE	Hemagglutinin-esterase
LAMP	Loopmediatedisothermal amplification
LDH	Lactate dehdrogenase
LFIA	Lateral flow immunoassay
MAP	Mobile analysisplatform
MARS-CoV	Middle East respiratory syndrome CoV
MCP1	Monocyte chemoattractantprotein 1
MIP	Macrophage inflammatoryprotein
MOD	Multi-organdysfuntion
NP	Nasopharygeal

NPs	Nanoparticles
OP	Oropharyngeal
ORF1a/b	Open reading frame 1a/b
PCR	Polymerase chain reaction
PCT	Procalcitonin
PDGFB	Platelet-derivedgrowth factor subunit-B
POC	Point-of-care
PRNA	Plaque reductionneutralizatonassay
RBD	Receptor binding domain
RdRp	RNA-dependent RNA polymerase
RPA	Recombinasepolymerase amplification
RT-PCR	Real-time reverse transcriptase-PCR
SARS-CoV	Severe acute respiratory syndrome CoV
SHERLOCK	Specifichigh-sensitivityenzymaticreporterunlocking
SISPA	Sequence-independent single primer amplification
SNP	Single nucleotidepolymorphisms
Th1	T-helper-1
Th2	T-helper-2
VEGFA	Vascularendothelialgrowth factor-A
WBC	White bloodcells
WHO	World HealthOrganizations

CONSENT FOR PUBLICATION

Not applicable.

CONFLICT OF INTEREST

The author declares no conflict of interest, financial or otherwise.

ACKNOWLEDGEMENTS

The instrumentation facility of CSIR-IMTECH and Nirma University is duly acknowledged. Authors express their gratitude towards the funding agencies, CSIR, New Delhi and DBT, New Delhi for supporting this study. Nikunj Tandel thanks Indian Council of Medical Research (ICMR), New Delhi, Govt. of India for providing fellowship for his research (ICMR-SRF No.: 2020-7623/CM--BMS).

REFERENCES

Ai, JW, Zhang, Y, Zhang, HC, Xu, T & Zhang, WH (2020) Era of molecular diagnosis for pathogen identification of unexplained pneumonia, lessons to be learned. *Emerg Microbes Infect,* 9, 597-600.
[http://dx.doi.org/10.1080/22221751.2020.1738905] [PMID: 32174267]

'COVID-19 Rapid POC CE-IVD Test. [Online] (2020) Available from: https://www.assaygenie.com/covid-19-rapid-poc-test/'

BioMedomics (2020) Available from: https://www.biomedomics.com/products/infectious-disease/covid--9-rt/'

Broughton, JP, Deng, X, Yu, G, Fasching, CL, Servellita, V, Singh, J, Miao, X, Streithorst, JA, Granados, A, Sotomayor-Gonzalez, A, Zorn, K, Gopez, A, Hsu, E, Gu, W, Miller, S, Pan, CY, Guevara, H, Wadford, DA, Chen, JS & Chiu, CY (2020) CRISPR-Cas12-based detection of SARS-CoV-2. *Nat Biotechnol,* 38, 870-4.
[http://dx.doi.org/10.1038/s41587-020-0513-4] [PMID: 32300245]

Cai, XF, Chen, J, Li Hu, J, Long, QX, Deng, HJ, Liu, P, Fan, K, Liao, P, Liu, BZ, Wu, GC, Chen, YK, Li, ZJ, Wang, K, Zhang, XL, Tian, WG, Xiang, JL, Du, HX, Wang, J, Hu, Y, Tang, N, Lin, Y, Ren, JH, Huang, LY, Wei, J, Gan, CY, Chen, YM, Gao, QZ, Chen, AM, He, CL, Wang, DX, Hu, P, Zhou, FC, Huang, AL & Wang, DQ (2020) A Peptide-Based Magnetic Chemiluminescence Enzyme Immunoassay for Serological Diagnosis of Coronavirus Disease 2019. *J Infect Dis,* 222, 189-93.
[http://dx.doi.org/10.1093/infdis/jiaa243] [PMID: 32382737]

Carter, LJ, Garner, LV, Smoot, JW, Li, Y, Zhou, Q, Saveson, CJ, Sasso, JM, Gregg, AC, Soares, DJ, Beskid, TR, Jervey, SR & Liu, C (2020) Assay techniques and test development for COVID-19 Diagnosis. *ACS Cent Sci,* 6, 591-605.
[http://dx.doi.org/10.1021/acscentsci.0c00501] [PMID: 32382657]

Cascella, M, Rajnik, M, Cuomo, A, Dulebohn, SC & Di Napoli, R (2020) Features, evaluation and treatment coronavirus (COVID-19). *Statpearls.* StatPearls Publishing.

CDC-Fact-Sheet (2019) Guidelines-proposed use of point-of-care (POC) testing platform for SARS-CoV-2 (COVID-19). https://www.cdc.gov/coronavirus/2019-ncov/downloads/OASH-COVID-19-guidance-testing-platforms.pdf, assessed on 15th June 2020.

Chan, JFW, Yuan, S, Kok, KH, To, KKW, Chu, H, Yang, J, Xing, F, Liu, J, Yip, CCY, Poon, RW-S, Tsoi, HW, Lo, SK, Chan, KH, Poon, VK, Chan, WM, Ip, JD, Cai, JP, Cheng, VC, Chen, H, Hui, CK & Yuen, KY (2020) A familial cluster of pneumonia associated with the 2019 novel coronavirus indicating person-t--person transmission: a study of a family cluster. *Lancet,* 395, 514-23.
[http://dx.doi.org/10.1016/S0140-6736(20)30154-9] [PMID: 31986261]

Che, XY, Qiu, LW, Pan, YX, Wen, K, Hao, W, Zhang, LY, Wang, YD, Liao, ZY, Hua, X, Cheng, VC & Yuen, KY (2004) Sensitive and specific monoclonal antibody-based capture enzyme immunoassay for detection of nucleocapsid antigen in sera from patients with severe acute respiratory syndrome. *J Clin Microbiol,* 42, 2629-35.
[http://dx.doi.org/10.1128/JCM.42.6.2629-2635.2004] [PMID: 15184444]

Cheng, MP, Papenburg, J, Desjardins, M, Kanjilal, S, Quach, C, Libman, M, Dittrich, S & Yansouni, CP (2020) Diagnostic testing for severe acute respiratory syndrome–related coronavirus-2: A narrative review. *Ann Intern Med,* 172, 726-34.
[http://dx.doi.org/10.7326/M20-1301] [PMID: 32282894]

Cheng, MS, Ho, JS, Tan, CH, Wong, JPS, Ng, LC & Toh, C-S (2012) Development of an electrochemical membrane-based nanobiosensor for ultrasensitive detection of dengue virus. *Anal Chim Acta,* 725, 74-80.
[http://dx.doi.org/10.1016/j.aca.2012.03.017] [PMID: 22502614]

Chu, DKW, Pan, Y, Cheng, SMS, Hui, KPY, Krishnan, P, Liu, Y, Ng, DYM, Wan, CKC, Yang, P, Wang, Q, Peiris, M & Poon, LLM (2020) Molecular diagnosis of a novel coronavirus (2019-nCoV) causing an outbreak of pneumonia. *Clin Chem,* 66, 549-55.
[http://dx.doi.org/10.1093/clinchem/hvaa029] [PMID: 32031583]

Corman, VM, Landt, O, Kaiser, M, Molenkamp, R, Meijer, A, Chu, DK, Bleicker, T, Brünink, S, Schneider, J, Schmidt, ML, Mulders, DG, Haagmans, BL, van der Veer, B, van den Brink, S, Wijsman, L, Goderski, G, Romette, JL, Ellis, J, Zambon, M, Peiris, M, Goossens, H, Reusken, C, Koopmans, MP & Drosten, C (2020) Detection of 2019 novel coronavirus (2019-nCoV) by real-time RT-PCR. *Euro Surveill,* 25, 2000045.
[http://dx.doi.org/10.2807/1560-7917.ES.2020.25.3.2000045] [PMID: 31992387]

Corman, VM, Rasche, A, Baronti, C, Aldabbagh, S, Cadar, D, Reusken, CB, Pas, SD, Goorhuis, A, Schinkel, J, Molenkamp, R, Kümmerer, BM, Bleicker, T, Brünink, S, Eschbach-Bludau, M, Eis-Hübinger, AM, Koopmans, MP, Schmidt-Chanasit, J, Grobusch, MP, de Lamballerie, X, Drosten, C & Drexler, JF (2016) Assay optimization for molecular detection of Zika virus. *Bull World Health Organ,* 94, 880-92.
[http://dx.doi.org/10.2471/BLT.16.175950] [PMID: 27994281]

Creamer, AW, Kent, AE & Albur, M (2019) Procalcitonin in respiratory disease: use as a biomarker for diagnosis and guiding antibiotic therapy. *Breathe (Sheff),* 15, 296-304.
[http://dx.doi.org/10.1183/20734735.0258-2019] [PMID: 31803264]

Cui, F & Zhou, HS (2020) Diagnostic methods and potential portable biosensors for coronavirus disease 2019. *Biosens Bioelectron,* 165, 112349.
[http://dx.doi.org/10.1016/j.bios.2020.112349] [PMID: 32510340]

de Souza Luna, LK, Heiser, V, Regamey, N, Panning, M, Drexler, JF, Mulangu, S, Poon, L, Baumgarte, S, Haijema, BJ, Kaiser, L & Drosten, C (2007) Generic detection of coronaviruses and differentiation at the prototype strain level by reverse transcription-PCR and nonfluorescent low-density microarray. *J Clin Microbiol,* 45, 1049-52.
[http://dx.doi.org/10.1128/JCM.02426-06] [PMID: 17229859]

DiaSorin (2020) Available from: https://www.diasorin.com/en/immunodiagnostic-solutions/clinica--areas/infectious-diseases/covid-19'

F. hoffmann-la roche ltd (2020) Media Release - Roche develops new serology test to detect COVID-19 antibodies. *Media Release.* https://www.roche.com/media/releases/med-cor-2020-04-17.htm

Freije, CA, Myhrvold, C, Boehm, CK, Lin, AE, Welch, NL, Carter, A, Metsky, HC, Luo, CY, Abudayyeh, OO & Gootenberg, JS (2019) Programmable inhibition and detection of RNA viruses using Cas13. *Molecular Cell,* 76, 826-37.
[http://dx.doi.org/10.1016/j.molcel.2019.09.013]

Goldsite SARS-CoV-2 IgG/IgM diagnostics kit (2020) Available from: http://en.goldsite.com.cn/prod_view.aspx?TypeId=139&Id=275&Fid=t3:139:3'

Gonzalez, RM, Seurynck-Servoss, SL, Crowley, SA, Brown, M, Omenn, GS, Hayes, DF & Zangar, RC (2008) Development and validation of sandwich ELISA microarrays with minimal assay interference. *J Proteome Res,* 7, 2406-14.
[http://dx.doi.org/10.1021/pr700822t] [PMID: 18422355]

Gootenberg, JS, Abudayyeh, OO, Kellner, MJ, Joung, J, Collins, JJ & Zhang, F (2018) Multiplexed and portable nucleic acid detection platform with Cas13, Cas12a, and Csm6. *Science,* 360, 439-44.
[http://dx.doi.org/10.1126/science.aaq0179] [PMID: 29449508]

Gootenberg, JS, Abudayyeh, OO, Lee, JW, Essletzbichler, P, Dy, AJ, Joung, J, Verdine, V, Donghia, N, Daringer, NM, Freije, CA, Myhrvold, C, Bhattacharyya, RP, Livny, J, Regev, A, Koonin, EV, Hung, DT, Sabeti, PC, Collins, JJ & Zhang, F (2017) Nucleic acid detection with CRISPR-Cas13a/C2c2. *Science,* 356, 438-42.
[http://dx.doi.org/10.1126/science.aam9321] [PMID: 28408723]

Grant, BD, Anderson, CE, Williford, JR, Alonzo, LF, Glukhova, VAS, Boyle, DS, Weigl, BH & Nichols, KP (2020) SARS-CoV-2 Coronavirus Nucleocapsid Antigen-Detecting Half-Strip Lateral Flow Assay Toward the Development of Point of Care Tests Using Commercially Available Reagents. *Anal Chem,* 92, 11305-9.
[http://dx.doi.org/10.1021/acs.analchem.0c01975] [PMID: 32605363]

Guo, L, Ren, L, Yang, S, Xiao, M, Chang, D, Yang, F, Dela Cruz, CS, Wang, Y, Wu, C, Xiao, Y, Zhang, L,

Han, L, Dang, S, Xu, Y, Yang, QW, Xu, SY, Zhu, HD, Xu, YC, Jin, Q, Sharma, L, Wang, L & Wang, J (2020) Profiling early humoral response to diagnose novel coronavirus disease (COVID-19). *Clin Infect Dis,* 71, 778-85.
[http://dx.doi.org/10.1093/cid/ciaa310] [PMID: 32198501]

Guo, X, Geng, P, Wang, Q, Cao, B & Liu, B (2014) Development of a single nucleotide polymorphism DNA microarray for the detection and genotyping of the SARS coronavirus. *J Microbiol Biotechnol,* 24, 1445-54.
[http://dx.doi.org/10.4014/jmb.1404.04024] [PMID: 24950883]

Harapan, H, Itoh, N, Yufika, A, Winardi, W, Keam, S, Te, H, Megawati, D, Hayati, Z, Wagner, AL & Mudatsir, M (2020) Coronavirus disease 2019 (COVID-19): A literature review. *J Infect Public Health,* 13, 667-73.
[http://dx.doi.org/10.1016/j.jiph.2020.03.019] [PMID: 32340833]

Hardick, J, Metzgar, D, Risen, L, Myers, C, Balansay, M, Malcom, T, Rothman, R & Gaydos, C (2018) Initial performance evaluation of a spotted array Mobile Analysis Platform (MAP) for the detection of influenza A/B, RSV, and MERS coronavirus. *Diagn Microbiol Infect Dis,* 91, 245-7.
[http://dx.doi.org/10.1016/j.diagmicrobio.2018.02.011] [PMID: 29550057]

Herold, T, Jurinovic, V, Arnreich, C, Lipworth, BJ, Hellmuth, JC, von Bergwelt-Baildon, M, Klein, M & Weinberger, T (2020) Elevated levels of IL-6 and CRP predict the need for mechanical ventilation in COVID-19. *J Allergy Clin Immunol,* 146, 128-136.e4.
[http://dx.doi.org/10.1016/j.jaci.2020.05.008] [PMID: 32425269]

Hesselink, DA, Bosmans-Timmerarends, H, Burgerhart, J-S, Petit, PL & van Genderen, PJ (2009) Procalcitonin as a biomarker for a bacterial infection on hospital admission: a critical appraisal in a cohort of travellers with fever after a stay in (sub)tropics. *Interdiscip Perspect Infect Dis,* 2009, 137609.
[http://dx.doi.org/10.1155/2009/137609] [PMID: 20016801]

Holshue, ML, DeBolt, C, Lindquist, S, Lofy, KH, Wiesman, J, Bruce, H, Spitters, C, Ericson, K, Wilkerson, S, Tural, A, Diaz, G, Cohn, A, Fox, L, Patel, A, Gerber, SI, Kim, L, Tong, S, Lu, X, Lindstrom, S, Pallansch, MA, Weldon, WC, Biggs, HM, Uyeki, TM & Pillai, SK Washington State 2019-nCoV Case Investigation Team (2020) First case of 2019 novel coronavirus in the United States. *N Engl J Med,* 382, 929-36.
[http://dx.doi.org/10.1056/NEJMoa2001191] [PMID: 32004427]

Horlock, C (2016) *Enzyme-linked immunosorbent assay (ELISA).*

Huang, C, Wang, Y, Li, X, Ren, L, Zhao, J, Hu, Y, Zhang, L, Fan, G, Xu, J, Gu, X, Cheng, Z, Yu, T, Xia, J, Wei, Y, Wu, W, Xie, X, Yin, W, Li, H, Liu, M, Xiao, Y, Gao, H, Guo, L, Xie, J, Wang, G, Jiang, R, Gao, Z, Jin, Q, Wang, J & Cao, B (2020) Clinical features of patients infected with 2019 novel coronavirus in Wuhan, China. *Lancet,* 395, 497-506.
[http://dx.doi.org/10.1016/S0140-6736(20)30183-5] [PMID: 31986264]

Ivaska, L, Niemelä, J, Heikkinen, T, Vuorinen, T & Peltola, V (2013) Identification of respiratory viruses with a novel point-of-care multianalyte antigen detection test in children with acute respiratory tract infection. *J Clin Virol,* 57, 136-40.
[http://dx.doi.org/10.1016/j.jcv.2013.02.011] [PMID: 23490399]

Iyer, M, Jayaramayya, K, Subramaniam, MD, Lee, SB, Dayem, AA, Cho, S-G & Vellingiri, B (2020) COVID-19: an update on diagnostic and therapeutic approaches. *BMB Rep,* 53, 191-205.
[http://dx.doi.org/10.5483/BMBRep.2020.53.4.080] [PMID: 32336317]

Jin, Y-H, Cai, L, Cheng, Z-S, Cheng, H, Deng, T, Fan, Y-P, Fang, C, Huang, D, Huang, L-Q, Huang, Q, Han, Y, Hu, B, Hu, F, Li, BH, Li, YR, Liang, K, Lin, LK, Luo, LS, Ma, J, Ma, LL, Peng, ZY, Pan, YB, Pan, ZY, Ren, XQ, Sun, HM, Wang, Y, Wang, YY, Weng, H, Wei, CJ, Wu, DF, Xia, J, Xiong, Y, Xu, HB, Yao, XM, Yuan, YF, Ye, TS, Zhang, XC, Zhang, YW, Zhang, YG, Zhang, HM, Zhao, Y, Zhao, MJ, Zi, H, Zeng, XT, Wang, YY & Wang, XH for the Zhongnan Hospital of Wuhan University Novel Coronavirus Management and Research Team, Evidence-Based Medicine Chapter of China International Exchange and Promotive Association for Medical and Health Care (CPAM) (2020) A rapid advice guideline for the diagnosis and treatment of 2019 novel coronavirus (2019-nCoV) infected pneumonia (standard version). *Mil Med Res,* 7, 4.

[http://dx.doi.org/10.1186/s40779-020-0233-6] [PMID: 32029004]

Kang, S, Peng, W, Zhu, Y, Lu, S, Zhou, M, Lin, W, Wu, W, Huang, S, Jiang, L, Luo, X & Deng, M (2020) Recent progress in understanding 2019 novel coronavirus (SARS-CoV-2) associated with human respiratory disease: detection, mechanisms and treatment. *Int J Antimicrob Agents,* 55, 105950.
[http://dx.doi.org/10.1016/j.ijantimicag.2020.105950] [PMID: 32234465]

Kim, H, Park, M, Hwang, J, Kim, JH, Chung, D-R, Lee, KS & Kang, M (2019) Development of label-free colorimetric assay for MERS-CoV using gold nanoparticles. *ACS Sens,* 4, 1306-12.
[http://dx.doi.org/10.1021/acssensors.9b00175] [PMID: 31062580]

Koczula, KM & Gallotta, A (2016) Lateral flow assays. *Essays Biochem,* 60, 111-20.
[http://dx.doi.org/10.1042/EBC20150012] [PMID: 27365041]

Lee, CY-P, Lin, RTP, Renia, L & Ng, LFP (2020) Serological approaches for COVID-19: epidemiologic perspective on surveillance and control. *Front Immunol,* 11, 879.
[http://dx.doi.org/10.3389/fimmu.2020.00879] [PMID: 32391022]

Li, X, Geng, M, Peng, Y, Meng, L & Lu, S (2020) Molecular immune pathogenesis and diagnosis of COVID-19. *J Pharm Anal,* 10, 102-8. a
[http://dx.doi.org/10.1016/j.jpha.2020.03.001] [PMID: 32282863]

Li, Z, Yi, Y, Luo, X, Xiong, N, Liu, Y, Li, S, Sun, R, Wang, Y, Hu, B, Chen, W, Zhang, Y, Wang, J, Huang, B, Lin, Y, Yang, J, Cai, W, Wang, X, Cheng, J, Chen, Z, Sun, K, Pan, W, Zhan, Z, Chen, L & Ye, F (2020) Development and clinical application of a rapid IgM-IgG combined antibody test for SARS-CoV-2 infection diagnosis. *J Med Virol,* 92, 1518-24. b
[http://dx.doi.org/10.1002/jmv.25727] [PMID: 32104917]

Lippi, G & Plebani, M (2020) Procalcitonin in patients with severe coronavirus disease 2019 (COVID-19): a meta-analysis. *Clinica Chimica Acta; International Journal of Clinical Chemistry,* 505, 190.
[http://dx.doi.org/10.1016/j.cca.2020.03.004]

Long, Q-X, Liu, B-Z, Deng, H-J, Wu, G-C, Deng, K, Chen, Y-K, Liao, P, Qiu, J-F, Lin, Y, Cai, X-F, Wang, DQ, Hu, Y, Ren, JH, Tang, N, Xu, YY, Yu, LH, Mo, Z, Gong, F, Zhang, XL, Tian, WG, Hu, L, Zhang, XX, Xiang, JL, Du, HX, Liu, HW, Lang, CH, Luo, XH, Wu, SB, Cui, XP, Zhou, Z, Zhu, MM, Wang, J, Xue, CJ, Li, XF, Wang, L, Li, ZJ, Wang, K, Niu, CC, Yang, QJ, Tang, XJ, Zhang, Y, Liu, XM, Li, JJ, Zhang, DC, Zhang, F, Liu, P, Yuan, J, Li, Q, Hu, JL, Chen, J & Huang, AL (2020) Antibody responses to SARS-CoV-2 in patients with COVID-19. *Nat Med,* 26, 845-8.
[http://dx.doi.org/10.1038/s41591-020-0897-1] [PMID: 32350462]

Mavrikou, S, Moschopoulou, G, Tsekouras, V & Kintzios, S (2020) Development of a portable, ultra-rapid and ultra-sensitive cell-based biosensor for the direct detection of the SARS-CoV-2 S1 spike protein antigen. *Sensors (Basel),* 20, 3121.
[http://dx.doi.org/10.3390/s20113121] [PMID: 32486477]

Mehrotra, P (2016) Biosensors and their applications - A review. *J Oral Biol Craniofac Res,* 6, 153-9.
[http://dx.doi.org/10.1016/j.jobcr.2015.12.002] [PMID: 27195214]

Moitra, P, Alafeef, M, Dighe, K, Frieman, MB & Pan, D (2020) Selective naked-eye detection of SARS-CoV-2 mediated by n gene targeted antisense oligonucleotide capped plasmonic nanoparticles. *ACS Nano,* 14, 7617-27.
[http://dx.doi.org/10.1021/acsnano.0c03822] [PMID: 32437124]

Montesinos, I, Gruson, D, Kabamba, B, Dahma, H, Van den Wijngaert, S, Reza, S, Carbone, V, Vandenberg, O, Gulbis, B, Wolff, F & Rodriguez-Villalobos, H (2020) Evaluation of two automated and three rapid lateral flow immunoassays for the detection of anti-SARS-CoV-2 antibodies. *J Clin Virol,* 128, 104413.
[http://dx.doi.org/10.1016/j.jcv.2020.104413] [PMID: 32403010]

Moore, S C, Penrice-Randal, R, Alruwaili, M, Dong, X, Pullan, S T, Carter, D, Bewley, K, Zhao, Q, Sun, Y & Hartley, C (2020) Amplicon based MinION sequencing of SARS-CoV-2 and metagenomic characterisation of nasopharyngeal swabs from patients with COVID-19. *MedRxiv.*

Ngom, B, Guo, Y, Wang, X & Bi, D (2010) Development and application of lateral flow test strip technology for detection of infectious agents and chemical contaminants: a review. *Anal Bioanal Chem,* 397, 1113-35.
[http://dx.doi.org/10.1007/s00216-010-3661-4] [PMID: 20422164]

Notomi, T, Okayama, H, Masubuchi, H, Yonekawa, T, Watanabe, K, Amino, N & Hase, T (2000) Loop-mediated isothermal amplification of DNA. *Nucleic Acids Res,* 28, E63.
[http://dx.doi.org/10.1093/nar/28.12.e63] [PMID: 10871386]

Nuccetelli, M, Pieri, M, Grelli, S, Ciotti, M, Miano, R, Andreoni, M & Bernardini, S (2020) SARS-CoV-2 infection serology: a useful tool to overcome lockdown? *Cell Death Discov,* 6, 38.
[http://dx.doi.org/10.1038/s41420-020-0275-2] [PMID: 32501411]

O'Farrell, B (2009) *Evolution in Lateral Flow-Based Immunoassay Systems Lateral Flow Immunoassay.* Springer.

OCD-Vitros (2020) Available: https://www.fda.gov/media/136967/download'

Panning, M, Charrel, RN, Donoso Mantke, O, Landt, O, Niedrig, M & Drosten, C (2009) Coordinated implementation of chikungunya virus reverse transcription-PCR. *Emerg Infect Dis,* 15, 469-71.
[http://dx.doi.org/10.3201/eid1503.081104] [PMID: 19239767]

Patel, R, Babady, E, Theel, ES, Storch, GA, Pinsky, BA, George, KS, Smith, TC & Bertuzzi, S (2020) Report from the american society for microbiology COVID-19 international summit, 23 march 2020: value of diagnostic testing for SARS–CoV-2/COVID-19. *mBio,* 11, e00722-20.

Poon, LL, Leung, CS, Tashiro, M, Chan, KH, Wong, BW, Yuen, KY, Guan, Y & Peiris, JS (2004) Rapid detection of the severe acute respiratory syndrome (SARS) coronavirus by a loop-mediated isothermal amplification assay. *Clin Chem,* 50, 1050-2.
[http://dx.doi.org/10.1373/clinchem.2004.032011] [PMID: 15054079]

Roche (2020) Elecsys® Anti-SARS-CoV-2 Immunoassay for the qualitative detection of antibodies (incl. IgG) against SARS-CoV-2. Available in: https://diagnostics.roche.com/global/en/products/params/elecsys-anti-sars-cov-2.html'

Rut, W, Lv, Z, Zmudzinski, M, Patchett, S, Nayak, D, Snipas, SJ, El Oualid, F, Huang, TT, Bekes, M, Drag, M & Olsen, SK (2020) Activity profiling and structures of inhibitor-bound SARS-CoV-2-PLpro protease provides a framework for anti-COVID-19 drug design. *bioRxiv,* 2020.04.29.068890.
[PMID: 32511411]

Sakamoto, S, Putalun, W, Vimolmangkang, S, Phoolcharoen, W, Shoyama, Y, Tanaka, H & Morimoto, S (2018) Enzyme-linked immunosorbent assay for the quantitative/qualitative analysis of plant secondary metabolites. *J Nat Med,* 72, 32-42.
[http://dx.doi.org/10.1007/s11418-017-1144-z] [PMID: 29164507]

Schroeder, HR (1982) Luminescent immunoassay in clinical analysis. *Trends Analyt Chem,* 1, 352-4.
[http://dx.doi.org/10.1016/0165-9936(82)88022-9]

Schroeder, HW, Jr & Cavacini, L (2010) Structure and function of immunoglobulins. *J Allergy Clin Immunol,* 125 (Suppl. 2), S41-52.
[http://dx.doi.org/10.1016/j.jaci.2009.09.046] [PMID: 20176268]

Seo, G, Lee, G, Kim, MJ, Baek, S-H, Choi, M, Ku, KB, Lee, C-S, Jun, S, Park, D, Kim, HG, Kim, SJ, Lee, JO, Kim, BT, Park, EC & Kim, SI (2020) Rapid detection of COVID-19 causative virus (SARS-CoV-2) in human nasopharyngeal swab specimens using field-effect transistor-based biosensor. *ACS Nano,* 14, 5135-42.
[http://dx.doi.org/10.1021/acsnano.0c02823] [PMID: 32293168]

Sethuraman, N, Jeremiah, SS & Ryo, A (2020) Interpreting diagnostic tests for SARS-CoV-2. *JAMA,* 323, 2249-51.
[http://dx.doi.org/10.1001/jama.2020.8259] [PMID: 32374370]

Shen, M, Zhou, Y, Ye, J, Abdullah Al-Maskri, AA, Kang, Y, Zeng, S & Cai, S (2020) Recent advances and perspectives of nucleic acid detection for coronavirus. *J Pharm Anal,* 10, 97-101.

[http://dx.doi.org/10.1016/j.jpha.2020.02.010] [PMID: 32292623]

Shirato, K, Yano, T, Senba, S, Akachi, S, Kobayashi, T, Nishinaka, T, Notomi, T & Matsuyama, S (2014) Detection of Middle East respiratory syndrome coronavirus using reverse transcription loop-mediated isothermal amplification (RT-LAMP). *Virol J,* 11, 139.
[http://dx.doi.org/10.1186/1743-422X-11-139] [PMID: 25103205]

Shokri, E, Hosseini, M, Davari, MD, Ganjali, MR, Peppelenbosch, MP & Rezaee, F (2017) Disulfide-induced self-assembled targets: A novel strategy for the label free colorimetric detection of DNAs/RNAs *via* unmodified gold nanoparticles. *Sci Rep,* 7, 45837.
[http://dx.doi.org/10.1038/srep45837] [PMID: 28387331]

St John, A & Price, CP (2014) Existing and emerging technologies for point-of-care testing. *Clin Biochem Rev,* 35, 155-67.
[PMID: 25336761]

Suthar, MS, Zimmerman, MG, Kauffman, RC, Mantus, G, Linderman, SL, Hudson, WH, Vanderheiden, A, Nyhoff, L, Davis, CW, Adekunle, O, Affer, M, Sherman, M, Reynolds, S, Verkerke, HP, Alter, DN, Guarner, J, Bryksin, J, Horwath, MC, Arthur, CM, Saakadze, N, Smith, GH, Edupuganti, S, Scherer, EM, Hellmeister, K, Cheng, A, Morales, JA, Neish, AS, Stowell, SR, Frank, F, Ortlund, E, Anderson, EJ, Menachery, VD, Rouphael, N, Mehta, AK, Stephens, DS, Ahmed, R, Roback, JD & Wrammert, J (2020) Rapid generation of neutralizing antibody responses in COVID-19 patients. *Cell Rep Med,* 1, 100040.
[http://dx.doi.org/10.1016/j.xcrm.2020.100040] [PMID: 32835303]

Tahamtan, A & Ardebili, A (2020) Real-time RT-PCR in COVID-19 detection: issues affecting the results. *Expert Rev Mol Diagn,* 20, 453-4.
[http://dx.doi.org/10.1080/14737159.2020.1757437] [PMID: 32297805]

Tanaka, T, Narazaki, M & Kishimoto, T (2014) IL-6 in inflammation, immunity, and disease. *Cold Spring Harb Perspect Biol,* 6, a016295.
[http://dx.doi.org/10.1101/cshperspect.a016295] [PMID: 25190079]

Tang, Y-W, Schmitz, JE, Persing, DH & Stratton, CW (2020) Laboratory diagnosis of COVID-19: current issues and challenges. *J Clin Microbiol,* 58, e00512-20.
[http://dx.doi.org/10.1128/JCM.00512-20] [PMID: 32245835]

Ulhaq, ZS & Soraya, GV (2020) Interleukin-6 as a potential biomarker of COVID-19 progression. *Med Mal Infect,* 50, 382-3.
[http://dx.doi.org/10.1016/j.medmal.2020.04.002] [PMID: 32259560]

Vashist, SK (2020) *In vitro* diagnostic assays for COVID-19: Recent advances and emerging trends. *Diagnostics (Basel),* 10, 202.
[http://dx.doi.org/10.3390/diagnostics10040202] [PMID: 32260471]

Vidarsson, G, Dekkers, G & Rispens, T (2014) IgG subclasses and allotypes: from structure to effector functions. *Front Immunol,* 5, 520.
[http://dx.doi.org/10.3389/fimmu.2014.00520] [PMID: 25368619]

Wang, W, Xu, Y, Gao, R, Lu, R, Han, K, Wu, G & Tan, W (2020) Detection of SARS-CoV-2 in different types of clinical specimens. *JAMA,* 323, 1843-4.
[http://dx.doi.org/10.1001/jama.2020.3786] [PMID: 32159775]

Wei, X, Su, J, Yang, K, Wei, J, Wan, H, Cao, X, Tan, W & Wang, H (2020) Elevations of serum cancer biomarkers correlate with severity of COVID-19. *J Med Virol,* 92, 2036-41.
[http://dx.doi.org/10.1002/jmv.25957]

WHO (2007) Guidelines for plaque reduction neutralization testing of human antibodies to dengue viruses. *World Health Organization.*

Winter, AK & Hegde, ST (2020) The important role of serology for COVID-19 control. *Lancet Infect Dis,* 20, 758-9.
[http://dx.doi.org/10.1016/S1473-3099(20)30322-4] [PMID: 32330441]

Wong, YP, Othman, S, Lau, YL, Radu, S & Chee, HY (2018) Loop-mediated isothermal amplification (LAMP): a versatile technique for detection of micro-organisms. *J Appl Microbiol,* 124, 626-43.
[http://dx.doi.org/10.1111/jam.13647] [PMID: 29165905]

Wu, F, Wang, A, Liu, M, Wang, Q, Chen, J, Xia, S, Ling, Y, Zhang, Y, Xun, J & Lu, L (2020) Neutralizing antibody responses to SARS-CoV-2 in a COVID-19 recovered patient cohort and their implications. https://ssrn.com/abstract=3566211
[http://dx.doi.org/10.2139/ssrn.3566211]

Xu, Y, Xiao, M, Liu, X, Xu, S, Du, T, Xu, J, Yang, Q, Xu, Y, Han, Y, Li, T, Zhu, H & Wang, M (2020) Significance of serology testing to assist timely diagnosis of SARS-CoV-2 infections: implication from a family cluster. *Emerg Microbes Infect,* 9, 924-7.
[http://dx.doi.org/10.1080/22221751.2020.1752610] [PMID: 32286155]

Yang, T, Wang, Y-C, Shen, C-F & Cheng, C-M (2020) Point-of-care RNA-based diagnostic device for COVID-19. *Multidisciplinary Digital Publishing Institute "with "Diagnostics (Basel)* 165.
[http://dx.doi.org/10.3390/diagnostics10030165]

Yeh, H-W & Ai, H-W (2019) Development and applications of bioluminescent and chemiluminescent reporters and biosensors. *Annu Rev Anal Chem (Palo Alto, Calif),* 12, 129-50.
[http://dx.doi.org/10.1146/annurev-anchem-061318-115027] [PMID: 30786216]

Yolken, RH (1980) Enzyme-linked immunosorbent assay (ELISA): a practical tool for rapid diagnosis of viruses and other infectious agents. *Yale J Biol Med,* 53, 85-92.
[PMID: 6990637]

Zeng, J, Zhang, Y, Zeng, T, Aleisa, R, Qiu, Z, Chen, Y, Huang, J, Wang, D, Yan, Z & Yin, Y (2020) Anisotropic plasmonic nanostructures for colorimetric sensing. *Nano Today,* 32, 100855.
[http://dx.doi.org/10.1016/j.nantod.2020.100855]

Zhai, P, Ding, Y, Wu, X, Long, J, Zhong, Y & Li, Y (2020) The epidemiology, diagnosis and treatment of COVID-19. *Int J Antimicrob Agents,* 55, 105955.
[http://dx.doi.org/10.1016/j.ijantimicag.2020.105955] [PMID: 32234468]

Zhang, B, Zhou, X, Zhu, C, Feng, F, Qiu, Y, Feng, J, Jia, Q, Song, Q, Zhu, B & Wang, J (2020) Immune phenotyping based on neutrophil-to-lymphocyte ratio and IgG predicts disease severity and outcome for patients with COVID-19. *medRxiv.*
[http://dx.doi.org/10.3389/fmolb.2020.00157]

Zhang, J-M & An, J (2007) Cytokines, inflammation, and pain. *Int Anesthesiol Clin,* 45, 27-37.
[http://dx.doi.org/10.1097/AIA.0b013e318034194e] [PMID: 17426506]

Zhang, Y, Odiwuor, N, Xiong, J, Sun, L, Nyaruaba, RO, Wei, H & Tanner, NA (2020) Rapid molecular detection of SARS-CoV-2 (COVID-19) virus RNA using colorimetric LAMP. *MedRxiv.*

SUBJECT INDEX

A

Abdominal 117, 128, 143, 144
   discomfort 117
   pain 128, 143, 144
Abnormalities 119, 140
   autonomic 140
   polymorphonuclear 140
Acid(s) 24, 88, 89, 147, 167
   lactic 167
   reflux disease 147
   sialic 24, 88, 89
Acquired immune deficiency syndrome 43
Acute pancreatitis 136
Acute 27, 30, 31, 33, 34, 74, 118, 119, 120, 134, 143, 147 148, 151
   respiratory distress syndrome (ARDS) 27, 30, 31, 33, 34, 74, 118, 119, 143, 148, 151
   thromboembolic disease 147
   tubular necrosis (ATN) 134
   urticaria 120
Adenovirus 169
Adjuvant immunotherapeutic agent 151
Alanine aminotransferase 128, 167
Alphacoronavirus 8, 9, 10
Alveolar 168
   cavity 168
   septal capillary 168
Amoxicillin 126
Amplicon-based system 176
Anemia 134
Angiotensin 31, 87, 118, 148, 149
   converting enzyme 87, 118
Anosmia 117, 119, 131, 146
Antibodies 90, 91, 164, 165, 172, 180, 182, 184, 185, 186, 187, 188, 189, 190
   monoclonal 90, 91, 189
   viral 164
Anti FITC antibody 174
Antigen, carcinoembryonic 183
Apoptosis 24, 91, 92, 95, 97, 99, 100, 103

activation of 100, 103
   mitochondrial 97
   signaling pathways 99
Aspartic acid glutamic acid-alanine-aspartic acid 96
Aspirate 124, 167, 170
   endotracheal 170
   nasopharyngeal 124
Assays 170, 171, 173, 176, 177, 179, 181, 182, 184, 185, 186, 187, 188, 189, 190
   chemiluminescence 189
   colorimetric 176, 177
   developed LAMP-based 173
   direct ELISA 184
   immunological 184
   immunological/serological 181
   isothermal amplification 190
   qPCR-based 179
   rapid diagnostic test 186
   serum neutralization 187
AtilaBioSystems 177
ATP 96, 188
   binding 96
   dependent duplex RNA 96
Aztecs disease 3

B

Bacillus Calmette-Guerin (BCG) 151
Backward inner primer (BIP) 173
Betacoronavirus 8, 10
Bilateral 126, 142
   air space opacification 126
   patchy pulmonary infiltrates 142
Biventricular hypertrophy 126
Blood 3, 5, 6, 30, 83, 84, 141, 167, 170, 180, 181
   clotting 103
   gas analysis 167
   oxygen, low 103
Body mass index 145
Bovine coronavirus 12

monitoring programs 12
transfer 12
Bradycardia 133
Breast cancer 146
Bronchiolitis 7, 29, 31
Bronchitis 11, 13
Bronchi tissue 28
Bronchoscopic biopsy 135
Bronchoscopy 135

C

Calcium homeostasis 183
Cancer 1, 2, 42, 45, 54, 119, 150
  high grade prostate 150
Canine coronavirus 20
Cardiac 34, 119, 126, 131, 134, 145, 151
  arrest 126
  arrhythmias 119, 131
  biomarkers 134
  complications 145, 151
  diseases 143
  injury 34, 119
  marker-creatine kinasemyocardial band 131
  myopathies 126
Cardiomegaly 126, 148
Cardiomyopathy 145
Cardiopulmonary 140, 146
  abnormality 140
  arrest 146
Cardiovascular 54, 119, 166
  disease 54, 166
  problems 119
cDNA 90, 172, 175, 176
  translation 90
Ceftriaxone 126
Cell(s) 21, 23, 25, 27, 28, 29, 83, 84, 85, 86, 88, 89, 91, 92, 94, 96, 97, 100, 103, 137, 173, 180, 187
  cycle arrest 96
  dendritic 83, 84, 91
  fusion 27, 88
  growth arrest 100
  hepatic 27, 29

intestinal 28
lysate 173
neuroglial 29
neuronal 92
proliferation 96
white blood 137, 180
Central nervous system 11
Cerebral 148
  arteriosclerosis 148
  stroke 148
Cerebrovascular disease 143
Chemiluminescent immunoassay 179
Chemosis 119, 120
Chest 74, 119, 123, 125, 128, 130, 136, 138, 144, 147
  distress 128
  pain 74, 119, 130, 136, 138, 147
  radiographs 123, 125, 136, 139, 144
Chinese 62, 63
  embassies 63
  national health commission 62
Chromatography 185
Chronic 11, 45, 141, 143, 145, 146, 148
  coughs 143
  health problems 45
  kidney disease 141, 145, 146
  pancreatitis 148
  progressive neurologic disease 11
Ciliostatsis 27
Clarithromycin 126
Clotting disorders, frequent 167
Clustered regularly interspaced short palindromic repeats (CRISPR) 164, 174
CNS 11, 25, 29, 89, 92
  demyelination 11
  disease 25
  infiltration 11
  pathogenesis 92
Cohort study 148
Colorimetric-based biosensing applications 176
Colorimetric bioassays 176
Community 75, 76, 164, 169
  healthcare 164
Community transmission 33, 60, 65, 75, 180

Comorbid diseases 133
Comorbidities, cardiac 133
Computerized tomography angiography (CTA) 138
Confirmed cases of COVID-19 in India 59
Congenital heart defect 131
Conjugate, antibody-enzyme 185
Conjunctival 6, 119, 120
  hyperaemia 119, 120
  secretions 6
Conjunctivitis 3, 7, 29, 119
  hemorrhagic 119
Consolidation 117, 119, 126, 129, 131, 134, 136, 138, 139, 143, 144, 145, 147, 148
  bilateral pulmonary 144
Contagious diseases 2, 76, 121
  deadly 76
Convalescent plasma (CP) 180
Coronary 145, 148
  artery disease 145, 148
  heart disease 145
Coronavirus 6, 7, 9, 10, 11, 18, 19, 20, 21, 27, 43, 44, 45, 83, 101, 102
  respiratory 9
Coronavirus disease 7, 8, 11, 33
Coronaviruse(s) 1, 7, 8, 9, 10, 11, 12, 13, 18, 19, 33, 36, 43, 68, 71, 73, 83, 170
  infection 43, 73, 83
  outbreak 71
  pandemic 68
  RNA 170
Cough 7, 30, 32, 34, 35, 60, 117, 118, 125, 126, 127, 130, 131, 132, 133, 135, 136, 137, 141, 142, 143, 144, 145, 146, 147, 148, 166, 168
  dry 30, 32, 117, 118, 127, 130, 133, 136, 137, 143, 146, 147, 166, 168
  etiquette 32
  persistent 148
  productive 145, 146
CoV associated protein 99
COVID-19 44, 65, 66, 67, 68, 74, 118, 124, 125, 126, 127, 130, 131, 138, 143, 150, 152, 178, 180
  co-infections 127

Coronavirus 178
  disease symptoms 180
  epidemiology 44, 74
  infection 65, 66, 67, 68, 118, 124, 125, 126, 127, 130, 131, 138, 143, 150, 152
  PCR test 54, 141
  related deaths 54
  situation in Africa 68
COVID-19 pandemic 43, 44, 45, 60, 66, 73, 75, 77, 143, 152
  in France 66
  in Germany 73
  in India 44, 60
CoV 84, 85, 86, 88, 91, 97, 100, 102, 104
  infection 84, 85, 86, 88, 91, 97, 100, 102, 104
  proteins 97
C-reactive protein (CRP) 128, 134, 142, 167
  and procalcitonin 142
CRISPR 174, 190
  associated assays 190
  isothermal amplification based assays 174
Crohn's disease 145
Cystic fibrosis 124
Cytokine 141, 168, 183, 184
  mediated lung damage 183
  storm 141, 168, 184

D

Deltacoronaviruses 8
Dengue virus 189
Detection 164, 165, 167, 170, 173, 174, 176, 177, 178, 179, 181, 182, 184, 186, 188, 189, 190
  biosensor-mediated 189
  luminescence 188
  nucleic acid 165
  qPCR-based 179
  respiratory virus 190
  systems 188
Diabetes mellitus 136, 141, 143, 145, 146, 148
  and hyperlipidemia 136
Diaphoresis 136, 140

Subject Index

Diarrhea 27, 28, 30, 32, 35, 125, 130, 136, 143, 144, 146
Dipeptyl peptidase 32
Disease 1, 2, 4, 5, 11, 12, 30, 31, 33, 42, 44, 45, 73, 76, 169, 180, 183
   epidemiology 180
   modulation 183
   related conditions 44
Distress syndrome 18, 27, 30, 31, 33, 45, 74, 118
   acute respiratory 27, 30, 31, 118
   developed acute respiratory 74
   respiratory 18
   severe respiratory 33
Dizziness 119, 135
DNA amplification 173
Droplets, respiratory 6, 7
Dyslipidemia 141
Dyspnea 117, 118, 119, 125, 126, 130, 135, 136, 138, 142, 143, 144, 145, 146, 147, 166
   acute 147
   progressive 142
   severe 118, 166

E

Ebola virus 6
EBV and COVID-19 co-infections 127
Echocardiography 126
Edema 5, 30, 168
   hemorrhagic 5
   interstitial 168
Effective screening methods 64
Electrochemical 188, 189
   biosensors 188
   impedance spectroscopy (EIS) 188, 189
Electro-chemiluminescence Immunoassay 179
ELISA assays 184
Emergency, national 67
Encephalitis 11, 19, 29, 135
Encephalomyelitis 9
Encephalopathy 137
Encode ACE2 protein 149

Endonuclease 94
Endoribonuclease 25, 86
Enteric 9, 20, 27, 28
   infection 9, 20
   systems 27, 28
Enteritis 19, 27, 28
   viral 27
Enterocytes 148
Enzyme-linked immunosorbent assay (ELISA) 164, 172, 179, 184, 185, 189
Enzymes 25, 27, 84, 93, 94, 148, 167, 172, 174, 184, 185
   muscle 167
   myocardial 167
   proteolytic 27
   reverse transcriptase 172
   transmembrane 148
Enzyme-substrate reaction 184
Epidemic 1, 2, 32, 43, 62, 76
Epithelial cells 27, 28, 83, 84, 100, 101, 103, 148
   alveolar 27
   regeneration of 103
Epstein-Barr virus (EBV) 127
Erythrocyte sedimentation rate (ESR) 167
Esterase 20, 24, 87, 88, 89
   activity 89
   domain 87
   hemagglutinin 20, 24
Eukaryotic translation initiation factor 96
Exonuclease 25, 86

F

Factors 11, 25, 44, 54, 60, 103, 118, 120, 150, 166, 167, 181
   basic fibroblastic growth 167
   colony-stimulating 167
   epithelial growth 103
   immune response 25
   inflammatory 167
   platelet-derived growth 167

Fever 1, 4, 117, 118, 120, 123, 125, 126, 131, 135, 140, 142, 143, 144, 145, 146, 147, 148, 151, 166
   low-grade 120, 126
   mild 166
   yellow 1, 4, 151
Flu 1, 4, 6, 30
   swine 1, 4, 6
Focal status epilepticus 147
Functions 21, 83, 85, 93, 94, 100, 130, 180
   haematopoietic 130
   viral 180
Fusion, mediating membrane 88

G

Gastroenteric disease 12
Gastroenteritis 7, 123
Gastroesophageal reflux 123
Gastrointestinal symptoms 144
Gene 21, 170
   accessory 170
   replicase 21
Genome 8, 18, 21, 24, 25, 28, 43, 89, 170, 174
   respiratory virus 174
   single-stranded RNA 170
Genomic 36, 44, 92, 93
   analysis 36
   sequence 44
Global epidemiology 43, 45
Glomerulopathy, collapsing 141
Glucose-6-phosphate dehydrogenase deficiency 146
Glutathione S-transferase 94
Glycoprotein 20, 21, 22, 24, 27, 86, 88
   glycosylated 27
   peplomer 20
   receptors 24, 88
Glycosylated polypeptide 24
Gold nanoparticles-based colorimetric assay 176
Ground glass opacity (GGO) 119, 122, 123, 128, 130, 134, 136, 139, 143, 144, 145, 146, 147, 148

Grover disease 146
Guillain Barne syndrome (GBS) 145

H

Headache 3, 34, 60, 74, 118, 119, 128, 132, 135, 140, 144
Head CT scan 127
Health 42, 45, 73, 169
   circumstances 73
   emergencies, global 169
   system 42, 45
Healthcare 65, 68
   facilities, standard 68
   professionals 65
Health risk 18, 104
   factors 104
   global 18
Heamglutinin esterase protein 21
Helicase 18, 21, 25, 85, 95, 170
Hemaagglutinating encephalomyocarditis virus 20
Hemagglutinin 24, 88, 170
   esterase 24, 88, 170
   esterase protein 24
Hematological 119, 164, 165, 167
   analysis 164, 165, 167
   symptoms 119
Hematology reports for total white blood cell 125
Hemoperfusion 134
Hemoptysis 34, 138
Hemorrhagic 6, 132, 147
   fever 6
   infarct 132
   rash 147
   venous infarct 132
Hepatic infection 9
Hepatitis 11, 12, 19, 20, 25, 29, 92, 93, 97, 142, 150
   C virus (HCV) 97
   chronic 142
   developed acute 12
Hepatocytes 183

Herpes simplex virus (HSV) 137, 147
Human 5, 36, 97, 104, 136, 137, 169, 170, 175
   immunodeficiency virus (HIV) 5, 97, 137
   pancreatitis 136
   transmission 36
   viruses 104, 169, 170, 175
Human respiratory 9, 11, 20
   coronaviruses 11
   infections 9, 20
Hygiene, basic 1
Hyperglycemia 117
Hyperlipidemia 136, 147
Hyperplasia 141
Hypertension 1, 34, 117, 119, 141, 142, 143, 145, 146, 147, 148, 149
   arterial 145, 148
Hypertensive 143, 148
   cardiopathy 148
   nephropathy 143
Hyperthermia 18, 30, 32, 34
Hypoproteinemia 148
Hypotension 134
Hypothyroidism 145
Hypoxemia 35, 142

I

Illness, contagious 2
Immature immune systems 121
Immune 28, 101
   markers, preliminary 101
   -mediated pathology 28
Immune cells 5, 29, 31, 32
   innate 32
Immune reaction 27
   innate 27
   virus-mediated 27
Immune responses 29, 98, 101, 103, 164, 180, 183, 190
   acquired 103
   adaptive 164
   antiviral 98
   innate 183

Immune system 5, 29, 31, 34, 42, 45, 66, 77, 120, 121, 151, 152, 181
   compromised 166
   innate 120
   weak 45
Immunity 29, 76, 117, 121, 151, 181, 190
   acquired 121
   adaptive 97
   cell-mediated 29
   post-infection 181
Immunoassays 164, 179, 181, 186, 188, 189
   colorimetric enzyme 189
   serological 164, 181
Immunodeficiency 76
Immunoglobulins 31, 181, 186
Immunosuppressant 92, 127
Indian council of medical research (ICMR) 60
Infection 1, 11, 18, 20, 28, 29, 30, 31, 32, 34, 60, 65, 66, 69, 72, 73, 76, 91, 102, 118, 119, 121, 150, 151, 152, 167, 179, 181, 183, 190
   acute 11, 29
   bacterial 167
   chronic pulmonary 18
   conducting airways 102
   corona 65, 66
   hospital-acquired 34
   intestinal 30
   invasive bacterial 183
   neurologic 20
   respiratory virus 121
   severe systemic 28
   transmission 73
Infectious 1, 3, 9, 18, 20, 23, 28, 84, 165
   bronchitis virus (IBV) 9, 18, 20, 23, 28, 84
   diseases 1, 3, 165
Inflammation 28, 97, 119, 135, 183
   indicated patchy chronic 135
Inflammatory pathologies 183
Influenza virus 5, 190
Interferon(s) 25, 27, 91, 92, 96, 99, 100, 101, 167
   activation 99
   release 27
   signaling 99, 100

synthesis 96
International non-government organizations (INGOs) 73, 74
Intracellular signaling cascades 97

L

Left ventricular ejection fraction (LVEF) 145
Lesions 11, 168
   outspread demyelinating 11
Liver 11, 25, 30, 91, 92, 93, 127, 167
   damage 25, 92
   enzymes 167
   transplantation 127
Load, viral 31, 100, 187
Lockdown 44, 61, 62, 63, 64, 65, 68, 69, 70, 71, 72, 73, 77
   effect of 44, 69
   national 71
   nationwide 72
   measures 73
   partial 63
   period 71
   restrictions 73
Long-chain fatty acid 188
Luminescence-based immunoassays 188
Luminescent immunoassay 188
Lymphopenia 30, 34, 92, 126, 143

M

Malignancy 146
Maltose-binding protein (MBP) 94
Mediastinal lymphadenopathy 119
Membrane 27, 30, 185
   hyaline 27, 30
   nitrocellulose 185
Membrane protein 18, 21, 23, 24, 26, 27, 83, 87, 90
Mengovirus 152
Metabolic acidosis 146
Metagenomic 175
   approaches 175
   sequencing based methods 175

Methyltransferase 86
Microcytic anemia 132
Middle East respiratory 4, 10, 11, 13, 18, 31, 33, 35, 43, 177
   syndrome (MERS) 4, 10, 11, 13, 18, 31, 33, 35, 43, 177
   virus 31
MinION sequencing technique 175
Ministry of health and family welfare (MoHFW) 72
Mitochondrial antiviral signaling protein 99
Mitogen-activated protein kinase 100
Mobile analysis platform (MAP) 175
Monocyte chemo-attractant protein 167
Mounier-Kuhn Syndrome (MKS) 143
mRNA 25, 26, 86, 93, 95, 96, 97
   genomic 86
   subgenomic 93
   synthesis 25, 26, 86
   viral 96, 97
Murine 9, 11, 13, 19, 20, 23, 24, 27, 29, 38, 84
   coronavirus 11, 29
   hepatitis virus (MHV) 9, 11, 13, 19, 20, 23, 24, 27, 29, 38, 84
Musculoskeletal disturbance 119
Mutations 18, 20, 89, 91, 94, 95, 149, 175, 176
   unglycosylated M-protein 91
   viral gene 176
Mycobacterium bovis 151
Myocarditis 31, 119
Myopericarditis 119

N

Neurodegenerative diseases 117
Neurological disorders 28
Neurologic complications 132
Neuropathogenesis 89
Neutralization assays 187
Nikolaidis 103
Non-small cell lung cancer (NSCLC) 145, 146
Nucleic acid 124, 170
   amplification assays 124

Subject Index

tests 170
Nucleic acid detection 170
   kits 170
   strategies 170
Nucleocapsid 21, 24, 25, 27, 32, 83, 84, 85, 87, 92, 97, 166, 167, 170, 182
   protein (NP) 21, 24, 25, 27, 32, 83, 87, 97, 166, 167, 170

O

Obstructive sleep apnea 145
   syndrome 145
Olfactory dysfunction 119
Organ 31, 119
   dysfunction, multiple 119
   failure 31
Organisms, pathogenic 176

P

Pain 117, 136, 141, 143, 144, 145, 147
   epigastric 136, 143, 147
   hip 145
   muscle 136
Painel coronavírus 71
Pancytopenia 130, 134
Pandemic(s) 1, 2, 3, 4, 5, 6, 7, 31, 32, 33, 42, 43, 44, 61, 65, 66, 77, 165
   corona 66
   disease 165
   infectious 77
   influenza 3, 43
   real plague 4
Papain-like protease (PLP) 25, 85, 95
Parainfluenza virus 130
Pathogenesis 7, 25, 83, 86, 88, 89, 151
   influence 25
   viral 83, 88
Pathogenic 23, 169
   agents 169
   phenotype 23
Pathogens 13, 33, 121, 173, 175, 176, 187, 188

infectious 173
   respiratory 13
Pathophysiology of coronavirus 102
PCR-based 165, 173, 179
   detection 165
   methods 173
   techniques 179
Personal protective equipment (PPE) 68
Placental transmission 36
Plaque reduction neutralization assays (PRNA) 187
Pneumonia 7, 11, 13, 18, 29, 31, 32, 34, 117, 118, 127, 130, 143, 146, 147, 151, 152, 166
   acute 31
   interstitial 127, 147
   life-threatening 7, 32
   severe 117, 118, 130, 166
Pneumonitis 12, 31
Poliovirus 93
Polymerase 20, 21, 25, 170, 172, 176, 186
   chain reaction (PCR) 170, 172, 176, 186
   dependent RNA 20, 25
Processed recombinant proteins 94
Processing precursor proteins 93
Prognosis 120, 184
Properties 10, 23, 24, 94, 95, 98, 151
   endo-ribosomal 94
   entero-pathogenic 24
   immunomodulatory 151
   interferogenic 24
   phylogenetic 10
   pneumo-protective 23
Protease 21, 23, 25, 85, 88, 90, 93, 95, 98, 182, 183
   activity 95
   cellular 88
   cysteine 98, 182
   enzyme 23
Proteins 21, 23, 24, 25, 26, 27, 83, 84, 85, 86, 87, 88, 89, 90, 91, 92, 93, 94, 95, 97, 99, 104, 178, 179, 182
   accessory 21, 84
   cellular 97
   endogenous 83

endosomal 104
fibrinogen-link 92
hemagglutinin-esterase 83, 87
maltose-binding 94
viral 26, 85, 86, 99, 104, 182
Protein synthesis 96, 97, 100
cellular 100
Proteolytic degradation 27
Public health 5, 67, 83, 169
crisis 83
emergency 67
interventions 169
officers 5
Pulmonary 103, 135, 146, 147
disease 135
embolism 146, 147
toxin 103

R

Rapid 172, 189
antigen detection tests 189
detection test 172
Real-time RT-PCR assay 166
Receptor binding domain (RBD) 23, 31, 86, 87, 179, 182
Receptor-binding motif (RBM) 87
Recombinant viruses 99
Red blood cells (RBCs) 151
Renal 54, 137, 141
disease 54
functions deteriorate 141
injury 137
Renal failure 31, 143
chronic 143
Renin-angiotensin system 23, 88
Replicase 18, 25, 26, 93
proteins 25, 93
Replication proteins 83
Resin-angiotensin system 88
Respiratory 29, 37, 84, 117, 126, 131, 137, 127, 144, 145, 146, 166, 183
alkalosis 146
arrest 137

complications 127
distress 29, 37, 84, 117, 126, 131, 144, 145, 146, 166
dysfunction 183
Respiratory disease 6, 7, 8, 12, 13, 54
bovine 12
Respiratory illness 6, 7, 12, 124, 166
contagious 7
viral 6
Respiratory infections 19, 20, 28, 29, 151, 166, 169
acute 169
Respiratory syndrome 10, 18, 29, 83, 186
coronavirus, severe acute 83, 186
Respiratory tract infection 18, 32, 124
lower 32
upper 124
RNA 20, 21, 25, 27, 85, 86, 92, 93, 94, 96, 99, 176, 190
and DNA duplex 94
modification enzymes 21
genetic 86
multiple sub-genomic 25
small nucleolar 94
subgenomic 25
RNAaemia 34, 119
RNA binding 24, 95
motif 95
protein 24, 95
RNA-dependent 85, 93, 96, 170
ATPase activity 96
RNA polymerases 85, 93, 170
RT-LAMP-VF assay 174
RT-PCR 100, 134, 171, 175
real-time 175
assays 171
for viral RNA 100
test of nasopharyngeal swab 134

S

Sandwich ELISA 184
SARI infections 59, 60
SARS-associated coronavirus 6

SARSCoV-2 infection 168
SARS-CoV-2 23, 142, 149, 171, 173, 175, 181, 189
  infection, symptomatic 171
  proteins 181
  RNA 142, 171, 175
  S1 protein 189
  detection rates and LAMP assay sensitivity 173
  genomic mutations 175
  infection 23, 149
  spike protein 23
SARS disease 6
Senile heart valve disorders 148
Septic shock 37, 117, 126, 142, 143
  managing 37
Severe acute respiratory 1, 2, 3, 4, 6, 11, 18, 23, 24, 29, 30, 31, 32, 33, 43, 59
  infection (SARI) 59
  syndrome (SARS) 1, 2, 3, 4, 6, 11, 18, 23, 24, 29, 30, 31, 32, 33, 43
Sickle cell disease 134
Signs of anicteric cholestasis and cytolysis 127
Single nucleotide polymorphisms (SNP) 175
Sjogren-syndrome 141
Sleep-disordered breathing (SDB) 142
Spike proteins 21, 22, 23, 24, 25, 26, 27, 83, 85, 86, 87
Surface plasmon resonance (SPR) 97, 176, 188

T

Tachycardia 137
Techniques 164, 165, 166, 169, 170, 171, 172, 173
  efficient sampling 171
  non-PCR-related 170
  novel nucleic acid amplification 172
  nucleic acid amplification 173
  reliable laboratory detection 169
  serological testing 164
  serology-based 166

serology-based detection 165
Techniques-chromatography 188
Technology, surface plasmon resonance biosensor 97
Therapy 130, 145, 172, 180, 187
  convalescent plasma 180, 187
  oxygen 37
  radiation 145
Thoracic malignancy 145
Throat 30, 32, 35, 60, 74, 117, 118, 122, 128, 131, 133, 139, 144, 166, 168
  sore 30, 32, 35, 60, 74, 117, 118, 128, 131, 133, 139
  swab 122, 168
Thrombosis 83, 103, 132, 146
Thrombotic 142, 151
  complications 142
  disorders 151
Time-resolved fluorescence immunoassay 179
Traction bronchiectasis 172
Transcriptional regulatory sequences (TRS) 89, 92
Transmembrane 20, 88, 89, 150
  glycoprotein 20
  motifs 89, 90
  protease/subfamily 88
  serine protease 150
Transmembrane proteins 23, 148, 170
  integral 23
Transmissible 6, 27
  disease 6
  gastroenteritis virus 27

V

Vaccination 5, 76, 117, 121, 152
Vaccines 1, 5, 12, 31, 36, 43, 76, 77, 104, 151, 152, 175
  killed 12
Vaginal secretions 5
Vascular endothelial growth factor-A (VEGFA) 167
Venous thrombo embolism (VTE) 132

Viral 32, 34, 61, 66, 86, 88, 89, 92, 95, 96, 97, 98, 100, 135, 164, 166, 171, 173, 179, 182, 183, 184, 187
  diseases 32, 100
  genetic material 164
  genome translation 95
  infections 61, 66, 88, 89, 92, 96, 97, 166, 173, 179, 183, 187
  invasion 34
  key proteinase 98
  load kinetics 171
  memory 182
  pathology 84
  RNA 86, 100, 135, 164, 171
Viral RNA 165, 171
  load 171
  tests 165
Virions 20, 21, 23, 24, 25, 26, 27, 89, 90
Virulence factors 95, 99
Virus 5, 7, 9, 11, 12, 18, 19, 20, 21, 23, 24, 25, 27, 28, 29, 31, 33, 44, 64, 83, 84, 86, 89, 90, 91, 92, 97, 100, 104, 137, 149, 152, 169, 179
  diarrhea 9
  encephalomyocarditis 152
  human immunodeficiency 5, 97
  infectious 92
  infectious bronchitis 9, 18, 20, 84
  infectious peritonitis 19
  like particles (VLPs) 86, 90, 91
  live attenuated 12
  measles 97
  murine hepatitis 11, 19, 84
  porcine hemagglutinating encephalomyelitis 19
  recurrent Herpes Simplex 137
  single positive-sense RNA 7
  single positive-stranded RNA 83
  single-stranded positive RNA 104
  smallpox 5
  transmissible gastric enteritis 84
Vomiting 117, 123, 125, 126, 127, 130, 133, 136, 139, 141, 144

W

White 10, 125, 137, 167, 180
  blood cell (WBC) 125, 137, 167, 180
  eye coronavirus 10
World health organization (WHO) 1, 2, 3, 6, 7, 8, 31, 33, 34, 44, 55, 65, 68, 73, 84

X

Xenopus laevis 94

Z

Zika virus 169
Zinc finger configuration 94

www.ingramcontent.com/pod-product-compliance
Lightning Source LLC
Chambersburg PA
CBHW051144220526
45473CB00003B/654